PAIN AND BEHAVIORAL MEDICINE

THE GUILFORD CLINICAL PSYCHOLOGY AND PSYCHOTHERAPY SERIES

MICHAEL J. MAHONEY, EDITOR

Pain and Behavioral Medicine: A Cognitive–Behavioral Perspective
Dennis C. Turk, Donald Meichenbaum, and Myles Genest

Cognitive Processes and Emotional Disorders: A Structural Approach to Psychotherapy
V. F. Guidano and G. Liotti

Agoraphobia: Nature and Treatment
Andrew M. Mathews, Michael G. Gelder, and Derek W. Johnston

Cognitive Assessment
Thomas V. Merluzzi, Carol R. Glass, and Myles Genest, Editors

Cognitive Therapy of Depression
Aaron T. Beck, A. John Rush, Brian F. Shaw, and Gary Emery

IN PREPARATION

Relapse Prevention
G. Alan Marlatt and Judith Gordon

Insomnia
Richard Bootzin and Thomas Borkovec

Attributional Processes in Clinical Psychology
Lyn Abramson, Editor

PAIN AND
BEHAVIORAL MEDICINE
A Cognitive–Behavioral Perspective

DENNIS C. TURK
Yale University

DONALD MEICHENBAUM
University of Waterloo

MYLES GENEST
University of Saskatchewan

THE GUILFORD PRESS
New York and London

To Lorraine and Kenny, who helped me take time to stop and smell the flowers.—*D. C. T.*

To Marianne, Lauren, Michelle, David, and Danny, who help make life painless.—*D. M.*

To Sharon, Aaron, and Anna, for yesterday, today, and tomorrow.—*M.G.*

© 1983 The Guilford Press
A Division of Guilford Publications, Inc.

Printed in the United States of America

Last digit is print number 9 8 7 6 5 4

LIBRARY OF CONGRESS CATALOGING IN PUBLICATION DATA
Turk, Dennis C.
   Pain and behavioral medicine.
   (The Guilford clinical psychology and psychotherapy series)
   Includes bibliographical references and index.
   1. Pain—Psychological aspects. 2. Pain—Treatment.
3. Behavior therapy. I. Meichenbaum, Donald. II. Genest,
Myles. III. Title. IV. Series. [DNLM: 1. Behavioral
sciences. 2. Behavior therapy. 3. Pain—Therapy.
WL 704 T939p]
RB127.T87 1983   616'.0472   82-11695

ISBN 0-89862-917-9 (paperback)

PREFACE

So neither ought you to attempt to cure the body without the Soul, and this . . . is the reason why the cure of many diseases is unknown to the physicians of Hellas, because they are ignorant of the whole which ought to be studied also, for part can never be well unless the whole is well.—*Plato*

In writing this book we have two particular goals in mind. The first, our more general goal, is to make available to professionals in the health sciences an overview of the cognitive–behavioral perspective on human functioning. We believe this perspective has important implications and utility for health care professionals, particularly those in the emerging fields of behavioral medicine and health psychology. From our own laboratory and clinical work and the contributions of many others, we have distilled what we view as central issues of concern to a wide variety of practitioners and researchers, including family physicians, dolorologists, nurses, physical and occupational therapists, social workers, rehabilitation counselors, and psychologists.

Second, we want to describe the rationale, development, and utilization of cognitive–behavioral techniques in the promotion of health, the prevention of disease, and the treatment of illness. We will focus in particular on the management of pain, one of the health care system's most costly and perplexing problems. Our coverage of pain management includes theoretical, research, and clinical issues, as well as case material. It is our hope that this material will be specific enough to provide practitioners with a useful knowledge of how cognitive–behavioral techniques are employed. Although we highlight the management of pain, we believe that the approach we offer and the general issues we raise are equally applicable to the broader spectrum of health and illness.

We will view particular physical problems in the context of the person's life. From this perspective, we are interested in examining any changes in the patient's condition (further degeneration or amelioration) in relation to ongoing life events, relationships, cognitive and affective patterns, and behaviors. Clinical issues discussed in regard to the treatment of pain patients, such as patient motivation, adherence to treatment, maintenance of treatment effects, the therapist–patient relationship, and the role of the patient's significant others, are equally applicable to other medical and clinical problems. In short, our discussion of the cognitive–behavioral treatment of pain patients provides a prototype for the treatment of other clinical populations.

It is *not* our intention to represent cognitive–behavioral *techniques* as panaceas. Rather, we believe that this perspective provides an important *theoretical and heuristic approach* for health care professionals. It provides a model that can help guide our understanding of the impact of illness on patients and their families and on patients' social and psychological environments. Further, the specific therapeutic procedures suggested by this perspective can enhance the practitioner's armamentarium, in some circumstances providing alternatives to traditional medical practice, in others serving as useful adjuncts to existing treatment modalities.

We have organized this book into four sections. The first section presents the theoretical rationale for the cognitive–behavioral perspective, describes the therapeutic approaches that follow from this perspective, and examines the application of the cognitive–behavioral techniques in health promotion, disease prevention, treatment of disease, and coping with medical problems. The second section is more specific, dealing with the theoretical conceptualization of pain based on both laboratory and clinical studies with acute and chronic pain. The second section also deals with the contribution of psychological factors to the experience of pain and the response to pain. The third section of the book is designed to be both a practical guide to the clinical issues in pain management and a detailed description of the treatment components of the cognitive–behavioral approach. Although the approach described is designed specifically for the management of pain, it is applicable to other diseases and illnesses. The fourth section provides a statement of the needed future directions.

Despite our enthusiasm for the material we are presenting, we wish to encourage a healthy skepticism in the reader. Cognitive–behavioral research and behavioral medicine will be advanced more by cautious exploration than by premature and uncritical proselytizing. Much of what we will be offering is intended to be provocative and hypothesis-generating rather than in any sense definitive. If this book stimulates practitioners and researchers to entertain new hypotheses, experiment with new approaches, and engage in productive exchanges of ideas, it will have fulfilled its purpose.

We are grateful to a number of people and agencies for their support over the years. Many people helped us in the data-collection phase, others provided opportunities for us to develop our clinical and research experiences, and still others provided careful editorial assistance. To each of you we are most grateful. These include Kathy Bergstrom, Janet Boothe, Ken Bowers, William Bowen, Phil Bryden, Donald Cameron, Rosa Cascione, Ken Craig, Susan Davies, Stefan Demjen, R. J. Evans, Sharon Genest, J. Barnard Gilmore, Edith Herman, Arnie Holzman, Robert Kerns, Jack Levine, John Rayburn, Karen Rennert, Margie Speers, Peter Stenn, and Merilyne Waldo. We would particularly like to thank Roy Cameron for his careful reading and incisive comments on an earlier draft of the manuscript.

We also gratefully acknowledge the financial support offered by the National Institutes of Health, the U.S. Veterans Administration, the Ontario Mental Health Foundation, the Canadian Medical Research Council, and the Canada Council. The first author (D. C. T.) wishes to express his appreciation to Yale University, whose award of a Junior Faculty Fellowship facilitated completion of this book. The second author (D.M.) wishes to express his appreciation to the Social Sciences and Humanities Research Council, whose support of a sabbatical leave helped make this book possible.

CONTENTS

CONTENTS

THE NATURE OF COGNITIVE-BEHAVIOR MODIFICATION: APPLICATION TO BEHAVIORAL MEDICINE

CHAPTER 1

A COGNITIVE–BEHAVIORAL PERSPECTIVE OF THE THERAPY PROCESS[1]

All psychotherapeutic activities have a cognitive component which restructures the patient's perceptions so that the same feelings which formerly indicated despair or anxiety now convey a message of hope.—*Jerome Frank (1961)*

In this chapter we introduce the cognitive–behavioral perspective of human functioning and then provide a general overview of the therapy process that follows from this perspective. A much more detailed treatment guide is offered in Section III of this book; at this point our objective is to provide a brief overview, highlighting the sequence of treatment techniques, with emphasis on the clinical sensitivity required. An evidential theory of change is offered that integrates the treatment components.

AN OVERVIEW OF COGNITIVE-BEHAVIOR MODIFICATION

This chapter describes a cognitive–behavioral view of the therapy process. This description will be useful in understanding the assessment and treatment procedures offered in later chapters. Let us begin by putting cognitive-behavior modification in some perspective.

During the past decade, we have seen in the therapy literature the proliferation of research and clinical applications of cognitive–behavioral approaches (e.g., see A. Beck, Rush, Shaw, & Emery, 1979; Foreyt & Rathjen, 1978; Kendall & Hollon, 1979, 1980b; Mahoney, 1974a; Meichenbaum, 1977; Meichenbaum & Jaremko, 1982; Merluzzi, Glass, & Genest, 1981). This development has not been without its critics (Ledwidge, 1978; Wolpe, 1976), who have also met with a lively response (Locke, 1979;

---

1. We are indebted to Roy Cameron for his help in formulating the ideas for this chapter.

Mahoney & Kazdin, 1979; Meichenbaum, 1979). A detailed discussion of this debate is, however, beyond our present scope. Rather, we wish to note that the evolving literature on cognitive-behavior modification is *not merely* suggesting a host of new treatment procedures. More important, cognitive-behavior modification is evolving as a perspective, a model, or a theoretical account of behavior change. It is becoming increasingly clear, moreover, that this model can be useful in furthering research and practice with regard to a broad range of problems, as we will document in subsequent chapters.

Cognitive-behavior modification is a rubric that is applied to a wide variety of therapeutic techniques, based upon somewhat different conceptualizations. For example, a recent major review of cognitive-behavioral therapies (Mahoney & Arnkoff, 1978) covered such diverse approaches as rational-emotive therapy, cognitive therapy, coping skills therapies, problem-solving therapies, self-instructional training, and self-control approaches. All these approaches tend to be characterized as "cognitive-behavioral."

The differences among approaches are at least as striking as the similarities: Different theories (ranging from conditioning to cognitive information processing and social learning conceptualizations) underlie the approaches; different aspects of cognitive experience (beliefs, attributions, expectations, coping self-statements and images, problem-solving cognitions, etc.) are emphasized; different prescriptions may be offered regarding the best point of intervention in the cognition-affect-behavior-consequence complex; different strategies for intervention (ranging from direct frontal assaults on irrational beliefs to encouraging patients to produce adaptive behaviors before focusing on cognitions) are evident; different treatment rationales are offered to patients (if, indeed, a rationale is provided at all); different styles of intervention are used (ranging from highly directive to collaborative); and different emphases are placed upon the use of behavior therapy procedures. In short, the term "cognitive-behavior modification" has as its referents a rather broad assortment of bedfellows. This makes it difficult and potentially misleading to discuss cognitive-behavior modification in general terms. To do so is to impose what Kiesler (1966) has characterized as a "myth of treatment uniformity."

Even though cognitive-behavioral techniques are implemented in diverse ways, some common elements can be identified. Interventions are usually active, time-limited, and fairly structured, with the underlying assumption that affect and behavior are largely determined by the way in which the individual construes the world. Therapy is designed to help the patient identify, reality-test, and correct maladaptive, distorted conceptualizations and dysfunctional beliefs. The patient is assisted in recognizing the connections among cognition, affect, and behavior, together with their joint consequences, and is encouraged to become aware of and monitor the role that negative thoughts and images play in the maintenance of maladaptive behavior. He or she is encouraged to test out the effects of cognitions and beliefs through selected homework assignments. The therapist is concerned with the contribution of cognitions, affect, and behavioral patterns to the maintenance of psychological and physical problems. The common denominators across approaches appear to be (1) interest in the nature and modification of patients' cognitions and feelings, as well as behaviors, and (2) some commitment to the use of behavior therapy procedures in promoting change.

The therapies under the rubric of cognitive-behavior modification have generally adopted a view of change that Bandura has termed "reciprocal determinism" (Bandura, 1978; Meichenbaum, 1976c, 1977; Turk, 1982). This view holds that behavioral change is a reflection of the intimate interrelationships among the patient's cognitive structures (schemata, beliefs), cognitive processes (automatic thoughts, internal dialogue, images), interpersonal behaviors, and resulting intrapersonal and interpersonal consequences. We should also note that such a reciprocal deterministic view has been presented by theorists with different theoretical backgrounds (e.g., G. Klein, 1970; Lewin, 1935; H. Murray, 1938; Rapaport, 1960/1970; Staats, 1963; Wachtel, 1977).

An example of this approach can be drawn from the therapy of A. Beck *et al.* (1979). A depressed patient is asked, challenged, and encouraged to engage in graded behavioral acts that will have consequences incompatible with his or her prior expectations. The patient is taught to view his or her thoughts as hypotheses, the validity of which is assessed by means of personal experiments. The therapist will then ask the patient to examine the nature of those beliefs, assumptions, schemata, and current concerns that give rise to expectations, appraisals, attributions, automatic thoughts, and images (cognitive processes).

In general, cognitive–behavioral therapists use environmental manipulations, as do behavior therapists, but for the former such manipulations represent informational feedback trials, which provide an opportunity for the patient to question, reappraise, and acquire self-control over maladaptive cognitions, feelings, and behaviors. As noted, the variety of therapeutic interventions under the cognitive–behavioral rubric represents differences in both the style and the point of intervention in the chain of cognitive, affective, and behavioral events. That is, treatment can intervene at the point of cognitive structures (beliefs, meaning systems), cognitive processes (automatic thoughts and images, problem-solving coping skills), behavioral acts, and environmental consequences. Moreover, the intervention may influence both the content of thought and the style of thinking.

The increasing cognitive orientation of behavior therapy suggests some convergence with more psychodynamically oriented views. It is interesting to compare, for example, some of the psychoanalytically oriented comments of Bieber (1974) with the general cognitive–behavioral view we have outlined:

> Outside the analysis, patients become involved in various testing maneuvers related to reinforcing or relinquishing an irrational belief. In steps one and two, irrational beliefs are delineated and patients, hopefully, become convinced that their beliefs are irrational. I view these steps as the "working out" phase of therapy. These steps proceed concurrently though they may be sequential. Step three is the "working through" phase. The patient comes to identify the operations of his beliefs in his life situation and in his interpersonal transactions. If the analysis proceeds well, this phase will see the extinction of symptoms and an alteration from neurotic or maladaptive to appropriate behavior. (p. 98)

Thus the cognitive–behavioral approach is *integrative*. That such a treatment orientation can facilitate change is evident in a rapidly growing literature focusing on a wide range of populations, including clients with interpersonal anxiety (e.g., Goldfried, 1977; Heppner, 1978; Lange & Jakubowski, 1976; Thorpe, 1975), test anxiety (e.g., Denney, 1980; Wine, 1981), uncontrolled anger (Novaco, 1978), depression (e.g., A. Beck *et al.*, 1979), sexual dysfunction (Rook & Hammen, 1977), and addictions and substance abuse (e.g., Chaney, O'Leary, & Marlatt, 1978; Intagliata, 1978; Marlatt & Gordon, 1980; Rychtarik & Wollersheim, 1978). The proliferation of applications is exciting, although we sometimes fear that the enthusiasm is disproportionate to the data. The interested reader should see an annual cognitive-behavior modification newsletter (Meichenbaum, 1975–1979) for further details.

THERAPY: A COGNITIVE-BEHAVIORAL PERSPECTIVE

We can better appreciate the cognitive–behavioral perspective of the therapy process by briefly tracing the various stages of treatment. This three-stage process will be described in more detail in Section III.

Conceptualizing the Problem and Its Treatments

Entering the Patient's Perspective

People seldom seek help for their problems without much anguish. Seeking assistance implies that a good deal of worry, anxiety, depression, and preoccupation with the problem(s) has occurred. This cognitive and emotional activity is often prolonged, emotion-laden, and intense, especially if the problem is chronic. "Is it serious?" "Will it go away in time?" "What caused it?" "Am I going crazy?" are some of the questions that anyone who has sought treatment will recognize.

As a result, patients often arrive at the clinic or office already having made some preliminary attempts to understand their problems and to formulate possible treatments and outcomes. All of this is quite apparent in those patients who, upon entering the office, unrestrainedly burst into a lengthy explanation of the symptoms, the perceived etiology, and the treatment that should be employed. More taciturn patients may also have elaborate conceptions of their problems, although these may be more difficult to elicit or less clearly articulated.

With many patients, the understanding that has been arrived at has been shaped by a variety of sources, including prior contacts with health care providers, friends and relatives who have freely offered their advice, mass media reports, and many other sources of accurate and erroneous information. Furthermore, the more intense the problem, the longer it has lasted, and the more therapeutic contacts the patient has made, the more likely he or she has some fairly entrenched conceptions.

Of what relevance to the presenting complaint is all of this? We submit that maximum effectiveness of *any* treatment, as well as adherence to any therapeutic regimen, is in part mediated by the closeness of fit of the treatment with the patient's understanding of the problem and how it can be treated.

In other words, patients are not prepared to submit passively to whatever treatment is prescribed. This is usually called "resistance" or "noncompliance," and it is clearly evident in a substantial proportion of patients, regardless of their problems. What is often overlooked is that patients can be expected to resist treatment that does not coincide with their understanding and expectations. Such resistance does not have to present a problem, because the patient and therapist can work together to establish a similar understanding and common expectations. Even when patients' expectations do not concur with those of the therapist, patients are often prepared to defer to expert opinion and change their views. But not always. Such noncompliance can be understood to be at least partly the result of an incompatibility between patient's beliefs and attitudes and those of the therapist (Jones, Wiese, Moore, & Haley, 1981). Because of the importance of the issues of noncompliance and adherence in behavioral medicine, we will consider them separately in Chapter 8.

The first issue faced by the therapist is assessing both the presenting problem *and the patient's conceptions of the problem* and how these will affect the treatment. For example, M. Davis (1967) reported that farm workers suffering from cardiac disease held some of the following beliefs that contributed to treatment noncompliance: "If you wait long enough, you can get over any illness"; "Illness and trouble is one way God shows displeasure"; "Some of the old-fashioned remedies are still better than things you get at the drugstore"; "You need to give your body some rest from medicine once in a while; otherwise your body becomes dependent on it or immune to it" (p. 276).

Another example comes from our work with pain patients. Often such a patient has the belief (frequently shared by the referring physician; e.g., see Gillmore & Hill, 1981) that there is "real" pain as compared to "psychogenic" pain and that seeing a psychologist means that the validity of one's pain is being challenged: "You think it is only in my head." "You think I'm making it up." Such beliefs contribute to resistance, and when they are accepted by the therapist, they place him or her in a double bind. If treatment is purely physical, the patient's beliefs are substantiated, and the credibility of psychologically based interventions is undermined further. If, however, the therapy deals with psychological variables—for example, the patient's peremptory (although perhaps unvoiced) rejection of the approach—this also may predispose treatment to failure. Thus an important aspect of therapy is to assess the patient's expectations, beliefs, and attitudes about such matters at the outset and to address these openly.

In short, what could be labeled as resistance and nonadherence may merely reflect the natural consequences of the patient's holding beliefs that are incompatible with the interventions undertaken. Once the therapist understands the patient's perspective, then what appear to be self-defeating, irrational, and maladaptive forms of resistance may make a good deal of sense.

Changing the Patient's Perspective: Reconceptualization

At the same time at which the therapist begins to understand the patient's perspective, the patient's perspective generally begins to change. A key feature of cognitive–behavioral treatment is facilitating the emergence of a new conceptualization over the course of therapy, thereby translating the patient's symptoms into difficulties that can be pinpointed and viewed as specific, solvable problems rather than as problems that are vague, undifferentiated, and overwhelming. A good deal of emphasis is placed on laying the groundwork for the emergence of this therapeutic reconceptualization. In the same way that a lawyer carefully lays the groundwork for a brief to be presented to a jury, the patient and therapist collect the data to be considered as the basis for a reconceptualization of the presenting problem(s).

There are two primary activities by which patients are encouraged to adopt a new perspective of the presenting problem: (1) by being educated in a set of new terms and in a new framework within which to understand the problem and (2) by collecting data themselves, in such a way as to further the reconceptualization process. These, of course, often will occur simultaneously rather than sequentially.

Education. The educational aspect of therapy is a flexible component that is adaptable to the needs of particular patients, therapists, and problems. It is not generally didactic, although in some programs educational lectures and similar presentations have been useful (e.g., Gottlieb, Strite, Koller, Madorsky, Hockersmith, Kleeman, & Wagner, 1977). More often, a Socratic-type interaction (whereby the therapist attempts to guide the patient) is likely to be most effective in encouraging the emergence of a new conceptualization. Patients may be encouraged to offer their own views of evidence that fit or do not fit the evolving view. Objectives here are to help patients to view their presenting problems and reactions in a more differentiated manner and to avoid adversary positions between patients and therapists.

As the therapist selectively responds to the patient's statements, asks questions, gives homework assignments, offers interpretations, or provides explanations, he or she implicitly or explicitly encourages the patient to reconstrue the problems discussed. The therapist begins to impart his or her own theoretical constructs in lay terms so that the patient gradually comes to interpret events and experiences in terms of the words and concepts used by the therapist. We suggest that this translation process is inherent in *all* treatments, medical as well as psychological.

The translation process serves a number of therapeutically important functions. First, it provides patients with explanations for their problems that are likely to be considerably more benign than the patients' initial interpretations. Whereas a patient, for example, may have interpreted pain and accompanying depression as a symptom of a completely physical chain of events or as a sign of an impending "mental breakdown," the translation process may lead the patient to view the pain and depression as the result of a complex process in which his or her own reactions play an important role.

Second, the translation generally recasts the problem into a form that renders it more amenable to solution: The therapist is committed to conceptualizing the problem in terms that point the way to effective intervention. This provides a basis for patients to move from feeling helpless and hopeless to experiencing a sense of hope and positive anticipation. A number of observers (e.g., Frank, 1974; Seligman, 1975) have suggested that the fostering of hope is a central, vital ingredient in the therapeutic process. Helping the patients reconceptualize their problems in a form that suggests a viable solution may be one of the most effective ways of fostering hope and one of the key challenges that any therapist faces.

This point is particularly important when dealing with patients with chronic medical conditions, who generally have received many different treatments, each failing to ameliorate their distress and discomfort. For example, a patient with arthritis may arrive at a clinic disillusioned, demoralized, and depressed. He or she may have a strong belief, reinforced by popular literature, that the disease is inevitably degenerative and untreatable by current medical means, let alone psychological interventions. We will return to the concept of hope in later chapters.

We should emphasize at this point that we do *not* assume that *any* therapeutic conceptualization will prove to be as good as any other conceptualization for bringing about change. Practitioners have the responsibility of interpreting the relevant literature to arrive at their own conclusions regarding which conceptualizations and interventions are most appropriate for particular clinical problems. The actual scientific validity of the particular conceptualization, however, may be less important than the face validity it provides. We want to note, however, that the conceptualization plays a role that can be as dramatic as the intervention itself.

If our analysis has heuristic value, and if the translation process is central to therapeutic endeavors, as we suggest, then the practical challenge for the therapist is that of effectively orchestrating this translation process. Some therapists are very didactic and directive and seem to force upon patients a particular conceptualization by the power of their personalities, jargon, or positions. In some instances this hard-sell approach may prove successful. The health care provider must, however, be concerned with the patients' thoughts and feelings regarding not only the presenting problems, but also the therapist and the therapeutic process (see Cameron, 1978; Meichenbaum & Gilmore, 1982).

Patients who view the therapist as dogmatic and intimidating may be disinclined to express misunderstandings or reservations about the conceptualization and may "go through the motions" of therapy, terminate prematurely, or both. An alternative way to proceed is to establish a *collaborative relationship* among patients, significant others, and health care providers, in which they work together to identify and interpret pertinent data and in which they cooperate in evolving a common conceptualization of the problem. This way of proceeding increases the likelihood that therapists will develop a clearer understanding of patients' ideas, and it makes specific components of the treatment more personally relevant to patients.

To achieve this collaborative relationship, health care providers should be quite conscious of their therapy styles. For example, it would be better for a therapist not to present a conceptualization with certainty, but rather, to offer it as a reflection of the current view of what is going on. The therapist can carefully check with the patient to see if, indeed, this view makes sense and will not seem highly unlikely: "What I hear you saying is . . ."; "You seem to be telling me . . ."; "Am I correct in assuming that . . . ?"; "I get the feeling that . . . ; correct me if I'm wrong"; "We have covered a lot of territory so far in this interview. Is there anything I said that troubled you? . . . Do you think we left anything out?" Such queries provide the basis for involving the patient in the process of collaboration and reconceptualization.

The reconceptualization process receives a good deal of attention from cognitive–behavioral theorists because treatment intervention procedures will follow directly from the particular reconceptualization that has emerged over the course of the initial phases of therapy. It is not as if the patient must sign an explicit contract in therapy saying that "my problem now fits this reconceptualization"; instead, a conceptualization or a working framework is created and refined over the entire course of therapy. The initial educational phase of therapy is seen as a key time for the prevention of unnecessary patient resistance.

In short, the educational component of cognitive-behavior therapy attempts to help patients reconceptualize their problems, to change what they say to themselves about the presenting problems or initial stress reaction, and to begin to point the way toward intervention strategies. This translation process evolves over the course of treatment and follows from the type of questions the therapist asks, the kinds of tests administered, the homework assignments given, and the explicit rationale offered.

Data Collection. The reconceptualization can generally be facilitated by having patients collect data, either informally (e.g., by means of self-report aided by imagery procedure or by providing anecdotes as requested by the therapist) or more formally, by using various forms of record keeping (e.g., see review volumes by Ciminero, Calhoun, & Adams, 1977; Cone & Hawkins, 1977; Hersen & Bellack, 1976; Kendall & Hollon, 1980b; Merluzzi et al., 1981). Initially patients are taught to be better observers of their own thoughts, feelings, and behaviors. Virtually all forms of therapy encourage patient "self-exploration" or teach patients formally to monitor behavior, affect, and cognition. This process of data collection allows therapist and patient alike to define the problems and to formulate therapeutic possibilities.

As patients become aware of pertinent data that previously have been disregarded or distorted, they develop a more differentiated understanding of the problem. For instance, a patient may learn to specify the environmental conditions under which problematic behavior is manifest (e.g., psychophysiological symptoms, elevated blood glucose level, cigarette smoking). As the patient reviews the data over the course of therapy, he or she may redefine the presenting problem (e.g., "I'm beginning to see that my problem in being assertive might be contributing to my trouble. Headaches do not just come on themselves"). Thus the data collection can contribute to the reconceptualization that is emerging.

Altering Thoughts, Feelings, and Behaviors

Habitual ways of thinking and responding do not seem to change abruptly. As patients begin to redefine their problem, their internal dialogues or self-communications sometimes reflect the old ways of thinking and sometimes the new. They may have to learn to execute complex new behaviors (such as those called for in effective interpersonal communication) or to produce familiar behaviors in situations in which such behavior had previously been inhibited. It requires time and practice to execute these new ways of responding smoothly, consistently, and eventually automatically. The therapist's concern is not only response processes and failures, but also the patients' thoughts and feelings in response to these failures and successes.

The objectives of this aspect of therapy are (1) to continue the reconceptualization of the problems, (2) to ensure that patients can execute the necessary behaviors for dealing effectively with the problems, (3) to ensure that patients learn to monitor their thoughts and behaviors during daily activities, and (4) to establish the gradually more consistent implementation of new ways of thinking and responding. In short, the essential goal of this phase is to induce patients to change cognitions, feelings, and behaviors as they engage in daily affairs.

Patients are encouraged to employ existing skills, develop untapped resources, and learn new methods of coping as suggested by the new conceptualization. Therapy generally provides both direct action and cognitive coping techniques, which differ from one situation to the next. Direct action modes include such activities as changing the environment in some way, engaging in various therapeutic activities, and learning relaxation skills. Another important direct action intervention involves developing and using one's social networks and support systems, as will be discussed in Section III.

The cognitive coping modes include training in problem solving (e.g., definition of problems, anticipation of consequences, evaluation of feedback; altering appraisals, attributions, and self-labels; shifting of attention; imagery rehearsal; and so forth). The teaching of such cognitive coping skills is possible if one views such processes as sets of statements and images that individuals say to themselves or imagine. One can then help modify patients' internal dialogues by having them become aware of, monitor, and change the negative, problem-engendering, self-defeating self-statements and images they experience during exacerbations, relapses, or failures.

The reader may find that speaking about the patients' thoughts as self-statements and internal dialogues is somewhat unusual. But there is good reason for using these phrases. As we will suggest in later chapters, calling a thought a "statement to oneself" emphasizes the potential deliberateness of that particular thought and the fact that it is under the patient's own control. "Self-statements" are used simply to represent ideas. Patients are told that such self-statements function as reminders to use the coping skills. Use of the phrase "internal dialogue" has a long history:

> For a good part of their waking life, people monitor their thoughts, wishes, feelings and actions. Sometimes there is an internal debate as the individual weighs alternative courses of action and makes decisions. Plato referred to this phenomenon as an "internal dialogue." (A. Beck, 1976, p. 38)

In collaboration with the trainer, patients can generate sets of coping self-statements or strategies that encourage them to assess the situation, anticipate and evaluate what might happen and what has to be done, examine the bases for the inference regarding expected outcomes, postpone action and possibly relabel arousal, "psych" themselves up, tolerate frustration, and in some situations even convince themselves to maintain hope and a sense of self-worth.

One emphasis of the cognitive–behavioral perspective is to assist patients in developing a problem-solving, task-oriented set of coping strategies, in which they think of each stressful, painful, or symptomatic situation as a problem having response alternatives rather than as a threat or provocation. By encouraging patients to attend to their own thoughts, feelings, and behaviors and to the reactions of others, treatment generalization is built into the therapy regimen. During and following therapy, patients' heightened awareness of the early warning signs of pain and maladaptive behaviors becomes the cue to use the coping skills that were modeled, discussed, and rehearsed in therapy.

Learning to self-monitor closely and to use the incipient, low-intensity components of the maladaptive behavioral sequences as signals to initiate other cognitions and behaviors appear to be a key to successful therapeutic change. To achieve this, therapists may find it valuable to clarify with patients those aspects of the maladaptive behavioral sequences that might effectively serve to "cue" production of the new responses. Cues should be salient and should occur early in the maladaptive response sequences (i.e., before affect has intensified, before complete reversion to older maladaptive patterns has occurred, and before other persons in the environment have begun their usual complementary reactions to the patients' maladaptive response chains). It may also be helpful to develop specific reorienting self-statements that switch patients out of the old sequences and into the new. In this way, patients' responses remind them to employ adaptive self-care and coping responses.

Cognition, Affect, and Behavior

Although we will have more to say about the role of affect in later chapters, at this point it is important to recognize that there are complex interactions among cognitive, affective, and behavioral change. Positive change in one of these areas may promote positive change in the others. This is particularly important because change may be more readily and effectively accomplished in one area than in another. If, for example, a patient with a behavioral deficit acquires the capability to execute the behavior smoothly (learning to deliver assertive statements convincingly, cope with pain, inject insulin, etc., through modeling, role playing, or *in vivo* practice with coaching and feedback), the patient is almost certain to think of himself or herself as better able to deal with problems. This self-perception of increased resourcefulness heightens a sense of control (Frank, 1974; Seligman, 1975) and self-competence (Bandura, 1977, 1980). These cognitive and affective changes, coupled with the patient's newly established behavioral skills, increase the probability he or she will respond differently in problem situations.

R. Lazarus (1966) has theorized that the amount of stress we experience in response to a threatening stimulus is proportional not only to the threatening qualities of the stimulus situation, but also to the extent to which we see ourselves as possessing resources to cope with the threat. Lazarus's analysis suggests that the person who has acquired relevant coping behaviors will interpret previously threatening stimuli as less threatening. In brief, if the patient acquires new cognitive and behavioral skills, he or she is likely to experience an increased sense of optimism and self-efficacy, which in turn increases the likelihood of dealing with new problem situations directly and effectively. The patient also is likely to experience less stress in previously distressing situations, since these are now interpreted as less threatening because of the newly acquired behavioral resources.

Once new responses are acquired, it is crucial for the therapist to arrange, as far as possible, for the patients to try out the responses under conditions that will enhance a sense of competence and self-efficacy. Bandura (1977) suggested that self-efficacy requires not only a belief that the behavior will lead to the desired outcome, but also a belief that one can produce the required behavior. Ideally, patients should engage in the new behaviors (1) *in vivo*, (2) where there is a high probability that the behaviors will evoke the desired responses, (3) under conditions that lead to attributing success to one's own capability rather than in some external circumstances (see Bandura, 1977).

The preceding discussion was intended to make the general point that behavioral changes induced by the therapist may give rise to therapeutically desirable cognitive and affective changes. Cognitive–behavioral therapies emphasize that affect and cognition are most effectively modified by changes in behavior (Bandura, 1977; Mahoney, 1979; Meichenbaum, 1977). It seems clear, however, that cognitive changes also give rise to behavioral and affective changes. Cognitions can elicit feelings, can enhance emotion by generating uncertainty, and can reduce it by providing clarity as well as specifying ways to control feelings.

Consolidation, Generalization, and Maintenance of Change

According to a cognitive–behavioral model, the first phase of therapy is concerned with helping the patient to define his or her problems in terms of a framework that makes the problems amenable to solution. The second phase is concerned with actually promoting cognitive, affective, and behavioral change. The tasks of the third phase, to which we now turn, are to consolidate the changes, promote generalization, and lay a foundation for maintenance of the changes. Our assumption is that the way patients interpret the changes they have made will influence the degree to which changes are generalized and maintained.

In general, we would like to have patients regard themselves as having changed as individuals. This implies that patients (1) recognize that meaningful change has occurred and (2) attribute this change to an alteration in themselves rather than to external circumstances. Patients are more likely to see a "real" change if there are demonstrable differences not only in the relationship with the therapist (these changes can easily be attributed to the efforts of the therapist, the special relationship existing in therapy, etc.), but also in their daily functioning outside the treatment session. Even therapeutic approaches that focus on the relationship between therapist and patient generally recognize that patients are unlikely to consider change to be significant if it does not occur in the course of daily activity as well.

Even if changes *are* taking place outside therapy, it is not clear that patients will spontaneously notice this or attribute it to their own efforts. By encouraging patients to note and to discuss changes occurring in the "real" world, the therapist may foster attention to data that can lead patients to the conclusion that they are indeed changing. Behavior therapists have long emphasized that the collection of such data is valuable not only to patients, but also to the therapist in attempting to gauge whether the therapeutic strategy is promoting change.

It is not enough, however, for patients to be aware that change is occurring. Patients must attribute that change to themselves. The therapist may encourage such self-attribution in at least two ways. First, the therapist may lay the groundwork for such attributions early in treatment by conceptualizing therapy as an educational, skill-training process. Second, whenever a patient reports a positive change, it may be advantageous for the therapist to encourage the patient to consider how he or she brought about the change. The objective here is not only to encourage a self-attribution, but also to ensure a grasp of how the change occurred. A patient will be in a better position to engage in comparable performances in the future if he or she has developed coping strategies out of personal experience. When a patient reports failures (e.g., intense and debilitating episodes of pain, inability to stick to a diet, a return to cigarette smoking), this should also be the occasion for a reanalysis. When such episodes occur, what patients say to themselves about such setbacks will affect the generalization and maintenance of treatment effects.

Enhanced treatment maintenance is most likely to result if the patient can come to anticipate and prepare for any possible intermittent relapse. Pain, anxiety, marital conflict, depression, poor eating habits, and most presenting problems are pervasive, commonly shared experiences in our society. Even if our patients are successfully treated, they are likely to reexperience their problems to some degree after therapy ends.

Medical treatment, which ideally aims to provide permanent symptomatic relief by eradicating underlying pathology, represents the implicit model that most people probably have in mind when they seek "treatment" in our culture. If patients in cognitive–behavioral therapy expect to become and remain symptom-free, they are likely to react negatively to relapses that occur during and after treatment. It is easy to interpret such failures as evidence that "the treatment is not effective," or "the therapist is not competent," or "I am not capable of really changing. I must be my same old self. The pain will never go away." It may be helpful to have patients anticipate relapse and how they will cope with the problem behavior when it recurs (Marlatt & Gordon, 1980). Because the aim of therapy is to change patients' responses to problems as they arise, we want patients to interpret any relapses as signals for coping rather than as evidence of failure or as an occasion for "catastrophizing" (i.e., extreme, affectively intense, often self-derogatory thoughts and images).

In summary, what is being suggested is an *evidential* theory of change through which the therapist helps patients generate, collect, and reconstrue data. The focus of therapy is on training cognitive and behavior skills that lead to alterations in behavior and self-communications and ultimately to changes in cognitive structures (i.e., beliefs, meaning systems). Patients are encouraged continually to consider data that show they are changing and to attribute the change to alterations in their own behavior and cognitions. Thus the therapist is concerned with the patients' inferences, thinking styles, and conceptualizations and also with the adequacy of patients' behavioral and interpersonal repertoires. In this way, cognitive-behavior therapy reflects the integration of the clinical concerns of cognitive therapists and the technology of behavior therapy. A. Lazarus and Fay (1982) have nicely captured the approach:

> Our model is essentially educational and we [the therapists] liken ourselves to a music teacher or an athletic coach—we supply guidance, offer specific training exercises, correct misconceptions, try to modify faulty styles, provide up-to-date information, display caring, support and encouragement, but most of the responsibility rests with the "trainee" to practice between training sessions. (p. 11)

With this overview of the cognitive–behavioral orientation and treatment approach in mind, let us now consider how the approach can be applied more specifically to the area of behavioral medicine.

CHAPTER 2

BEHAVIORAL MEDICINE:
A COGNITIVE–BEHAVIORAL PERSPECTIVE

There are among us those who haply please
to think our business is to treat disease.
And all unknowingly lack this lesson still
'tis not the body, but the man is ill.
—S. Weir Mitchell (cited in Schofield, 1902)

This chapter begins with a review of the emerging themes in the field of behavioral medicine. Following that is a discussion of the concept of disease as an objective phenomenon and of illness and illness behavior as subjective experiences and responses to disease. The roles of cognitive and affective factors in the various stages of illness are outlined, followed by a discussion of a cognitive–behavioral approach to the assessment of stress and coping.

THE CASE FOR BEHAVIORAL MEDICINE

During the past 50 years, infectious diseases other than respiratory infection and venereal diseases have largely been brought under control. In 1900, infectious diseases were the leading causes of death; by midcentury, however, chronic diseases had emerged as the most common causes of death (Jonas, 1978). Although the likelihood of dying from an infectious disease in 1968 was one-sixth what it was in 1900, the death rate from heart disease had increased 268% in that same period.

According to Haggerty (1977), patterns of malnutrition (including an excess of poorly chosen foods), pathogenic inactivity, excessive use of drugs (ranging from coffee, tobacco, and alcohol to stimulants and depressants), and failure to reduce environmental hazards constitute the major known causes of avoidable illness in Western society today. The recent U.S. Surgeon General's report on health promotion and disease prevention (1979) supports Haggerty's assessment. This report suggests that as much as half of the mortality in the United States may be due to unhealthy behavior or life-style. It further suggests that of the ten leading causes of death in the United States, at least seven could be substantially reduced if persons at risk altered just six habits—poor diet, smoking, lack of exercise, alcohol abuse, maladaptive responses to tension and stress, and use of antihypertensive medications. If these risk-producing habits could be changed to health-promoting ones, there is good reason to believe that morbidity and mortality due to heart disease, neoplastic disease, stroke, arteriosclerosis, emphysema, diabetes mellitus, cirrhosis of the liver, and psychological disabilities would be reduced (Lalonde, 1974; U.S. Surgeon General, 1979). It is the realization that behaviors and life-styles contribute to health and illness that has contributed to the evolution of the discipline *behavioral medicine*.

These observations have led to a shift in focus with regard to improving the quality of health—a shift from external factors, such as microorganisms and poor sanitation, to behavioral problems determined by the interaction among factors internal to individuals, the social environment, and the physical environment. Individuals require education in order to change behavioral patterns, including patterns of eating, excessive drinking, and tobacco and drug use, as well as other maladaptive behaviors that may be responses to stress. In recent years cognitive–behavioral techniques have been used to modify several of these contributors to disease and illness (e.g., hypertension, smoking, obesity, coronary-prone behavior pattern, and maladaptive responses to stress). We will consider examples of the application of a cognitive–behavioral approach to prevention, assessment, treatment, and rehabilitation in the next chapter. Before we examine how these techniques can be applied to behavioral medicine, we will consider several concepts that have been emerging in medicine.

CONCEPTS OF DISEASE, ILLNESS, AND ILLNESS BEHAVIOR

Pathology as Multifaceted and Multidetermined

In earlier times disease was generally attributed to a single pathogenic agent—a toxin, a germ, an endocrine imbalance, or a vitamin or nutritional deficiency. Recent immunological research (reviewed by L. Thomas, 1978) has indicated that in most instances infectious disease is due to the misreading of signals between an invading agent or pathogen and the host. It is often the organism's own bodily reactions or defense mechanisms that cause the disease (e.g., bronchial asthma, allergic reactions). L. Thomas provided several examples in which disease and death are due to an immunological system's overreaction.

Furthermore, a number of authors (e.g., J. Cassel, 1976; Dodge & Martin, 1970; S. Friedman & Glasgow, 1974; Mason, Buescher, Belfer, Artenstein, & Mougey, 1979; Syme, 1967, 1975) have argued that psychosocial stress may be one of a set of etiological factors in almost all diseases and especially in chronic diseases. These studies have contributed to an increased recognition that the etiology of poor health is multidimensional, involving the interaction among physical, psychological, social, and environmental factors.

The mere presence of stressful events or stimuli may, however, be less significant in the etiology of disease than the manner in which these events are interpreted. For example, migraine headaches have been described as resulting from prolonged, excessively stressful situations. Henryk-Gutt and Rees (1973), however, found that the life stresses to which migraine sufferers and headache-free individuals are exposed are practically identical. In another study, Katz, Weiner, Gallagher, and Hellman (1970) determined the stress level in 30 women hospitalized for breast tumors several days before biopsies were performed. The patients evidenced a *broad range* of stress responses, as indicated in assayed 17-hydroxycorticosteroid (17-OHCS) secretion, despite the fact that they all faced the same stressors: the biopsy and a potential diagnosis of breast cancer.

Still another example of the important role of the appraisal process was offered by R. Lazarus (1975b), who reported that a physiological stress pattern was initiated by injuries to conscious organisms only, not to unconscious ones. This raises the possibility that the psychological significance of the noxious agent in conjunction with bodily damage is the crucial factor in many diseases.

It has been suggested that both physiological and psychological stress have a final common pathway, *the perception of threat* (R. Lazarus, 1966; Mason, 1971). This perception appears to be the antecedent of various biochemical stress reactions.

Another recent emphasis is the distinction between disease, illness, and illness behavior. "Illness" refers to the patient's *subjective experience* of the *objective disease*. Mechanic (1968) noted that "illness behavior," in comparison to disease, involves three components: (1) the patient's attentiveness to physical or mental symptomatology; (2) the processes affecting how symptoms are defined and accorded significance; and (3) the patient's seeking help, altering life routines, and so on. (For extended discussions of differences among health behavior, illness behavior, and sick-role behavior, see Kasl & Cobb, 1966a, 1966b; Parsons, 1951, 1958.)

The course and outcome of a disease depend not only on the physical and psychological state of the patient, but also on the ways clinical staff, family, employers, and friends react to the situation. The form and magnitude of illness and illness behaviors are products of both subjective experience and social definitions, as well as of the severity and quality of actual symptoms and physical incapacity.

Disease onset may be associated with a number of factors, including "presence of stressful environmental conditions, perceptions by the individual that such conditions are stressful, the relative ability to cope with or adapt to these conditions, genetic predisposition to a disease and the presence of a disease agent" (Rabkin & Struening, 1976, p. 1014).

One theme arising from recent work, then, is that disease should be viewed as both multifaceted and multidetermined and not simply as a function of an isomorphic relationship between an external pathogenic agent and the body. Furthermore, how the individual responds to the disease will influence the course of the disease.

Cognitive Factors

A second theme emerging in behavioral medicine is the central role of cognitive factors. Cognitive factors are viewed as (1) determining the ways in which individuals define health, disease, and illness; (2) influencing decisions regarding the utility of engaging in either health-promoting behaviors or risk-related behaviors; (3) determining how individuals respond to symptoms and incapacities; (4) influencing how individuals utilize the health care system; and (5) contributing directly and indirectly to disease and illness.

Reciprocal Determinism

The continuous reciprocal interaction between the individual and the environment that influences what individuals think, feel, and do, and consequently their relative health or illness, constitutes a third theme. To appreciate the relevance of reciprocal determinism (Bandura, 1978), consider the following example: A man awakens one morning and notes a dull throbbing in the frontal region of his head. The intensity of the stimulus may focus his attention on the sensations, and he may attempt to evaluate them, to decide what is the cause, probable course, and so on. He may, then, regard the head pain simply as a minor inconvenience resulting from his excessive alcohol intake the night before or as a deserved punishment for irritable behavior directed toward his wife; alternatively, he may regard it as a sign of a brain tumor, from which his father died.

These different evaluations would likely lead to different emotions, such as anxiety, guilt, depression, or a sense of helplessness, which in turn would partially determine behavior. The man with the head pain may ignore the sensations and distract himself by attending to other tasks, take an aspirin, resolve to give up drinking, apologize to his wife, bear the discomfort stoically, take a cold shower, call his physician or psychiatrist, or go out for a vigorous jog. His choice will depend in part upon his prior history. If past episodes of drinking resulted in headaches, and if aspirin alleviated the distress, the most likely course of action might be to take an aspirin. However, if he does not relate the throbbing sensations to drinking but instead to a possible brain tumor, then his action might be to contact the same physician who treated his father for a brain tumor.

Whichever course of action the man chooses, he will create a unique environment. He will be setting the stage for a particular subset of future events that will be different from the subset any other choice would have induced. The particular environment he shapes for himself in this way will, in turn, have effects on his thoughts, feelings, and actions. Each environmental route will have its own consequences. This complex chain of events may, of course, occupy no more than an instant of reflection, be quite automatic and involve little conscious awareness, and have minimal impact upon the man's life, especially if the pattern is familiar to him. On the other hand, it might involve a much longer period of time and have a powerful impact upon other aspects of his life.

Thus individuals not only respond to impinging stimuli and observe the consequences of their behavior, but also actively select from the array of potential stimuli available, transform and categorize stimuli in idiosyncratic fashions, and partially determine some of the stimuli that impinge upon them. The environment only partially influences what people attend to, perceive, and think. By altering the immediate environments, by creating cognitive self-inducements, and by assigning conditional incentives for themselves, people can exercise influence over their environments and their responses. The experiences generated by behavior also partially determine what individuals think, feel, and do, which in turn influences subsequent behavior. The relative influence exerted by the environment and by cognition, affect, and behavior will vary in different individuals under different circumstances.

In sum, we suggest that recent research and theory concerning health, disease, and illness can be accommodated well within a *transactional model*, as described by Lazarus and his colleagues (R. Lazarus & Cohen,

1977; R. Lazarus & Launier, 1978; Roskies & Lazarus, 1980) and by Mason (1975c). The transactional model highlights the nature of the fit or the lack of fit between the person and the environmental demands. The discrepancy between the perceived demands upon a person (whether those demands are internal or external, whether challenges or goals) and the way the individual perceives his or her potential responses to these demands constitutes stress and has an impact upon the individual's health and the course of disease.

STAGES OF ILLNESS

Illness may be viewed as being composed of five stages: (1) symptom perception, (2) medical contact, (3) acute illness, (4) convalescence and rehabilitation, and (5) chronic illness and/or disability. Each stage presents unique challenges to the patient, and each challenge requires one or more coping responses on the part of the patient. The response the patient makes at any stage may influence subsequent perceptions and responses as well as how he or she is responded to or treated. Not all patients move through each of these stages, and a patient may cycle back to an earlier stage.

Symptom Perception and Medical Contact

Responses to physiological symptoms are influenced by the perception and appraisal of those symptoms (Mechanic, 1968; Meichenbaum, 1977; Rodin, 1978). For example, Katz et al. (1970) observed that one of the most common ways women coped with breast lumps was by avoidance and denial, which resulted in delay in seeking medical examination. Excessive delays could result in metastasis and a much poorer prognosis if the growth were malignant. Similarly, Gentry (1975) has estimated that as many as 70% of individuals suffering from myocardial infarction misinterpret or deny the source of their symptoms, which may result in disastrous consequences.

Certain information is required in order to appraise symptoms accurately, yet in most human affairs, especially those involving threat, unclear or insufficient information is common. When information is ambiguous or insufficient, it is more difficult to evaluate the likely outcomes of different response alternatives. R. Lazarus (1966) noted that "the more ambiguous are the stimulus cues concerning the nature of the confrontation, the more important are general belief systems in determining the appraisal process" (p. 134, original emphasis).

This point may be particularly important in health and illness since many physiological symptoms are ambiguous and thus likely to be interpreted largely on the basis of currently held beliefs and attitudes (Janis & Rodin, 1979). It is during the unorganized phases of the illness that patients attempt to assess their symptoms, conceptualize possible causes, and begin to formulate decisions about whether help is necessary and what types of help to seek. One final, dramatic example underscores this point. T. Hackett and Cassem (1975) observed that when some men experienced symptoms of heart attack, they performed vigorous pushups or ran up flights of stairs, reasoning that they could not be having a heart attack since the exercise did not kill them!

Acute Illness, Convalescence and Rehabilitation, Chronic Illness and Disability

Cognitive factors have been found to be important in recovery from acute disorders, response to noxious diagnostic medical procedures, and adaptation to chronic illnesses (Turk, 1979; Turk & Genest, 1979). Recovery from acute illness often depends upon adherence to therapeutic regimens. However, Marston (1970) estimated that nonadherence to medication regimens ranges from 4% to 92%. Patients' *attitudes* regarding their symptoms, their susceptibility to illness, their physicians, and the efficacy of treatments have been thought to be related to failures to adhere to medical recommendations (Maiman, Becker, Kirscht, Haefner, & Drachman, 1977). We will consider this important topic further in Chapters 3 and 8.

Several reviews (Garrity & Klein, 1971; R. Klein, 1975; Krantz, 1980; Pranulis, 1975) indicate that the ways coronary patients cope with hospitalization and recuperation may influence the chances of survival (see also Cousins, 1976). Cognitive appraisals and coping strategies in a variety of diagnostic and therapeutic situations have been related to such outcomes as early release from the hospital, reductions in analgesic medication, return to work, and reduced emotional distress (Garrity, 1973a, 1973b; Leventhal, Meyer, & Nerenz, 1980; Krantz, 1980). One study (R. Klein, Dean, & Willson, 1965) found that among a sample of myocardial infarction patients, the subjective meaning of the heart attack was an important determinant of the degree of disability. An important consideration was how this disorder was going to affect their roles as providers, parents, and husbands, as well as their activities.

There are significant differences in the psychological impact of chronic, as opposed to acute, illness. Chronic disease is, however, a poorly defined category that includes such diverse conditions as congenital defects, acquired injuries, diseases leaving residual damage, and incurable diseases with a progressive or unremitting course (McDaniel, 1969; Shontz, 1975; Turk, 1979).

Despite the range of conditions and disabilities encompassed by the category of chronic disease, a number of common features exist. Chronic diseases represent assaults on several areas of functioning, not just physical well-being. Patients with various chronic diseases may face separation from family and friends; loss of key roles; disruption of plans for the future; assaults on self-images and self-esteem; uncertain and unpredictable futures; distressing emotions such as anxiety, depression, resentment, and helplessness; and such illness-related factors as permanent changes in physical appearance or in bodily functioning (Turk, 1979; Turk, Sobel, Follick, & Youkilis, 1980). The presence of a chronic disease challenges both patients and the health care system.

Nonetheless, a substantial proportion of chronically ill patients make satisfactory adjustments. (For extended discussion of this topic, the interested reader should see Bieber & Drellich, 1963; Mattson & Gross, 1966; Tavormina, Kastner, Slater, & Watt, 1976; Turk, 1979; Weisman, 1979; and Weisman & Sobel, 1979.) For example, in an investigation of patients' coping with poliomyelitis, Visotsky, Hamburg, Goss, and Lebovits (1961) concluded the following:

> Many patients are remarkably resourceful even in the face of a catastrophic situation. Though our patients were deprived for long periods—and sometimes permanently—of abilities which are part of basic human equipment, most of them nevertheless showed an impressive resiliency and the ability to work out new patterns of living. (p. 445)

Turk (1979) reported observations on individuals who had been able to accommodate successfully to their diseases and those who had made less satisfactory adjustments. According to Turk, the factors that differentiated the patients making satisfactory adjustments from those having more difficulty were the following: (1) information concerning different aspects of the disease; (2) knowledge of appropriate coping resources, including individual coping strategies and social support systems; (3) a problem-solving attitude, including a perspective of active resourcefulness, and flexible and constructive behavior in contrast to premature resignation and passive helplessness; (4) a sense of personal mastery; and (5) motivation to keep working despite the prolonged nature of their diseases. Recently, Weisman and Sobel (1979) reached similar conclusions in their observations of high- and low-emotional-distress cancer patients. In the papers cited previously, the patients' cognitive appraisals markedly influenced the overt and covert behaviors and the quality of these responses for adjustment, adaptation, and rehabilitation. And how the patient responds to the challenges of illness is likely to determine, at least to some extent, how others respond to the patient (sympathy, avoidance, hostility).

What we have been proposing is that an individual's conceptual and affective systems are intrinsically involved with health, disease, and illness. These conceptual systems are composed of the patient's (1) values, beliefs, and goals regarding health, disease, and illness; (2) information about the disease and sense of perceived competence; and (3) role expectations and sets of action plans for responding to situational demands. Such cognitive and affective factors not only contribute to patients' responses to disease, but also determine the ways people define health and illness, respond to symptoms and incapacity, and utilize the health care system.

Our emphasis on conceptual and affective processes in health, disease onset, and illness suggests that it is important for behavioral medicine to assess these dynamic events. A recent study involving coping with job-related stress illustrates this assessment (Dewe, Guest, & Williams, 1979). We will briefly outline the method of that investigation and will then present a general coping assessment model.

ASSESSMENT OF OCCUPATIONAL STRESS AND COPING

Occupational Stress: An Illustration

To examine the methods people use to cope with work-related stress, Dewe *et al.* (1979) used an open-ended interview. They asked middle managers in a transport industry: "Can you think of a particular time at work when you have felt under stress? Can you tell me what happened and how you managed to cope with it?" They were able to group the answers to these questions according to what R. Lazarus (1975b) has categorized as direct action (altering the sources of discomfort) and palliative (reducing the feelings of discomfort) coping techniques.

Interviews with other employees (clerks, administrators, and white-collar supervisors) indicated that primarily four direct-action responses were used to cope with stress. These included facing the situation head-on, working harder, setting priorities, and talking things over with management. Avoiding the subject of contention and forgetting work when finished for the day were the two common palliative coping responses used. On the basis of these interview data, Dewe *et al.* developed a questionnaire to assess coping behavior that yielded four styles of coping.

The first style reflected task-oriented coping behaviors. Dewe *et al.* indicate that this style consisted of three elements. The first included analyzing and getting rid of the causes of stress ("Find out more about the situation," "Take immediate action," "Set priorities"). The second element involved actions to avoid and reduce panic (e.g., "Tackle routine work to get composure back," "Try not to worry," "Try to reassure yourself," "Take a break and come back to it later," "See the humor in the situation"). The third element of this task-directed coping behavior included action designed to prevent subsequent repercussions ("Let people know where you stand," "Make sure people are aware of what you are doing," and "Follow proper channels to cover yourself").

The second coping style focused on the expression of feelings coupled with a search for social support at work. The ability to let off steam, to get rid of tension by expressing some irritability and frustration, and to remove oneself temporarily from the stressful situation, plus the ability to seek advice from others or talk it over with someone else (i.e., use social supports), constituted the second constellation of coping skills.

The third major way the employees coped with work-related stress was to use outside activities. These included physical exercise, nonwork activities (e.g., hobbies), and family life, as well as talking over the problem at home. This latter coping activity reflected the desire to sort out the problem while away from the stressful environment.

Dewe *et al.* described the fourth coping style as involving mainly a passive attempt to ride out the situation, to ignore the sources of the stress for the time being. Such statements as "Let the feeling wear off," "Drop what you are doing and take up something totally unrelated," "Move into something you know you can get satisfaction from," "Do nothing," and "Try to carry on as usual," illustrate this coping style.

Although individuals may have a tendency to use one class of coping responses more than others, they often combine various coping responses (direct action, social support, and emotional control). Which combination will work will surely depend upon the job and the setting (e.g., the willingness of management or supervisors to change). Moreover, in the Dewe *et al.* study, employees did not readily report ways in which they cope by means of antisocial behaviors.

The Dewe *et al.* study illustrates how one can use open-ended interviews to have individuals enumerate coping responses. From such a clinical assessment, one can generate assessment devices that can be validated against external criteria and, in turn, can develop a training approach tailored to the specific population and setting. Although one should be knowledgeable about the findings for other populations, one should also be cautious in transferring assessment procedures and treatment programs to a specific population. The coping styles described by Dewe *et al.* for middle-class workers in the transportation industry may be quite inappropriate for workers in other sectors of the work force. What *is* transferable is the strategy used to identify and measure coping behavior. How these coping behaviors or styles relate to various behavioral and physical disorders is grist for the mill of behavioral medicine.

AN ASSESSMENT MODEL

Turk and his colleagues (Turk, 1979; Turk, Sobel, Follick, & Youkilis, 1980) have recently detailed a general model that applies the strategies used in the Dewe *et al.* (1979) investigation, which are an extension of the original behavior-analytic approach designed by Goldfried and D'Zurilla (1969). The emphasis of the approach is on a functional analysis of the relationship between thoughts, feelings, and behaviors and the disease-related threats, problems, and demands. These assessment procedures can be administered several different times.

Problem Identification

The first step in the model calls for a systematic assessment of the range of problems confronting patients and their significant others. A number of techniques (questionnaires, interviews, diaries, role playing, etc.) can be employed with patients, significant others, and health care providers in order to compile a comprehensive list of the variety of both practical (e.g., self-care) and psychosocial (e.g., dysphoric affect) problems.

Gordon and his colleagues (Gordon, Freidenbergs, Diller, Hibbard, Wolf, Levine, Lipkins, Ezrachi, & Lucido, 1980) surveyed 135 cancer patients and identified 122 psychosocial problems covering 13 areas of life functioning: "physical discomfort, medical treatment, medical service, mobility, housework, vocation, finances, family, social concerns, worry regarding the disease, affect, body image, and communication" (p. 744). A list of these problems was presented to new groups of cancer patients, who were asked to indicate (on a rating scale) the perceived severity of each of the problems listed. Gordon *et al.* (1980) used these data to identify major problematic areas for patients and to pinpoint specific problems for individual patients. The psychosocial treatments provided to patients were based on the material obtained from the questionnaire. We will examine the intervention developed by Gordon *et al.* in the next chapter.

Follick and Turk (1978) conducted a similar problem-identification procedure. In this study, however, significant others and health care providers (e.g., nurses, social workers, and enterostomal therapists) were also included. Additionally, Follick and Turk focused this assessment process on groups of patients with a very specific medical condition— patients who had had ostomies. An ostomy is a surgical procedure that results in an artifical opening in the abdominal wall through which bodily waste is excreted. An individual with an ostomy must wear a collection bag or appliance over the artificial opening because there is a loss of control over the process of elimination.

Six problem clusters were identified by Follick and Turk (1978): technical management (e.g., leakage, skin irritation); occupational adjustment (e.g., change in occupation, requirement of additional toilet breaks); social adjustment (e.g., reduction in or alteration of recreational or social activities); marital/sexual adjustment (e.g., reduction in the frequency of sexual activity, diminished sexual drive); family adjustment (e.g., alteration in family members roles, discussion of ostomy with family members); and emotional adjustment (e.g., depression, anxiety, feelings of being different). Follick and Turk emphasized the importance of including significant others and health care providers—not just patients—in order to generate a more comprehensive list of problems and to identify discrepancies between patients' perceptions of problems and the perceptions of those involved with their care. Important discrepancies between patients' and health care providers' perceptions have been noted by several authors (e.g., Blank, 1979; Hanson & Franklin, 1976).

Response Enumeration

The second step in the model presented by Turk, Sobel, Follick, and Youkilis (1980) is designed to identify the range of responses that are employed to cope with the problems, threats, and demands cataloged during the initial problem identification. Since overt behavioral responses designed to address problems are not always possible or appropriate, Turk et al. emphasized the importance of enumerating both overt and covert coping responses, that is, both the actual mode of responding and the thoughts and feelings that patients experience before, during, and following specific problem situations.

A number of papers have described procedures (e.g., imagery, role playing, sampling of thoughts) that may be employed to elicit such cognitive behaviors (e.g., Ericsson & Simon, 1980; Genest & Turk, 1981; Kendall & Hollon, 1980a; Meichenbaum & Butler, 1979). This assessment should enable the investigator to identify a patient's cognitive appraisal of problems and their personal meanings to the patient. Such an analysis should be of help in developing an individualized treatment program.

An individualized approach based on problem identification and response enumeration has recently been employed by Sobel and his colleagues (Sobel, 1981; Sobel & Worden, 1981; Weisman & Sobel, 1979). They presented cancer patients with TAT-type (thematic apperception test) pictorial cards displaying various problem situations identified by earlier groups of cancer patients and asked the patients to report the thoughts and feelings of characters depicted on the cards, as well as how the characters would respond. Through this projective technique, Sobel sought information about the coping responses of the cancer patients and incorporated this information in the treatment of cancer patients (Sobel & Worden, 1981). We will examine the treatment approach developed by Weisman and his colleagues in the next chapter.

Response Evaluation

How effective are different responses for a particular problem? To what extent do the various thoughts and feelings exacerbate or ameliorate the problem? These questions are typically evaluated by health care providers based on theoretical orientation, a priori beliefs, or face validity. The perceptions of patients and significant others have rarely been examined in a systematic manner.

The third step in the model is specifically designed to determine the relative efficacy of different responses from the perspective of patients, significant others, and health care providers. This strategy is designed to determine the perceived utility of alternative responses. Weisman, Worden, and Sobel (1980) have conducted such a response evaluation with cancer patients. Currently, several investigators are conducting assessments of the coping responses of chronic pain patients (e.g., Genest, 1982; Keefe & Rosenstiel, 1980; Turk & Kerns, in progress). These investigators are examining how patients' coping responses and their cognitions concerning their coping responses (metacognitions) affect the range and success of adaptation.

Usefulness of the Model

This assessment strategy, which includes problem identification, response enumeration, and response evaluation, should enable better understanding of problems and coping strategies of patients with different chronic diseases. This procedure can also be used to develop screening instruments to identify "high-risk" patients in need of psychosocial interventions and to pinpoint the content and direction of such interventions. Finally, the procedure should be of use in assessing the relative efficacy of treatment interventions.

SUMMARY

The development of preventive or remedial programs requires detailed knowledge of the process of adaptation specific for each disease or chronic condition, including relevant adaptive tasks and strategies for task accomplishments. Thus, prior to the implementation of therapeutic regimens, it is necessary to identify the problems posed by each disease, the range of response options, and information concerning the relative efficacy of coping strategies and resources.

By the nature of their work, clinicians in the field of behavioral medicine tend to see only those patients who are having difficulty adjusting to their plight. Although health care providers are expected to help patients learn to cope more effectively, they often possess little knowledge of how coping and adaptation are accomplished by more successful patients. The approach described by Turk, Sobel, Follick, and Youkilis (1980) should be helpful in remedying this deficiency in our knowledge. The systematic approach to assessment of coping and the transactional emphasis are hallmarks of the cognitive–behavioral approach.

In this chapter we have emphasized the importance of cognitive process and affective factors in the entire spectrum of problems encompassed by the field of behavioral medicine. We have tried to show how these cognitive and affective factors contribute to health, disease, and illness and how they cannot be isolated from purely physiological factors specific to a disease. In the next chapter we will focus more specifically on representative research that has examined the contribution of psychological mediation to health, disease, and illness.

CHAPTER 3

BEHAVIORAL MEDICINE: COGNITIVE–BEHAVIORAL APPLICATIONS IN HEALTH PROMOTION, DISEASE, AND ILLNESS

We should be bold in what we attempt but cautious in what we claim.
—*Neal Miller* (*1975*)

This chapter focuses on the applications of cognitive–behavioral approaches in the facilitation of disease prevention, of health maintenance, and of the process of coping with disease, aversive medical procedures, convalescence, and rehabilitation. Studies are reviewed that illustrate the role of cognitive and affective factors in facilitating or inhibiting disease as well as in coping with and adapting to diverse medical procedures, diseases, and the illness process.

APPLICATIONS

In recent years psychological techniques have been employed (1) to modify self-imposed risks to health (e.g., obesity, substance abuse, maladaptive life-styles); (2) to alleviate distress related to aversive diagnostic and noxious therapeutic medical and surgical procedures (e.g., pelvic examinations, cardiac catheterization, endoscopic examinations, postsurgical distress and discomfort, debridement of burns); (3) to enhance adaptive coping with stress (e.g., tension and migraine headaches, irritable bowel syndrome, gastric and duodenal ulcers, mucous colitis); and (4) to assist patients to live more satisfactory lives despite chronic medical conditions (e.g., low back pain, diabetes, cancer). Let us consider how cognitive–behavioral procedures have been used to achieve each of these objectives. The studies chosen for review are illustrative and in many cases reflect the pioneering and tentative nature of the "state of the art."

As we will see, a common feature of cognitive–behavioral treatments is that the patient is viewed as an important agent in guiding, directing, and controlling his or her own health, disease, and illness. To the extent that the person has learned to engage in maladaptive or ineffective behaviors, he or she can be taught to manage responses so that they are more adaptive and effective. Moreover, if many maladaptive behaviors are learned, then they can be prevented through the acquisition of more adaptive behaviors. A host of procedures has been employed to accomplish change (e.g., coping skills training, problem-solving training, cognitive restructuring, self-control training; see Cameron, 1980; Mahoney & Arnkoff, 1978; Meichenbaum, 1977; Turk, 1982). These techniques will be described in Section III.

Modification of Health "Risk" Factors

A factor considered to be a "risk" factor is one, such as obesity, that is associated with the development of a disease, such as diabetes mellitus. For example, a number of risk factors have been related to the development of coronary heart disease (CHD), the number one cause of death in the United States. A major direct factor associated with the incidence of CHD is hypertension. Other factors that are considered to be direct risk factors for CHD are obesity and cigarette smoking. Hypertension has, in turn, been related to a factor that may be considered an "indirect" risk, labeled Type A coronary-prone behavior. The Type A behavior pattern is characterized by high competitiveness, aggressiveness, and a hostile response to frustration. In addition to the association with CHD, hypertension has been implicated as a risk factor for kidney disease and cerebrovascular accidents (strokes).

In the next section, we will briefly examine several risk factors for a variety of diseases and will present interventions that have been employed to reduce morbidity and mortality.

Essential Hypertension

"Essential hypertension" is defined as sustained, elevated blood pressure of unknown etiology. No subjective symptoms are present, and diagnosis is usually made during routine physical examinations. Elevated blood pressure is a major risk factor for cardiovascular and other diseases. In the now-famous Framingham longitudinal study (Kannel, 1976), hypertension was found to be one of the most robust predictors of such life-threatening disorders as myocardial infarction, congestive heart failure, stroke, and kidney disease. Risk of such medical problems was found to be elevated with increases in blood pressure, with hypertensives three times more likely to develop cardiovascular diseases than normotensives.

There is a growing recognition that the pharmacological treatment of essential hypertension has many undesirable side effects (Bulpitt & Dollery, 1973) and is less effective than drug advertisements might lead one to believe (Kannel & Dawber, 1973; LoGerfo, 1975). Such evidence has resulted in a number of attempts to employ psychological interventions to reduce high blood pressure.

Psychological treatments of essential hypertension have been based on a model in which it is hypothesized that repeated and prolonged elicitation of the "emergency reaction" (Cannon, 1932), with its characteristic blood pressure lability, leads to hypertension in predisposed individuals (Gutmann & Benson, 1971; Henry & Cassel, 1969; Stoyva, 1976). Treatment techniques focus on reducing the sympathetic nervous system reaction that mediates the so-called emergency reaction. Approaches have included biofeedback, relaxation, and meditation—all designed to reduce the symptom, namely, high blood pressure. After an extensive review of these techniques, Seer (1979) concluded the following:

> At the present time we have no convincing indication that essential hypertensives can achieve clinically relevant and persistent blood pressure reductions through blood pressure feedback training . . . it is safe to say that in contrast to blood pressure biofeedback training, relaxation/meditation has produced small but significant reductions in blood pressure with essential hypertension. (p. 1037)

The relatively meager results of biofeedback and relaxation are likely partly a function of the focus of these treatments on modifying sympathetic nervous system activity, with insufficient attention to cognitive variables. Little attention is paid to the likelihood that sympathetic arousal reflects the idiosyncratic ways that patients perceive, appraise, and interact with their environments. One could, on the other hand, evaluate and modify the hypertensive patient's maladaptive appraisal and coping patterns in order to prevent increased sympathetic arousal, as well as attempt to decrease directly sympathetic overreactivity. This can be accomplished through assessment of the situations and events associated with a patient's blood pressure elevation and through analysis of dysfunctional patterns of thoughts, emotions, and behaviors. Once these dysfunctional patterns are identified, treatment may be designed to teach active stress-managing coping skills, including problem-solving training, cognitive restructuring, and relaxation exercises to reduce physical arousal.

Patel and North (1975), for example, developed a comprehensive treatment for hypertensives that consisted of an educational program, controlled breathing, relaxation, meditation, biofeedback, and a number of self-control procedures for coping with everyday stresses. Reductions of systolic and diastolic blood pressure of 26 mm Hg and 15 mm Hg, respectively, were obtained following 6 weeks of training. These clinically significant improvements were maintained at a 3-month follow-up. This result was a significantly greater reduction than that achieved by a control group of subjects who were taught only to relax. These control subjects later underwent the full treatment, reducing systolic blood pressure a further 28 mm Hg and diastolic 16 mm Hg.

It is impossible to determine the contributions of the various components to the treatment efficacy in the Patel and North (1975) study. One additional study, however, does lend some support for the importance of the coping-skills-training component. Frankel, Patel, Horowitz, Friedwald, and Gaardner (1978) employed a treatment package similar to Patel and North's, but omitted the coping-skills-training component. After 4 months of training, Frankel *et al.* found no significant reduction in blood pressure.

In another study Novaco (1976b) employed a stress-inoculation procedure (originally developed by Meichenbaum and his colleagues; Meichenbaum & Cameron, 1972b; Meichenbaum & Turk, 1976) with a group of individuals having problems of anger control. (Anger has been related to the coronary-prone behavior pattern discussed in the next section.) The stress-inoculation program incorporated cognitive coping skills training, self-instructional training, and relaxation training. Novaco found changes in the behavior patterns of hyperangry patients and also significant decreases in both systolic and diastolic blood pressure relative to control treatment groups.

Treatments that focus on teaching cognitive, behavioral, affective, and interpersonal skills provide encouraging data. Further research with these techniques is needed to demonstrate whether a significant clinical reduction in blood pressure will be maintained by hypertensive patients.

Type A Coronary-Prone Behavior Pattern

Since the pioneering work of M. Friedman and Rosenman in the 1950s, growing evidence has pointed to a relationship between CHD and a pattern of behavior (Type A coronary-prone behavior) characterized by intense ambition, constant preoccupation with occupational deadlines, a sense of time urgency, and competitive drive (M. Friedman & Rosenman, 1959; Rosenman, Brand, Jenkins, Friedman, Straus, & Wurm, 1975; Rosenman, Brand, Scholtz, & Friedman, 1976).

The relationship between Type A behavior and the development of CHD was indicated in the prospective Western Collaborative Group study. In this study 3154 initially well, middle-class men classified according to behavior pattern (Type A or Type B, indicating the absence of coronary-prone behavior) were followed for 8½ years to determine their subsequent cardiac morbidity and mortality (Rosenman, Friedman, Straus, Wurm, Kositchek, Hahn, & Werthessen, 1964). The results indicated that, even controlling for the effect of other risk factors (e.g., smoking, obesity), Type A men had twice the risk of developing or dying from CHD than did the men classified as Type B and, within the age range of 39 to 49 years, were six times more likely to develop CHD (Rosenman, Rahe, Borhani, & Feinlieb, 1975). Moreover, following a first myocardial infarction, the incidence of a subsequent infarction among Type A men was approximately twice that observed among Type B men (Jenkins, Zyzanski, & Rosenman, 1976).

At a recent conference on CHD, the conclusion was drawn that for the first time in medicine a behavioral method—one that did not tap subclinical signs and symptoms—was capable of successfully and independently predicting the future emergence of a somatic disease (Dembroski, Caffrey, Jenkins, Rosenman, Spielberger, & Tasto, 1977). Many recent reviews of the research supporting the relationship between Type A behavior and CHD have been presented (e.g., Dembroski, 1977; Glass, 1977; Jenkins, 1976; Roskies, 1980). Some recent studies, however, have not confirmed this association. For example, Dimsdale and his colleagues (Dimsdale, Hackett, Catanzano, & White, 1979; Dimsdale, Hackett, Hutter, & Block, 1980; Dimsdale, Hackett, Hutter, Block, Catanzano, & White, 1979) failed to find a relationship between the Type A behavior pattern and coronary vessel disease, angina symptoms, or history of myocardial infarction.

One explanation for the somewhat inconsistent findings may be related to the range of behaviors that have been associated with the Type A behavior pattern. For example, eagerness to compete, self-imposed deadlines, desire for recognition, quickness of mental and physical functioning, intense drive toward self-selected but poorly defined goals, impatience at the rate of progress of events, thinking about or acting upon multiple tasks simultaneously, vague guilt or unease at relaxing, scheduling more things in less time, rapid talking and moving, accentuating words in speech, hostility, and the perception of challenges where none exists have all been identified as components of the Type A behavior pattern. Reconciling the inconsistent data may be accomplished by identifying which components of the Type A behavior pattern actually predict CHD (Roskies, 1980, 1982).

In their original formulation, M. Friedman and Rosenman (1959) viewed the Type A behavior pattern as only a surface manifestation of a global life-style and an underlying philosophy of life. Thus they tended to view the behavior pattern as representative of a recalcitrant underlying trait or disposition. They suggested that any attempt to modify the trait would require a major modification of life-style and philosophy. Perhaps because of difficulties seen in bringing about such a major reorganization of thinking, behaving, and feeling, only one study adopting the Friedman and Rosenman conceptualization has been conducted to modify the Type A pattern.

Rosenman and Friedman (1977) developed a complex intervention designed to modify personality, life-style, and attitude and thus effect a major philosophical change. The intervention program included philosophical discussions, group meditation, biofeedback, and autogenic training, as well as a host of self-management techniques (e.g., rational restructuring, self-monitoring). The authors reported that this therapeutic regimen was successful. Their claim for success, however, was based solely on the subjects' self-reports of their feelings of "enhanced well-being." Furthermore, the authors' report is of limited value because it was anecdotal, did not employ control groups, did not indicate the length of the treatment, and did not include a follow-up.

From a behavioral perspective, Type A behavior is viewed as a learned pattern subject to modification rather than as an enduring and inflexible manifestation of a personality trait. Type A behaviors are hypothesized to be acquired by societal reinforcement of achievement, competitiveness, assertiveness, and aggressive drive. Glass (1977) has proposed that the Type A individual is one who has internalized all too well Western society's emphasis on the ability to master and control the environment. In a sense, the individual manifesting Type A behavior has adjusted to society and is rewarded accordingly.

Glass (1977) suggests that Type A behavior is elicited in susceptible individuals by uncontrollable stressful situations. Additionally, there is some evidence that Type A individuals may tend to be more sensitive to certain stressors (Rosenman & Friedman, 1977; Scherwitz, Berton, & Leventhal, 1977). And, finally, Dembroski, McDougall, and Shields (1977) and Glass (1977) have indicated that Type A individuals may create much of their own distress by perceiving challenges where others do not.

Suinn and Bloom (1978) based a behavioral intervention on the possible interaction among stress, Type A behavior, and CHD. Their treatment was designed to teach new ways of coping with stress to substitute for the less adaptive Type A behaviors.

The stress-management program developed by Suinn and Bloom (1978) was conducted with volunteer subjects who considered themselves as having Type A characteristics. This referral process may have confounded the results with self-selection biases. The training program, which consisted of two sessions per week for 3 weeks, included the use of imagery to precipitate stress. The imaginal stress served to facilitate the identification of muscular signs of stress onset. Finally, training in stress reduction through relaxation was conducted. Additional emphasis was placed on practicing stress management in response to feelings of time urgency. These subjects were compared with control subjects who only discussed factors related to stress. Suinn and Bloom reported that the stress-management training group reported comparatively less anxiety following the training. Cholesterol, triglycerides, and blood pressure, however, were not significantly reduced. No follow-up was reported, nor was the credibility of the attention-placebo group established. Thus the Suinn and Bloom data must be interpreted with caution.

Roskies and her colleagues (Roskies, Kearney, Spevack, Surkis, Cohen, & Gilman, 1978, 1979) contrasted two treatments for Type A behaviors: One, a psychodynamically oriented approach, focused on resolving the behavior pattern by elucidating unconscious conflicts. A second, cognitive–behavioral approach focused on increasing awareness of control over behavior, relaxation training, and self-monitoring. These treatments included 14 therapy sessions spread over 5 months. The two groups of subjects were composed of healthy volunteers (no CHD); a third group consisted of subjects who already had signs of CHD. This last group received the cognitive–behavioral treatment.

All three groups showed significant reductions in anxiety and other psychological symptoms, as well as reductions in serum cholesterol (psychodynamic group: 237.1 mg/ml to 221.0 mg/ml; cognitive–behavioral group: 238.2 mg/ml to 197.5 mg/ml) and blood pressure (psychodynamic group: systolic 127.9 mm Hg to 122.6 mm Hg, diastolic 83.2 mm Hg to 83.4 mm Hg; cognitive–behavioral group: systolic 122.5 mm Hg to 117.9 mm Hg, diastolic 83.4 mm Hg to 81.4 mm Hg) following treatment. The cognitive–behavioral treatment groups showed greater, but not significantly different, reduction in serum cholesterol than the psychodynamic psychotherapy group. At 6-month follow-up all groups showed good maintenance of treatment effects; the cognitive–behavioral treatment groups tended to demonstrate better maintenance than the psychodynamic psychotherapy group, although, once again, not significantly so. Interestingly, these changes occurred without modification of diet, exercise, smoking, or work load. Thus it appears that psychological interventions without modification of some risk factors can result in decreased CHD incidence. The long-term clinical validity of these results, however, remains an open question.

Jenni and Wollersheim (1979) conducted a study in which they contrasted Suinn and Bloom's stress-management program with a cognitive therapy treatment that was based on modifying stressful appraisals of events. Additionally, "irrational beliefs" (Ellis, 1962) believed to be relevant for Type A individuals (e.g., "I must be perfect, thoroughly competent, and achieving in everything I do") were presented, with the goal of having subjects become aware of how maladaptive such ideas might be. Finally, subjects were taught to reinterpret situations associated with time pressure, competitiveness, and hostility.

Subjects in the Jenni and Wollersheim (1979) study either were referred by physicians or responded to a newspaper advertisement. All subjects received six weekly 90-minute sessions. Compared to the stress-management group, the cognitive–behavioral therapy group reduced self-reports of Type A behavior and of anxiety, but failed to demonstrate reductions in cholesterol or blood pressure. These results were evident at a 6-week follow-up as well. Thus, in both the Suinn and Bloom (1978) study and the Jenni and Wollersheim (1979) study, self-reports of change following cognitive–behavioral training were obtained, but no changes were evident on physiological measures. In contrast, the Roskies studies reported changes in both psychological and physiological measures.

Although these studies indicate the potential of cognitive–behavioral techniques for modifying Type A behavior, they must be regarded as tentative because they have failed to report extended follow-up morbidity and mortality data. Obviously, modifying subjects' self-reports and even Type A behaviors is not sufficient. There is a need to establish that such treatments have long-term physiological effects. (See Roskies, 1982, for a more detailed discussion of these issues.)

Obesity

Medical researchers have identified obesity as a major health problem and as a major risk factor for both CHD and diabetes. The most traditional approaches to weight reduction have included suggestions to exercise, to follow a diet designed to reduce caloric intake, to use stimulant drugs (amphetamines), and in some cases to undergo psychodynamic psychotherapy. After reviewing this research, Stunkard (1958) concluded that "most obese persons will not stay in treatment for obesity, of those who stay in treatment most will not lose weight, and of those who lose weight, most will regain it" (p. 85). Because of such pessimistic conclusions, and because of the rapid development of behavior therapy, investigators have applied behavior modification techniques to the refractory problem of obesity.

The major assumption in behavioral treatments of obesity is that obesity is due to a combination of excessive food consumption (resulting from faulty eating habits) and low energy expenditure. It has been hypothesized, but not actually confirmed, that several behaviors contribute to overweight, including rapid rate of consumption, taking large bites of food, frequent feeding, ingestion of large quantities at a given meal, frequent snacking, and excessive eating during times of stress. These behaviors are regarded as operants, reinforced by the pleasure of eating and under partial control of environmental cues associated with eating.

A common explanation of "overeating" is that reinforcing consequences are immediate, whereas aversive consequences are delayed. This formulation has led to treatment strategies that (1) provide immediate reinforcement for "appropriate" eating or abstinence from food (money, social approval, self-reward), (2) diminish the strength of pleasure as a reinforcement for eating (aversive conditioning to high caloric foods, covert conditioning), (3) make long-term negative consequences more salient at time of eating (e.g., consideration of the undesirability of being fat and the value of thinness), and (4) eliminate food cues that trigger eating (e.g., ridding the house of fattening foods or restructuring the time and place in which eating occurs).

Over the last decade, a wide range of behavior modification techniques have been employed in the treatment of obesity. Extensive reviews of the efficacy of specific procedures have appeared elsewhere (Jeffery, Wing, & Stunkard, 1978; Leon, 1976; Stunkard & Mahoney, 1976; Wilson, 1978b; Yates, 1975). Generally, behavioral treatments have been significantly effective compared to nonbehavioral treatments (e.g., S. Hall & Hall, 1974; Leon, 1976; Ost & Gotestam, 1976; Stunkard, 1972a; Stunkard & Mahoney, 1976). Nevertheless, recent critical reviews of long-term behavioral follow-up studies of obesity (6 months or longer) have concluded that maintenance *has not clearly been demonstrated* (Brightwell & Sloan, 1977; Mahoney & Mahoney, 1976; Stunkard, 1977a). Furthermore, most weight loss results do not appear to be clinically significant, averaging only about 11 lb. (Jeffery *et al.*, 1978).

Most, if not all, of the studies on obesity in the literature report group differences, but these group data mask tremendous individual differences: Changes following behavioral treatment range from losses of up to 40 lb. to *increases* of 50 lb.! Individual differences also are demonstrated in the attrition rates in the behavior modification studies of obese patients. In a review of behavioral treatments, S. Hall and Hall (1974) reported that dropout rates ranged from 0% to 83%. The lack of maintenance, the high attrition rates, and the limited clinical significance of the reported weight loss raise questions of how behavioral treatments can be extended or modified.

One important factor is the recognition that obesity is not a uniform phenomenon, nor is it likely to be treated successfully by a uniformly standardized treatment program. Studies attempting to modify obesity have promulgated both subject and treatment uniformity myths (Kiesler, 1966). Individuals may become obese or maintain excessive weight for a number of reasons, including a sedentary life-style, eating as a coping technique to deal with tension, excessive snacking of high-caloric foods, or eating rapidly. Such individual behavior patterns emphasize the need to assess carefully individual eating patterns, including both internal and external antecedent and consequent events (e.g., thoughts and feelings that precede, accompany, and follow eating) as well as situational factors and behavioral patterns that affect exercise.

Another important factor in planning a treatment regimen is to consider the patient's social support systems. Is the environment of the obese person sufficiently reinforcing? How do significant others respond to the problem of obesity? How are significant others likely to respond to losses of weight? A consideration of these questions will increase the sensitivity of the treatment program.

Successful treatment programs should attend not only to eating behaviors, but also to the individuals' thoughts and feelings regarding themselves, obesity, the treatment program offered, and the likelihood that they will be able to lose weight and maintain the loss. In several studies obese subjects have been asked to monitor weight-relevant internal dialogues (e.g., Leon, Roth, & Hewitt, 1977; Mahoney, Moura, & Wade, 1973; Sjoberg & Persson, 1979). Mahoney (1975) classified weight-relevant thoughts into five categories: (1) thoughts about pounds lost (e.g., "I've starved myself and only lost 2 lb."), (2) thoughts about capabilities (e.g., "I just don't have the willpower"), (3) excuses (e.g., "If I weren't under so much pressure at my job, I would lose weight"), (4) standard setting (e.g., "Well, I blew it with that doughnut—my day is shot"), and (5) thoughts about actual food items.

Sjoberg and Persson (1979) studied the conditions under which thoughts and feelings lead to deviations from the weight-control regimen. They reported that, in the majority of cases, episodes of overeating were preceded by maladaptive and distorted thinking, for example, "An extra sandwich now helps me to eat less later," or "I've already lost a lot of weight, so I can indulge myself this once." Sjoberg and Persson (1979) also noted a "domino effect" such that initial deviation often resulted in complete relapse. Leon *et al.* (1977) asked people on diets to record the behaviors they engaged in to avoid overeating when they had the urge to eat. Two patterns were identified, namely, active behaviors that served as distractions from eating (e.g., doing the laundry, starting to sew) and covert activities such as visualization of positive and negative self-images.

Poor self-esteem often constitutes a problem for obese people. Contributing to this poor self-esteem is the general belief that the obese are responsible for their condition (Wooley, Wooley, & Dyrenforth, 1979). Cultural stereotypes of the obese as lacking ambition and discipline and as being sloppy, lazy, ugly, and stupid, for example, are often adopted by the obese individual. Self-defeating attitudes and histories of unsuccessful attempts to lose weight tend to reinforce beliefs held by obese individuals that they are not capable of adhering to and following weight-loss programs (Loro, Levenkron, & Fisher, 1979).

The data presented regarding covert self-statements, images, attitudes, beliefs, and feelings underscore the importance of attention to cognitive and affective processes related to body image, self-control, self-esteem, maladaptive urges, maladaptive cognitions associated with eating and exercise, low self-efficacy, and learned helplessness following multiple failures, as well as to patterns of eating and energy expenditure. Meaningful treatment suggestions will need to take into consideration such factors as these: (1) knowledge of nutrition, exercise, and the physiology of metabolism; (2) the patient's attitudes concerning obesity, dieting, and exercise; (3) social factors related to caloric intake and expenditure, prior dieting experience, and current eating and exercise patterns; and (4) tailoring the treatment regimen to the individual patient.

Such a treatment regimen for obesity was developed by Mahoney and Mahoney (1976). This program relies heavily on cognitive variables, self-monitoring, and energy expenditure. Self-control is taught through extensive self-monitoring of the time, place, and amount of food eaten; monitoring of food-related thoughts; and development of social supports. Patients are instructed to specify maladaptive cognitions associated with eating and to replace these cognitions with more adaptive thoughts and images. The program advocated by Mahoney and Mahoney (1976) emphasizes setting reasonable goals for behavior change, goals that are flexible enough that they can be modified if the patient has difficulty meeting them. Patients are encouraged to take responsibility for their own environments. Emphasis is placed on self-control of choices and decisions in relation to food consumption and energy expenditure.

The preliminary results of cognitive–behavioral approaches to management of obesity appear promising (Mahoney, 1974b; Mahoney et al., 1973). More systematic, controlled investigation, however, needs to be conducted before firm conclusions regarding efficacy can be drawn.

Smoking

The deleterious effects of smoking cigarettes have been suspected for some time, and recent reports have linked smoking directly with cardio-vascular disease, chronic bronchopulmonary disease, various cancers, and low birth weight among children born to mothers who smoked during pregnancy. Smoking has been identified as one of the major causes of the current health care crisis (Abelson, 1976; Kristein, 1977; Lalonde, 1974; Pollin, 1977; U.S. Surgeon General, 1979). Attempts to reduce smoking by removal of advertising on television, antismoking ads, and mass education have had some success. It has been estimated that 30 mil-lion Americans have quit smoking since 1964. However, 47 million Ameri-cans continue to smoke, with many of these expressing the desire to quit. Of those who desire to quit, 64% of the males and 60% of the females surveyed had already tried unsuccessfully to quit on their own (USPHS, 1976).

As noted in the case of obesity, the immediate positive pleasures of smoking (e.g., pleasurable experiences, reduction of craving) outweigh the delayed aversive consequences (long-term health problems). Addi-tionally, children and adolescents may find smoking reinforced by ap-proval of peers and by a sense of rebellion against parents and authority. Smoking may thus be viewed as a learned pattern of behavior (e.g., Hunt & Matarazzo, 1970, 1973).

This view has led to the development of a host of behavior-management programs to reduce smoking. For example, behavior therapists have paired smoking with immediate aversive events such as electric shock (e.g., Carlin & Armstrong, 1968), aversive noise (R. S. Greene, 1964), and hot smoke blown into the smoker's face (Best & Steffy, 1971; Franks, Fried, & Ashem, 1966), or they have tried to change the reinforcing value of smoking by using satiation procedures (i.e., having the client smoke 200% to 300% more cigarettes during a period of days prior to treatment sessions; e.g., Best, Owen, & Trentadue, 1978).

Another behavioral procedure that has been used to make the conse-quences of smoking more immediately aversive has been increasing the immediate *response cost* (e.g., the smoker's tearing up a dollar bill each time a specified number of cigarettes are smoked; Axelrod, Hall, Weis, & Rohrer, 1974). The converse of response cost, *contingency contracting*, makes valued consequences contingent upon progressively longer periods of abstinence (Winett, 1973). Still another technique is *stimulus control*, whereby the client avoids the situation in which smoking usually occurs, for example, being in a bar or in front of the television (D. Shapiro, Tursky, Schwartz, & Shnidman, 1971).

Extensive reviews of the relative efficacy of behavioral treatments for smoking reduction have appeared in the literature (e.g., Bernstein & McAlister, 1976; Best & Block, 1979; Lichtenstein & Danaher, 1976; Pechacek & McAlister, 1979). Each of these reviews concludes that treatment programs result in significantly reduced smoking behavior during the initial behavioral intervention stage, but that this is followed by rapid relapse during follow-up. Hunt and Bespalec (1974) reviewed 89 smoking cessation studies and reported that approximately 70% of initial abstainers relapsed within the first 6 months.

During the discussion of obesity, we raised concerns about treating all patients or all treatments alike. These concerns can be echoed here. Individuals engage in smoking behaviors for diverse reasons (e.g., social approval, to cope with negative affect), each tied to a wide variety of discriminative stimuli (e.g., social situations, studying, after meals, driving a car). To examine the variety of covert processes related to smoking and maintenance of smoking cessation, several studies have asked successful and unsuccessful "quitters" to report on the nature of their smoking-related thoughts and coping techniques (Best, 1980; Jacobs, Spilken, Norman, Wohlberg, & Knapp, 1971; Pederson & Lefcoe, 1976; Perri, Richards, & Schultheis, 1977; Sjoberg & Johnson, 1978; Wax & Wax, 1978).

Perri *et al.* (1977), for example, interviewed 24 successful and 24 unsuccessful quitters, concluding that successful quitters used more stimulus control techniques for a longer period and made more frequent use of self-reinforcement and problem-solving procedures. Wax and Wax (1978) reported that successful quitters used a variety of techniques to help them suppress the urge or impulse to smoke. Some subjects accomplished this by reminding themselves of the pain in their chests when they had last smoked. Others said that, whenever they felt like smoking, they consciously put the idea out of their minds: "You will have to do it [withdraw] all over again, and it was so hard." And still others used thoughts as self-reinforcements: "I just tell myself how good I feel about having stopped."

Sjoberg and Johnson (1978) noted the presence of both positive and negative mood preceding abstinent smokers' relapse and of distorted reasoning similars to that observed in obese individuals: "I've been doing so well. I'll treat myself to just one cigarette." Relapsed smokers reported fatalistic attitudes about the results of treatment and a low sense of self-efficacy related to their repeated failures to quit: "Once a smoker, always a smoker" (Blittner, Goldberg, & Merbaum, 1978; Tamerin, 1972). Finally, Best (1980) noted that, at the 6-month follow-up of a smoking cessation study, 55% of the reasons given for relapse were related to coping with stress, five times more than any other reasons for relapse.

These observations suggest that treatment approaches for smoking reduction and maintenance might be more effective if they altered not only the reinforcing effects of smoking, but also the individual's internal dialogue, and enabled the individual to develop alternative coping skills for dealing with stress or smoking urges. A number of interventions have successfully combined traditional behavioral approaches with various cognitive techniques (Best, Bass, & Owen, 1977; Blittner *et al.*, 1978; Brengelmann & Sedlmayr, 1977; Lando, 1977; Pomerleau, Adkins, & Pertschuk, 1978; Steffy, Meichenbaum, & Best, 1970).

For example, Pechacek and Danaher (1979) used a multicomponent cognitive–behavioral approach consisting of three stages: preparation, cessation, and maintenance. Specific treatment strategies included (1) a cognitive–behavioral rationale, (2) self-monitoring, (3) behavioral self-control (e.g., stimulus control, response costs), (4) aversive smoking (e.g., satiation, rapid smoking), (5) target termination dates, (6) massed or daily treatments, (7) skills training (e.g., relaxation, problem solving), (8) behavioral rehearsal of alternatives, and (9) graded spacing of treatment sessions. Although the data from this and other related cognitive–behavioral treatment programs are promising, they are preliminary. We describe the training regimen in order to convey the complex nature of treatment.

If only bioactive factors were involved in smoking, physical habituation would be the major problem and could be resolved by a variety of behavioral approaches leading to abstinence. But smoking is also a social activity charged with affect and accompanied by complex symbolism and ritual, so that behaviors, as well as attitudes, beliefs, and other cognitive and affective processes enter into consideration.

Alcoholism

The recent U.S. Surgeon General's report (1979) cites misuse of alcohol as a factor in more than 10% of all deaths in the United States. Excessive alcohol consumption has been implicated as a direct risk factor for cancer of the larynx, oral cavity, liver, and esophagus. It is also an indirect risk factor in accidents, suicides, and homicides. Additionally, alcohol abuse is known to contribute to family disruption and poor school and job performance, and it is believed to be related to low birth weight in neonates and to birth defects.

It is estimated that 68% of adult Americans consume alcohol at least on some occasions, with 12% of these estimated to be heavy drinkers. Heavy drinking is usually defined as drinking alcohol daily or consuming large quantities of alcohol intermittently. It is further estimated that there are 10 million alcoholics in the United States (U.S. Surgeon General,

1979). "Alcoholism" is defined as compulsive, habitual, or addictive drinking that poses a serious threat to the individual's health and well-being (Cahalan, Cisin, & Crossley, 1974; Cahalan & Room, 1974).

Alcoholism was once considered amoral behavior. Since the 1900s, however, the prevailing view has been that alcoholism should be attributed to a constitutional or genetic defect and thus should be considered a disease. The treatment of alcoholism based on a disease model typically consists of a program designed to produce total abstinence (Jellinek, 1960; Keller, 1976). Perhaps the most popular approach to treatment based on a disease model has been Alcoholics Anonymous (AA), a self-help approach. Approximately 10% of the alcoholics in the United States are members of AA.

It has been estimated that only 10% of alcoholics treated in abstinence-based programs such as AA remain abstinent at follow-ups of 18 months or longer (Armor, Polich, & Stambul, 1976), with an additional 26% reporting moderate drinking at follow-up. We should note that, although the AA programs make explicit reference to a disease model of alcoholism, the support the groups offer is complex and multifaceted, often including the variables we have been noting. We do not wish to downgrade the value of these groups to the people they successfully serve. Attention to the key components of success, however, may serve to increase efficacy for a large proportion of patients.

In contrast to the disease model, a behavioral perspective treats alcohol consumption as a learned behavior. Adherents to the behavioral viewpoint are particularly interested in the determinants of drinking behavior, including situational and environmental antecedents, the individual's prior history and experience with alcohol, and the consequences of drinking (e.g., reinforcing as a reducer of stress or as a social facilitator).

The behavioral intervention that follows from the learning conceptualization is designed to alter drinking patterns through the use of behavioral technology similar to that employed with termination of cigarette smoking and obesity (e.g., aversive conditioning, contingency contracting, stimulus control). As in the cases of weight reduction and cessation of smoking, it appears that modification of the maladaptive behavior can be readily achieved by a host of treatment procedures; the long-term maintenance, however, has been disappointing.

Recent views of the role of cognitive factors in reactions to alcohol have emphasized the critical contribution of drinkers' appraisals, expectations, and sense of self-efficacy (Marlatt, 1976, 1978; Marlatt & Rohsenow, 1980; G. Wilson, 1978c). For example, several investigators have demonstrated that for both social drinkers and alcoholics, prior expectations about the presence or absence of alcohol in a drink exert a stronger influence than the actual physical effects of the alcohol (Abrams & Wilson, 1979a; Engle & Williams, 1972; Maisto, Lauerman, & Adesso, 1977; Marlatt, Demming, & Reid, 1973; G. Wilson & Abrams, 1977; G. Wilson & Lawson, 1976).

The role of cognitive and affective factors is highlighted in the work of Marlatt (1978), who examined the causes of relapse among subjects who had been successful in various alcohol treatment studies. He found that relapse situations could be classified into four types: (1) frustration and inability to express anger; (2) inability to resist social pressure to drink; (3) negative emotional states; and (4) inability to resist temptation to drink. Interestingly, subjective perceptions of physiological craving were not identified as a cause of relapse. Similar findings were reported by Ludwig (1972), lending support to Marlatt's analysis. Based on this evidence, it seems likely that environmental factors and the emotional and cognitive factors that accompany them are among the determinants of relapse following successful completion of any treatment program.

These findings suggest that a successful program for treating alcoholics might include not only traditional behavioral techniques to bring alcohol consumption under control, but also coping skills training to deal with high-risk-of-relapse situations. The drinkers' expectations about the effects of alcohol and how to construe and cope with failures (violation) of abstinence need to be addressed for treatment success to be maintained (Higgins & Marlatt, 1975; P. Miller, Hersen, Eisler, & Hilsman, 1974), because these are potential hazards to all impulse-control programs (food intake or cigarette smoking as well as alcohol consumption).

In one illustrative study, Chaney et al. (1978) compared three groups in an abstinence treatment program: a cognitive–behavioral treatment group; a discussion group emphasizing feelings associated with relapse and related situations, but not including any coping skills training; and a control group that received the standard abstinence program based on the AA model. The cognitive–behavioral training incorporated modeling of appropriate behaviors, behavioral rehearsal, and attention to the factors that contribute to relapse. Subjects were taught how to identify problematic situations (i.e., potential high-risk-of-relapse situations), generate response alternatives, and consider both short- and long-term consequences. Finally, there was practice in carrying out adaptive responses in the natural environment. (Marlatt, 1979, has presented a detailed description of this experimental treatment program.)

At the end of treatment and at a 1-year follow-up, the cognitive–behavioral group showed significantly fewer days intoxicated (mean number of days intoxicated 11.1 vs. 64.0), less alcohol consumed (total number of drinks 400 vs. 1593), and shorter periods of excessive alcohol consumption than a group provided with the more traditional inpatient treatment. The Chaney *et al.* data demonstrate that training alcoholics to cope with a variety of standardized high-risk relapse situations may prove to be an effective component of treatment for alcoholism.

As noted in the discussion of high-risk behaviors, these initial encouraging results for cognitive–behavioral treatments bear replication and extension. The notion of teaching patients ways of handling potential relapses, however, will be considered in more detail in the treatment of pain patients in Section III.

PREVENTING MALADAPTIVE BEHAVIORS

So far we have been emphasizing the utility of a number of psychological approaches to the modification or elimination of existing behavioral health-risk factors (e.g., cigarette smoking, obesity, alcohol consumption). If, however, the assumption is made that risk factors are related to specific learned behavioral patterns, then the acquisition of such learned behaviors should be preventable.

Recently, a number of preventive programs have been developed. Three general strategies have been employed. One has been to try to teach school-aged children and adolescents about potential risk factors (e.g., Coates & Perry, 1980; R. Evans, Rozelle, Mittelmark, Hansen, Bane, & Havis, 1978; Hurd, Johnson, Pechacek, Bast, Jacobs, & Luepker, 1980). The second, more extensive strategy, has attempted to address risk factors at the community level (e.g., Maccoby, Farquhar, Wood, & Alexander, 1977; Meyer, Nash, McAlister, Maccoby, & Farquhar, 1980). The third approach has focused attention on high-risk occupational groups (e.g., police officers: Novaco, 1977; Sarason, Johnson, Berberich, & Siegel, 1979; teachers: Ayalon, 1982; Coates & Thoresen, 1976; Turk, Meeks, & Turk, 1982; nurses: Brief, Alday, Sell, & Melone, 1979; business executives: Howard, Rechnitzer, & Cunningham, 1975; Newman & Beehr, 1979; Roskies, 1982). We must be cautious in drawing conclusions from these recent studies because there are few long-term follow-up data.

Several studies have attempted to prevent children from beginning to smoke because smoking is addictive and early smoking predicts later smoking (M. Russell, 1971). Traditional health education programs have an adult focus and emphasize the long-term dangers of smoking to health. Children and adolescents seem to be oriented much more to the present and to conforming to group norms and peer pressures (Dekker, 1975; R. Evans *et al.*, 1978). Recently, the programs that have been directed to children and adolescents have taken these observations into consideration (e.g., Coates & Perry, 1980; R. Evans *et al.*, 1978; Hurd *et al.*, 1980; McAlister, Perry, & Maccoby, 1979).

Each of these programs has focused on the short-term consequences of smoking (social consequences), especially peer pressure and conformity. The most successful programs have attempted to "inoculate" the children against peer pressure through the use of visual media, role playing, practice in combating peer pressure, and nonsmoking role models. Preliminary results reported by McAlister *et al.* (1979) and Hurd *et al.* (1980) are encouraging because they demonstrate that smoking prevention programs aimed at junior and senior high school students can reduce the number of students who begin smoking.

Coates and Perry (1980) describe programs designed (1) to reduce weight and increase physical activity among adolescents and (2) to modify the consumption of foods related to CHD (e.g., saturated fats, cholesterol, sodium, sugar) among elementary school children. These programs incorporated problem-solving training to assist children in planning activities and meals; behavioral techniques, such as contingency contracting, to increase adherence; and behavioral rehearsal of techniques to resist peer and media pressure to overeat or ingest risk-related foods (e.g., those high in cholesterol). The preliminary results (Coates & Perry, 1980) suggest that these prevention programs do lead to weight reductions and alterations in maladaptive eating and exercise habits.

Although these demonstration programs seem to offer promise, much more research is required before any one of them is adopted on a large scale. Prevention of risk-related behaviors deserves much more attention and is one area in which behavioral medicine may contribute to health promotion.

The second, community-wide strategy has been given major impetus by the Stanford Heart Disease Prevention Project (Farquhar, Maccoby, Wood, Alexander, Breitrose, Brown, Haskell, McAlister, Meyer, Nash, & Stern, 1977; Maccoby *et al.*, 1977). This project examined the utility of a combination of extensive mass media and face-to-face instruction to modify smoking, exercise, and dietary behavior simultaneously. The face-to-face component incorporated self-control principles such as self-observation, modeling, and token reinforcement. Preliminary results suggest that the media plus face-to-face instruction program did lead to reduction in cardiovascular risk factors. Although the Stanford project has received some criticism (e.g., Kasl, 1980; Leventhal, Safer, Cleary, & Gutmann, 1980), the effort given to this major undertaking must be applauded. Refinements and continued examination of the utility of such community-oriented approaches deserve increased attention.

A vast literature concerned with occupational stress and coping with job stresses stems from many diverse disciplines, primarily psychology, sociology, psychiatry, and occupational medicine (e.g., Kahn, Wolfe, Quinn, Snoek, & Rosenthal, 1964; Levi, 1979; McKay & Cox, 1979; McLean, 1974, 1979; McLean, Black, & Colligan, 1978). Concern for employees under stress is increasing among both management and unions. Social science research has led to the enactment of legislation in the Scandinavian countries, where employers must attend to job satisfaction and the presence of stress (McLean, 1979). The legal system in the United States, beginning with workers' compensation and more recently augmented by the Occupational Safety and Health Act, mandates examination of both psychological and physical stressors in places of employment.

Much effort has been expended in altering the working environment to eliminate some aspects of occupational stress, but the very nature of some occupations makes them stressful (e.g., health care providers, law enforcement officers, air traffic controllers). In these occupations total elimination of stress may be impossible, and the workers may have to learn more effective strategies for coping with stress (see Meichenbaum, in press; Turk et al., 1982).

A recent study by Sarason et al. (1979) illustrates the potential of a preventive occupational-stress-management program. Sarason et al. (1979) developed and assessed the effectiveness of a program designed to help police officers cope with stress. In this study nine police academy trainees received six, 2-hour training sessions that included practice in the self-monitoring of reactions to stressful situations, muscular relaxation, and the development of adaptive self-statements. Emphasis of the training was placed on both anxiety and anger, problems identified by Novaco (1977) as major causes of stress among law enforcement officers. Trainees in the stress-management group were compared to a control group that did not receive the training.

Although the relative effectiveness of this program on some measures was equivocal, it was evaluated by police academy personnel as superior in several of the simulated police activities. What is particularly surprising is not so much the results of the study as the observation by Sarason et al. that, despite the general agreement that the law enforcement profession is stressful, no systematic studies, prior to the one described, had been conducted to examine stress-management programs for police officers. The same comment is true of many stressful occupations. This is one area in which controlled, empirical research is essential. For example, see a recent study by Novaco, Cook, and Sarason (1982) using cognitive–behavioral techniques with marine recruits.

PSYCHOPHYSIOLOGICAL DISORDERS

As we noted earlier, within the transactional model, perceptions of threat and coping resources are central to the experience of stress. Stress is one of a set of etiological and maintaining factors in physicological dysfunction that also includes biological and environmental factors (cf. Weiner, 1977). Coping with threat has emerged as an important construct in stress research. There is a growing consensus that the way people cope with stress can be a more important determinant of maladaptive physiological response than the frequency and character of stressful events confronted (Antonovsky, 1974; Frankenhaeuser, 1980; Roskies & Lazarus, 1980).

Dysfunctional coping may contribute to or maintain diseases in at least three ways (R. Lazarus & Launier, 1978). First, different coping responses may be associated with different underlying physiological mechanisms, each with its own characteristic hormonal profiles. This may, in turn, predispose individuals to develop some psychophysiological disorders and not others (Mason, 1971, 1975a; Obrist, 1976).

For example, several investigators have shown that various components of the immunological system are responsive to stress (T cells, B cells, macrophages; Palmblad, Cantell, Strander, Froberg, Karlsson, Levi, Granstrom, & Unger, 1976; Solomon, Amkraut, & Kasper, 1974). It has been suggested that a slight imbalance in the immunological system may dramatically influence an individual's susceptibility to pathogens in the external environment and within the body (Amkraut & Solomon, 1975; Cassel, 1976). After reviewing this literature, Bowers and Kelly concluded:

> When a situation is perceived as threatening, and/or when psychological defenses are unable to contain the emotional reactions to the perceived stress, the person's biological defenses may be diminished as well, making him/her potentially more vulnerable to infectious diseases, as well as to cancer. (1979, p. 493)

A second way dysfunctional coping may affect physiology is by directly exposing the body to pathogens, as in the example of smoking, drinking alcohol, or overeating in response to the threat (e.g., Horowitz, Hulley, Alvarez, Reynolds, Benfari, Blair, Borhani, & Simon, 1979; Katz, Weiner, Gutmann, & Yu, 1973). And third, the actual strategies for coping with symptoms of illness (e.g., denial, minimization, persistent attempts at mastery) can influence the course and maintenance of the illness, as in the case of women who denied the significance of lumps in their breasts (Katz *et al.*, 1970), or men who denied that they were having a heart attack (T. Hackett & Cassem, 1975).

If physiological reactions depend upon the perception of threat and the cognitive and behavioral responses to demands, then successful treatment programs need to be designed to modify not only the physiological response, but also the environmental demands and the affective, cognitive, and behavioral responses (Holroyd, 1980; Meichenbaum & Turk, 1981; N. Miller, 1976; Turk, Meichenbaum, & Berman, 1979). A number of comprehensive treatment programs have been developed to alleviate a range of psychophysiological disorders (e.g., peptic ulcers, irritable bowel syndrome, mucous colitis, bronchial asthma, migraine and tension headaches). The literature on such programs is quite extensive, and we will examine only a few illustrative studies in this chapter. In later chapters we will give additional attention to migraine and tension headaches when we specifically discuss pain treatment programs.

One of the earliest investigations of the efficacy of a psychological approach designed to alter both cognitive and behavioral responses to stress in ulcer patients is reported by Chappell and his colleagues (Chappell, Stefano, Rogerson, & Pike, 1936; Chappell & Stevenson, 1936). Chappell *et al.* describe the efficacy of a program consisting of (1) information about the relationship between emotions and gastric physiology, (2) suggestions that participants should disrupt worry and ruminative thinking by employing specific imaginal and self-instructional coping strategies (e.g., pleasant recollections whenever one finds oneself worrying), (3) advice and training in how to avoid conflicts and use relaxation, and (4) advice and encouragement to reduce discussion of symptoms with friends. This treatment program was combined with medication and dietary regimens typically employed with ulcer patients.

The patients receiving the treatment program were compared to a group of patients who were treated exclusively with medication and controlled diet. At the end of 2 months, only one of the patients receiving the combined treatment reported any recurrence of ulcer symptoms, whereas 19 of the 20 control patients had serious recurrences. At a 3-year follow-up, 10 of the patients who had received the combined treatment were symptom-free, whereas none of the control subjects was free of recurrences.

In a more recent study with duodenal ulcer patients, Brooks and Richardson (1980) examined the efficacy of a treatment regimen similar to that described by Chappell and Stevenson (1936). Brooks and Richardson provided 11 ulcer patients with a treatment that included (1) information about the relationships among anxiety, emotional inhibition, and ulcers; (2) information about the perpetuating cycle of anxiety, worry, and ulcers; (3) discussions of the relationship of irrational beliefs and worry; (4) discussions of the impact of negative and positive thoughts and images; (5) training in the use of coping imagery; (6) cognitive restructuring focusing on erroneous beliefs about expressive emotions and assertiveness; (7) relaxation training; and (8) behavioral rehearsal in the patients' natural environments. This training was provided in eight 60- to 90-minute sessions.

Patients who received the treatment were compared to an attention-control group whose treatment focused on support and the expression of emotion. Over a 60-day follow-up period, patients receiving the comprehensive training regimen reported less severe ulcer symptomatology, experienced fewer days of symptomatic pain, and consumed less antacid medication than the attention-support group. A comparison of the groups 3½ years after termination of the program revealed significantly lower rates of ulcer recurrence in the cognitive–behavioral treatment group. Thus the Brooks and Richardson study provides a replication of the Chappell and Stevenson (1936) study.

What is particularly impressive about both of these studies is the maintenance of beneficial effects at long-term follow-up. Training programs similar to those described here have proved to be beneficial in case studies of patients with mucous colitis (Youell & McCullough, 1975) and irritable bowel syndrome (Bowen & Turk, 1979; Harrell & Beiman, 1978). And finally, Creer and Burns (1978) have developed similar stress-management programs for use with patients with bronchial asthma; however, no data are as yet available with which to assess the efficacy of the training regimen. Although the results describing the utility of programs based on the transactional model of stress are preliminary, the findings, especially with essential hypertension and ulcers, seem most promising.

AVERSIVE MEDICAL DIAGNOSTIC PROCEDURES

Many surgical and medical procedures (e.g., gastroendoscopic examinations, debridement of burns), as well as natural physiological processes (e.g., childbirth), may produce considerable pain, discomfort, and suffering. We will review the cognitive–behavioral techniques employed to alleviate the pain and distress accompanying such procedures and natural processes in Section III. At this point we will examine the utility of distress-prevention strategies for a number of aversive, but common, medical diagnostic procedures (e.g., cardiac catheterization, coronary cineangiography, gastrointestinal endoscopy, pelvic examinations, induction of anesthesia) and hospitalization itself.

With recent advances in medical technology, many invasive diagnostic procedures have been developed and are now routinely employed. For example, gastroendoscopic examinations, designed to identify lesions in the gastrointestinal tract, require the patient to swallow a flexible fiberoptic tube 12 mm in diameter and 90 cm long. This tube must be retained by the patient from 5 to 90 minutes. The cardiac catheterization procedure involves the insertion of small catheters into a large vein and a large artery in the groin. Measures of blood pressure in the heart chambers and pictorial images of the main pumping chambers to the coronary arteries are obtained through the catheters.

Such procedures may actually involve minimal nociception, but are, however, often viewed as quite distressing by patients. It is not uncommon for patients facing aversive procedures to report and evidence disproportionate amounts of anxiety and stress. Perception of threat and unpleasantness may result in avoidance of routine elective procedures such as pelvic examinations (Fuller, Endress, & Johnson, 1978). Moreover, tense patients may experience more discomfort than necessary (Kendall, Williams, Pechacek, Graham, Shisslak, & Herzoff, 1979), or patients may actually interfere with the procedures (e.g., Auerbach & Kilmann, 1977).

The important role that cognitive and affective variables play is illustrated in a study of patients undergoing cardiac catheterization (Kendall *et al.*, 1979). The investigators constructed a 20-item self-statement inventory specifically designed for the cardiac catheterization procedure. After undergoing the procedure, subjects completed the inventory, which included 10 positive and 10 negative self-statements that the patient might have experienced during the procedure. Positive self-statements were conceptualized as self-verbalizations that would likely facilitate coping behavior during the catheterization (e.g., "I was thinking that the procedures could save my life"). Negative self-statements were conceptualized as self-verbalizations that might inhibit coping behavior during the catheterization (e.g., "I keep thinking that the procedure might cause complications that might never go away"; "I was listening and expecting them to say something bad about my heart"). Patients were asked to indicate how much each of these positive and negative self-verbalizations was characteristic of their thoughts during the procedure. Kendall *et al.* (1979) found that the patients' negative self-statement scores were correlated with both the physician's and the technician's ratings of patient adjustment during the procedures. The more frequent the negative thoughts, the poorer the adjustment.

Since the threat created by these medical procedures is quite common, since the procedures are often scheduled well in advance, and since many of the sensations and specific features of the procedures are predictable, a number of approaches to reduce distress and unpleasantness have been attempted. Cooperative and relaxed patients facilitate rapid and successful completion of the examinations. Thus, reducing patient distress is beneficial to the health care provider as well as to the patient.

Attempts have been made to reduce distress by providing patients with sensory and/or procedural information (e.g., Fuller et al., 1978; J. Johnson & Leventhal, 1974; J. Johnson, Morrissey, & Leventhal, 1973; Kendall et al., 1979; Mills & Krantz, 1979; L. Peterson & Shigetomi, 1981); information describing particular coping strategies designed either to reduce stress or to assist in more rapid completion of the procedures (Fuller et al., 1978; J. Johnson & Leventhal, 1974; L. Peterson & Shigetomi, 1981); or a combination of both types of information (Fuller et al., 1978; L. Peterson & Shigetomi, 1981; Shipley, Butt, & Horowitz, 1979; Vernon & Bailey, 1974). Additionally, a comprehensive intervention that focused on training patients to discriminate anxiety-producing cues and to apply their *own* coping strategies in response to such cues was conducted by Kendall et al. (1979). Because the literature on preparation for medical procedures and hospitalization is voluminous (cf. reviews by Auerbach & Kilmann, 1977; Turk, 1978a; Turk & Genest, 1979), we will only examine several examples and draw some general conclusions about the utility of preparatory approaches.

J. Johnson and Leventhal (1974) examined the relative efficacy of sensory information, behavioral instructions, and a combination of these types of information on reducing distress and enhancing cooperation of patients undergoing an endoscopic examination. The procedural information described the various stages of the examination, including where the examination would be performed, throat swabbing with a topical anesthetic, intravenous puncture, passage of the fiberoptic tube, time for the procedure to be completed, position on the examination table, lighting of the room, and pumping of air into the stomach. This procedural information was provided to all patients. The group receiving the sensory information was provided with the procedural information as well as with information related to specific sensations that the patients would likely experience during the examination (i.e., needle stick, drowsiness, feeling of fullness in the stomach).

A third group of patients received behavioral coping instructions plus the procedural information described. The coping information included specific instructions for rapid mouth breathing and panting to reduce gagging during throat swabbing, instructions regarding swallowing motions with the mouth open and chin down while the tube was being inserted, and so on. These instructions were designed to facilitate more rapid and less distressing experiences during the examination. No information was provided to help the patient deal with increased emotional arousal (i.e., the sort of negative thoughts and feelings that Kendall *et al.* assessed).

J. Johnson and Leventhal reported that the sensory instructions and the combined sensory and coping instructions were more effective than the procedural information alone and that the combination was the most effective in reducing distress and enhancing cooperation. Cassell (1965) modified the presentation of information for children who had to undergo the endoscopic examination by using puppets to convey sensory and procedural information. Cassell reported results similar to those of J. Johnson and Leventhal (1974), as did Finesilver (1978).

Kendall *et al.* (1979) examined the relative efficacy of a regimen comprising cognitive and behavioral coping strategies in contrast to procedural information, an attention placebo, and no treatment with patients undergoing the cardiac catheterization procedure. The cognitive–behavioral intervention consisted of a series of procedures that focused on labeling stress, identifying stress-related cues, discussing coping, cognitively rehearsing coping strategies, and the trainer's self-disclosing information on how to handle negative thoughts and feelings. One point that deserves emphasis in the Kendall *et al.* program is the encouragement and reinforcement of the patient's *own* cognitive coping strategies. No cognitive coping strategies were imposed upon the patient.

The cognitive–behavioral group and the procedural information group demonstrated the highest ratings of cooperation by physicians and technicians who were "blind" to the treatment condition. Patients in these groups also reported less anxiety than the attention-placebo and no-treatment control groups. On both ratings and self-reports of anxiety, the cognitive–behavioral group was superior to the procedural information group.

Fuller *et al.* (1978) examined the utility of sensory information, a behavioral coping strategy (relaxation), and a combination of both procedures with patients who were to undergo routine pelvic examinations. The sensory information group demonstrated less overt distress and lower pulse rates than the other groups; the sensory information, however, seemed to have no effect on self-reports of fear. The combined sensory information and relaxation group showed significant differences from the control group in self-reported fear. No significant effects were found for the relaxation-only group.

The relative ineffectiveness of relaxation is somewhat surprising in light of many studies that have reported that relaxation reduces stress (e.g., Benson, Greenwood, & Klemchuk, 1975; Deffenbacher, Mathis, & Michaels, 1979; Goldfried & Trier, 1974; Taylor, Farquhar, Nelson, & Agras, 1977). The relaxation training provided by Fuller *et al.*, however, consisted of only a 2-minute taped instruction, and this may not have provided patients sufficient training.

In the Fuller *et al.* study, 10 of the 12 patients who received relaxation instructions indicated that training was indeed helpful, but this was not evident on the behavioral measures. In contrast, patients who received the sensory information were much less enthusiastic. Because such routine pelvic examinations are desirable, the effect of the limited relaxation training on self-reports of fear and the patient's enthusiasm may be particularly important in increasing the likelihood that patients would return for future examinations. The combination of sensory and relaxation instruction appears to be a valuable intervention to employ with patients who require pelvic examinations.

The studies reviewed illustrate the potential value of preparation of patients for aversive diagnostic medical procedures. The generally positive results reported in these studies are consistent with many other studies that have developed distress-prevention procedures for a variety of distressing medical events (e.g., orthopedic cast removal: J. Johnson, Kirchhoff, & Endress, 1975; injections to children: Hedberg & Schlong, 1973; blood donation: Mills & Krantz, 1979; stress related to children's hospitalization: Melamed & Siegel, 1975; L. Peterson & Shigetomi, 1981; Vernon & Bailey, 1974; and the stress of adult hospitalization: Elms & Leonard, 1966).

Despite generally positive results, treatments interact with patient characteristics. For example, Shipley and his colleagues (Shipley *et al.*, 1979) found that individuals who characteristically cope with stress by means of careful attention to threatening cues, information seeking, and cognitive preparation benefited from provision of information. In contrast to these "sensitizers," a group of patients who are called "repressors," namely, those who characteristically cope with stress by not thinking about it, denying it, and simply not recognizing any potential stressfulness, benefited most from distraction procedures (Shipley, Butt, Horowitz, & Fabry, 1978). Similarly, J. Wilson (1977) recently reported that several personality variables interacted with preparation for elective surgery (cholecystectomy and abdominal hysterectomy) in affecting postoperative recovery. Patients who evidenced less fear and aggression on questionnaire measures benefited more from treatments (relaxation and information, alone or in combination) designed to prepare them for surgery. Significantly, however, J. Wilson found that even patients who used denial to deal with the impending operation were not harmed by the preparation.

Patients do not respond to psychological procedures in a uniform fashion. Furthermore, information provided to patients is likely to have little effect on distress unless it (1) results in a more accurate assessment of the potential harm (i.e., corrects a previously unrealistic appraisal of threat), (2) reduces uncertainty and hence anxiety, or (3) suggests a certain mode of coping with the situational demands and distress (Averill, 1973). The apparent efficacy of patient preparation programs is very encouraging, and such programs represent an area in which behavioral medicine seems to have much potential for health care practice.

CONVALESCENCE AND REHABILITATION

Periods of convalescence and rehabilitation are particularly important in helping patients recover from physical traumas (e.g., myocardial infarction, cerebrovascular accidents, spinal cord injuries). Yet for many patients these are periods of extreme dysphoria, and after the hospitalization period, many are reluctant to resume many normal activities or to participate actively in the rehabilitation process. One common reaction following hospitalization for myocardial infarction patients has been termed "cardiac invalidism," characterized by dependency, helplessness, and restriction of activity (Garrity, 1975). Similar reactions have been noted among stroke and spinal-cord-injured patients (Grzesiak & Zaretsky, 1979), mastectomy patients (Meyerowitz, 1980), and chronic pain patients (Pilowsky & Spence, 1976a, 1976b).

Feelings of dependency and helplessness contribute to the restriction of activity, which may contribute to a worsening of medical status as a result of physiological deconditioning, muscle atrophy, and increased edema. There is a large literature concerning psychological factors in rehabilitation (e.g., A. Cobb, 1974; Fordyce, 1976; Ince, 1981; R. Murray & Kijek, 1979), and we will return to this problem in discussing chronic pain in Section III. We will therefore not review this literature here, but will take up the issue of prevention.

Although we know a great deal about the potential problems that may arise during the posthospitalization period, surprisingly little attention has been given to prevention of invalidism. A study conducted by Gruen (1975) will illustrate the potential value of prevention in rehabilitation of physical disorders.

Gruen (1975) provided 35 myocardial infarction patients with a brief, cognitively oriented therapy designed to facilitate coping with myocardial infarction. The treatment focused on acknowledgment of the normality of negative reactions (e.g., fear, anxiety, depression), reflections of feelings, reinforcement of patients' strengths and positive coping strategies, and encouragement of appropriate information seeking. Patients who received this counseling were seen for one-half hour, five to six times per week for the duration of the hospitalization period. These patients were contrasted with a matched control group of myocardial infarction patients. Gruen's data showed that treated patients had shorter stays in the hospital (22.5 days vs. 24.9 days), were less likely to develop medical complications in the form of arrhythmias (7 vs. 18), showed fewer manifestations of depression and anxiety, and were more able to return to normal activities at a 4-month follow-up than the control group of patients.

CHRONIC DISEASE

In considering the topic of chronic disease, it is important first to provide a caveat concerning the notion of adjustment. Since any treatment program is designed to nurture *adaptation*, satisfactory criteria for successful adaptation are necessary. Defining "satisfactory adjustment" is complicated by the fact that adaptation is not a static state, but a dynamic, evolving process (e.g., Hamburg, Coelho, & Ådams, 1974; R. Lazarus & Launier, 1978; Turk, 1979).

There has been a tendency to conceive of adaptive behavior in terms of dichotomies—good–bad, satisfactory–unsatisfactory, adaptive–maladaptive. It might be more appropriate to consider such adjectives as extreme points. It is quite feasible that, at any point, an individual might be responding quite adaptively in relation to a specific problem, moderately successfully to a second, and marginally to a third. The quality of adjustment will vary, also, during the course of an illness. In short, adaptation is a *process*, not an outcome, with progressive changes and refinements occurring over time and in multiple contexts. Thus we must be cautious in making broad generalizations about how well patients have adapted to their conditions.

A second point to note is that "adaptation" tends to connote mastery or the surmounting of some obstacle in contrast to surrender or capitulation to the inevitable. But because chronic disease may require individuals to relinquish certain goals and restrict the range of their activities, persistent efforts at mastery may be frustrating, inappropriate, and in a sense, maladaptive. Successful coping with a given problem will not always involve active mastery over the environment. Retreat, toleration, or disengagement may be the most appropriate response in certain circumstances. As R. White (1974) suggested, the adaptive process might be more appropriately conceptualized as "a striving towards acceptable compromise" (p. 52).

With these concerns in mind, the descriptive criteria for "satisfactory adjustment" that we will employ in the remainder of this book are those outlined by Hamburg and Adams (1967):

> Keeping distress within manageable limits; maintaining a sense of personal worth; restoring relations with significant other people and increasing the likelihood of working out a personally valued and socially acceptable situation after maximum physical recovery has been obtained. (p. 278)

Because adjustive demands vary significantly from one disease to another, it is necessary to identify the problems posed by each disease and the range of coping response options available (Moos & Tsu, 1977). Even subtypes of a general class of disease create unique problems, threats, and demands. For example, although all forms of cancer are life-threatening, subtypes such as breast cancer, cancer of the bowel, and lung cancer present the patient and their families with varying problems and threats. For example, surgery for breast cancer creates a demand for exercises that may be painful at first, whereas a colostomy creates a demand for a range of self-care behaviors that may be distasteful and emotionally charged (Follick & Turk, 1978; Meyerowitz, 1980). It would be a mistake to identify problems and coping strategies of patients with one type of cancer and assume that these are consistent across subtypes (Weisman & Worden, 1977).

Interventions for the Chronically Ill: An Example, Cancer

The diversity of diseases and conditions encompassed under the general class of chronic disease makes a complete examination of treatment regimens for each specific disease prohibitive. Thus we will examine the cognitive–behavioral approach to coping with only one disease, cancer, in order to illustrate the general approach.

Cancer is our example for three reasons. Epidemiological studies reveal that approximately 25% of all individuals will receive a diagnosis of cancer at some point in their lifetimes, and many others will be directly affected by the presence of cancer in a significant other (American Cancer Society, 1978; USDHEW, 1975b). Second, increasing numbers of cancer patients either are cured or have their life span expanded substantially, thus increasing the numbers of patients who will have to learn to live with cancer (USDHEW, 1975a, 1975b). And, finally, a substantial body of literature has recognized the importance of psychosocial factors in coping with cancer (e.g., Cullen, Fox, & Isom, 1976; Gordon *et al.*, 1980; Meyerowitz, 1980; Weisman, 1970; Wortman & Dunkel-Schetter, 1979).

Many of the psychosocial intervention programs designed for cancer patients have focused on death and dying. The literature is replete with reports on how the health care provider might interact with the dying patient to facilitate "appropriate" death. In contrast, many fewer reports have addressed the major problem, that of living with cancer (e.g., Gordon *et al.*, 1980; Weisman, 1972). Those authors who have considered patients' coping with factors other than the threat of death have largely provided only anecdotal data describing the efficacy of their approach. These studies have been largely descriptive, relying on minimal outcome information other than patients' self-reports of the helpfulness of programs. Until recently, many studies did not employ any control groups, thereby not permitting statements regarding specific ingredients of an approach in comparison to increased attention by the health care provider (e.g., Euster, 1979; E. Johnson & Stark, 1980; Simonton, Matthews-Simonton, & Sparks, 1980).

Recently, two studies that included control groups examined the relative efficacy of psychosocial interventions with cancer patients (Gordon *et al.* 1980; Weisman *et al.*, 1980). We will consider these studies, because they generally fit within the cognitive–behavioral perspective that we have been presenting.

Gordon *et al.* (1980) developed a psychosocial intervention for cancer patients based on information obtained from the problem-identification survey described in the previous chapter. Three different, general types of cancer were investigated: breast, lung, and melanoma. A total of 157 patients were provided with a comprehensive psychosocial evaluation and a systematic program that consisted of three components: educational, counseling, and environmental. Although these general components were included in the intervention with each patient, the specific content for each patient was based on his or her responses to the problem-identification survey. The patients receiving the psychosocial intervention were contrasted with those in a no-treatment control group.

During the educational phase of the psychosocial intervention, patients were taught skills to assist them in coping with cancer. General information about the medical system and information on the patient's own medical condition were provided to each patient. Additionally, patients were taught about cancer, cancer treatment, and the side effects of both the disease and the treatment. Instruction was given in relief methods for both physical and emotional discomfort (e.g., relaxation training, cognitive reappraisal). Finally, patients were presented with information about the emotional reactions of patients and the possible responses of others.

The second component of the intervention, counseling, focused on the ventilation of feelings, verbal support, and help in clarifying feelings. Patients were also encouraged to act on their environment and to become more assertive.

The third component was not presented directly to the patients; rather, the therapist consulted with relevant health care providers in order to improve communications with the patients. The importance of communication to the adjustive process was recently presented cogently by Wortman and Dunkel-Schetter (1979), who emphasized the isolation and loneliness of cancer patients and their distress at avoidance by relatives and even health care providers. Many friends and relatives of cancer patients indicated that they tended to avoid the patients because they were unsure what topics should be excluded and feared making the patient more distressed.

Briefly, the results of Gordon *et al.*'s study were as follows: (1) The psychosocial intervention significantly ameliorated many of the patient's problems as identified on the psychosocial problem survey; (2) patients in the intervention group demonstrated a more rapid decline in dysphoric affect (anxiety, hostility, and depression); (3) patients in the intervention group showed a more realistic outlook on life; (4) a greater proportion of the patients in the intervention group returned to previous vocational status; and (5) patients in the intervention group evidenced a more active pattern of time usage than the patients in the control group. The authors also reported that each of the three types of cancer was associated with different clinical issues and different patterns of recovery, but that all responded favorably to treatment.

Although Gordon *et al.* (1980) viewed their intervention from a psychodynamic perspective, the specific components and the emphasis on the patient's thoughts, feelings, and behaviors, as well as on the patient's transactions with the environment, appear closely related to the cognitive–behavioral perspective. Regardless of the theoretical origin of therapy, the results seem to suggest the utility of specific cognitive and behavioral coping techniques. One problem with the Gordon *et al.* study was the failure to employ an attention-placebo control group. From the data presented, it is impossible to determine whether the results were a function of the specific components of psychosocial intervention or simply of the greater attention given to patients in this group. This is a major concern in light of the Wortman and Dunkel-Schetter (1979) article.

To our knowledge, only one study examining the relative efficacy of an intervention with cancer patients has incorporated active treatment comparison groups with a control group, and even in this case, more careful controls could have been included. This is the study, referred to in the previous chapter, that was conducted by Weisman and his colleagues (Weisman *et al.*, 1980) at the Massachusetts General Hospital. These investigators developed two somewhat different, yet overlapping, psychosocial interventions, which were subsequently employed with patients having cancer of several different types (breast, colon, Hodgkin's disease, lung, malignant melanoma, and gynecological).

On the basis of previous research, Weisman and Worden (1977) identified 125 patients who were predicted to be at "high risk" of emotional distress following a diagnosis of cancer. Of these patients, 59 actually received one of the two interventions, 28 refused to participate, and 38 were excluded because of mental status or because they were unavailable during follow-up (moved out of the Boston area or died). The percentage of refusal, 22%, is comparable to that of patients refusing to participate in the Gordon *et al.* (1980) study just described. One difference to note is that Weisman *et al.* carefully selected individuals who were predicted to have significant problems, whereas Gordon *et al.* did not employ such a selection procedure. Since Weisman *et al.*'s screening procedure has proved to be a good predictor of distress, this approach would seem to be more cost-effective than providing extensive intervention to all patients.

The two psychosocial interventions employed by Weisman *et al.* are not completely different, because both emphasize problem solving (i.e., emphasis on clarifying problems related to cancer and ways of coping with the problems identified). However, one of the interventions, consultation therapy, was "patient-centered," whereas the second intervention, cognitive skills training, was somewhat more didactic. A third group of patients who were not predicted to be highly distressed was followed and served as a control.

Weisman *et al.* reported that, compared to the control group, both interventions significantly reduced patients' distress at the end of treatment and at the 2- and 6-month follow-ups. This is particularly impressive, because the amount of distress experienced by the treatment-group patients, who were predicted to be highly disturbed, was significantly less than that of the patients who were *not expected to be highly distressed*. The three groups did not differ in the number of problems experienced following treatment; the intervention groups, however, obtained significantly higher problem-resolution scores (based on performance on a self-report developed by the authors) than the nonintervention group. The authors note that both interventions were equally effective. This is not surprising, since both focused on problem solving and the enhancement of perceived competence and self-mastery.

One problem with the Weisman *et al.* study is that no attempt was made to assess patients' expectancies for the program, nor was an attention-placebo group included. It is possible that the active ingredient of both treatments was an expectancy or placebo effect. The attention of the therapist may have been the active ingredient, rather than any of the specific, overlapping components of the interventions. Despite the problems noted, the Gordon *et al.* (1980) and Weisman *et al.* (1980) studies illustrate how cognitive–behavioral techniques can be employed in interventions with chronically ill patients.

SELF-CARE

Medical treatment is undergoing changes that have important implications. With the development of relatively inexpensive self-monitoring procedures (e.g., urine testing, blood glucose monitoring, blood pressure monitoring), patients have been given increasing responsibility for their own health care. But this practice creates problems concerning whether patients actually comply with and adhere to the prescribed treatment regimen. Interestingly, research has indicated that physicians greatly overestimate the degree to which patients comply with treatment (Charney, 1972). Moreover, physicians have been shown to be unable to judge which of their patients were adhering to treatment and which were not (Kasl, 1975b). We will consider the general issue of adherence in Chapter 8.

Because a number of recent review papers and books have carefully examined the research on compliance and adherence, we will not provide another comprehensive review. The interested reader should see Barofsky (1977); Blackwell (1976); Christensen (1978); Cohen (1979); Dunbar (1980); Dunbar and Stunkard (1979); Gillum and Barsky (1974); Haynes, Taylor, and Sackett (1979); Kasl (1975b); Marston (1970); Sackett and Haynes (1976); G. Stone (1979); and especially Leventhal *et al.* (1980). Research on the issue indicates that the failure to adhere is a function of a complex interaction among the patient, the disease process, the treatment environment, and the health care provider.

The major factors that have been identified as consistently being associated with nonadherence are characteristics of the treatment regimen (e.g., complexity, duration, and perceived effectiveness) and the quality of the patient–physician relationship. Despite this complexity, most attempts to enhance adherence have focused almost exclusively on the presentation of information to increase patient knowledge about the nature and importance of carrying out self-care behaviors and on skills training in the appropriate methods of self-care (e.g., Etzwiler & Robb, 1972; Hulka, Kupper, Cassel, & Mayo, 1975; Speers & Turk, 1982; D. Stone, 1964; Watts, 1980). Although these studies often demonstrate increased patient knowledge following participation in patient education programs, the relationship between increased knowledge and actual performance of necessary self-care behaviors has frequently *not* been demonstrated (e.g., Turk & Speers, 1982).

Additionally, Joyce, Caple, Mason, Reynolds, and Matthews (1969) found that, as the amount of information from physician to patient increased, the patient retained less information in both absolute and proportional amounts. In most programs little, if any, attention is given to how the patient appraises the information and to the impact of self-care efforts upon the patient and his or her social, recreational, marital, occupational, and family life.

In contrast, let us consider the issue of self-care from a cognitive–behavioral perspective. Given that nonadherence is such a major problem in chronic disease (Marston, 1970), we will confine our illustration to the self-care behaviors associated with diabetes mellitus, a problem that one of us (D. C. T.) is currently investigating.

Diabetes Mellitus: An Illustration of the Complexities of Self-Care

Diabetes mellitus is a chronic disease of uncertain course, characterized by chronic hyperglycemic and other disturbances of carbohydrate and lipid metabolism and associated with the development of vascular complications. These complications may affect specific organs such as the eyes (diabetic retinopathy, resulting in blindness) or the kidney (diabetic nephropathy, which may lead to kidney failure). Diabetes is associated with peripheral vascular disease (frequently leading to amputations) and increased frequency of CHD (Blakenship & Skyler, 1978; Levine, 1981; Pirat, 1978; Skyler, 1981). Based on preliminary results reported recently (cited in USDHEW, 1979), there are more than 4.8 million diagnosed diabetics in the United States and an estimated 5 million undiagnosed diabetics. In 1972–1973 alone, 612,000 persons were newly diagnosed as diabetics (USDHEW, 1979).

Diabetes is one of only a few diseases in which the patient must make independent therapeutic decisions based on daily clinical observations. The patient with diabetes must monitor urine or blood glucose levels to determine the dosage of the medication required. The quantity of medication required is influenced by diet, exercise, physical health, and emotional factors. The diabetic patient is required to make significant changes in all aspects of his or her life. The patient must regulate both diet and the spacing of food intake. In addition, the patient must constantly self-monitor all aspects of his or her life, attending to and treating physical signs of poor control (either high or low levels of blood glucose). The patient is constantly aware of the disease, the nearness of disaster, and potential complications.

The presence of diabetes in any family member has an impact on each of the other family members. Social events must be carefully arranged to make sure the patient is able to carry out self-care behaviors, and family members must be alert to signs of hyperglycemia and hypoglycemia and know the appropriate treatment.

The complexity and duration of the therapeutic self-care regimen would suggest that patients with diabetes are good candidates for failure to carry out necessary self-care behaviors. The available data confirm this and suggest that approximately 48% of diabetic patients do *not* carry out prescribed self-care behaviors (Watkins, Williams, Martin, Hogan, & Anderson, 1967) and that many others do so in an unsatisfactory manner. For example, the most thorough surveys of diabetic self-care (Watkins, Roberts, Williams, Martin, & Coyle, 1967; Williams, Martin, Hogan, Watkins, & Ellis, 1967) reveal that 80% of the patients surveyed administered self-care in an unhygienic and unacceptable way, 58% administered the wrong dosage of insulin, 77% tested urine inaccurately or interpreted the results "in a manner likely to be detrimental to their treatment," 75% were not eating prescribed foods, and 75% were not eating with satisfactory regularity.

Data such as these have led to an emphasis on patient education programs. Such programs, however, frequently do not lead to changes in behavior. Results from several studies (Beaser, 1956; Etzwiler & Robb, 1972; Hulka *et al.*, 1975; McDonald, 1968; D. Stone, 1964) reveal that, although general knowledge and skill training may be necessary, it is not sufficient to produce skill or information utilization in the patients' natural environment.

Analysis of diabetic self-care can be used as a prototype for other self-care programs. This analysis reveals a number of factors that are likely to contribute to the satisfactory production of the appropriate self-care behaviors (Turk & Speers, 1982). In the case of diabetes, it seems important for the patient

1. To have information on the nature of the disease and on the specific self-care required.
2. To have an understanding of the rationale underlying each of the self-care behaviors.

3. To remember the information provided.
4. To acquire the skills necessary to carry out the self-care appropriately (e.g., urine test, insulin injection, use of diabetic food-exchange lists).
5. To believe that proper self-care is likely to lead to better control of the disease.
6. To have the confidence to carry out the necessary self-care.
7. To believe that the "cost" of carrying out the self-care is outweighed by the benefits.
8. To retrieve information from memory as required (e.g., before meals).
9. To know how to deal with dysphoric affect in situations that are emotionally charged (e.g., reminders of the potentially devastating results of disease).
10. To self-reinforce and/or be reinforced for carrying out the self-care behaviors.
11. To know how to deal with problematic situations (problem solving and flexibility).
12. To know how to deal with the responses of others toward self-care behaviors (e.g., telling someone who invites him or her to dinner that a special meal is required).
13. To know how to deal with failures to carry out self-care behaviors.
14. To attribute the satisfactory completion of self-care to his or her own efforts (i.e., make self-attributions) rather than solely to the efforts of the health care provider (i.e., external attributions, leading to lesser maintenance).

Each of these factors is important, and a failure at any level may lead to the failure of self-care. A patient may fail to implement the necessary behaviors because he or she lacks information skills, may fail because the skills are utilized in an inappropriate manner (e.g., urine testing carried out inappropriately), may fail to remember how to carry out the behavior, or may fail to produce the behavior because of interference or response inhibition (dysfunctional emotional arousal, negative self-referent ideation).

A program designed to enhance patients' self-care behaviors has several concerns: presenting information in manageable chunks and in several formats, such as orally, written, or by visual media; emphasizing benefits to the patient; using a Socratic, rather than didactic, format; involving the patient as a collaborator in developing a self-care regimen that is most suitable to the patient's life-style; and using graded practice of self-care.

A variety of training techniques, including self-monitoring, problem-solving training, and stress-management training, can be included as part of the self-care regimen. For example, in the treatment protocol being tested by Turk and Speers (in progress), diabetic patients are encouraged to view self-monitoring and maintenance of good metabolic control as a reinforcement in order to remove some of the negative connotations of having to carry out self-care behaviors. Stress-management training is included to help patients deal with dysphoric affect and overresponse to situational events that have been related to poor metabolic control. Problem-solving training is incorporated to help patients learn how to approach new situations that might require alterations in self-care behaviors.

Patients are encouraged to establish cues in their environment to serve as reminders to carry out self-care behaviors. High-risk situations—those likely to interfere with the conduct of self-care behaviors—are examined (e.g., alteration of normal schedule), and ways of responding discussed.

Significant others are involved in the self-care program in order to provide necessary social supports and to act as reinforcing agents. They are encouraged to carry out specific tasks instead of constantly reminding patients to carry out self-care behaviors, which is often viewed as nagging (Brownell & Stunkard, 1979). And finally, periodic booster sessions are being incorporated. To whatever extent possible, the patient is included in the decision-making process regarding self-care behaviors. Thus self-care is a responsibility shared among patient, health care providers, and significant others. Similar approaches have been promoted by Baranowski (1979) and G. Stone (1979).

As yet, the relative efficacy of the approach has not been demonstrated, and modifications and additions may be required. We present the description here only to demonstrate how adherence, a major area of concern for behavioral medicine, is conceptualized from a cognitive-behavioral perspective. The specific details of these various components will be discussed in Section III, when we elaborate on the approach with chronic pain patients.

SUMMARY

In this chapter we have examined the applicability of the cognitive-behavioral perspective across the entire range of behavioral medicine, from health promotion to preparation for aversive medical treatments and coping with chronic disease. Our illustrations have included assessment, prevention, and intervention. We chose to discuss the range of applications rather than going into depth on each topic reviewed.

There are many other areas within the purview of behavioral medicine that we did not specifically address (e.g., medical decision making, sociological aspects of the "sick role," the health care system and societal change, the influence of the media on health perception). Some of these will be considered in later chapters when we examine the special case of chronic pain. Our major objective in this chapter was to foster the idea that the individual's covert processes (cognitions and affects) play an important role in all phases of health, disease, and illness and that a cognitive–behavioral treatment approach has potential with a range of behavioral medicine problems.

PAIN: A COGNITIVE–BEHAVIORAL PERSPECTIVE

CHAPTER 4

PAIN: ITS IMPACT

Pain—one of the most pressing issues of our time.—*John J. Bonica (1974)*

In this chapter we consider the personal, social, and economic costs of pain. The pain experience is complex, as is evident from a historical perspective and from the various models of pain. This chapter provides a backdrop for later chapters, which will discuss specific treatment interventions that follow from a multidimensional view of pain.

ECONOMIC AND SOCIAL COSTS

Perhaps the most universal form of stress encountered by humans is pain. No medical symptom is more ubiquitous. Many millions of Americans suffer from chronic pain, and a substantial proportion of those are classified as partially or completely disabled. The statistics on both chronic and acute pain are staggering. It has been estimated, for example, that there are 20 million to 50 million sufferers of arthritis, with 600,000 new victims each year (Arthritis Foundation, 1976), and 25 million migraine sufferers (Paulley & Haskell, 1975). Low back pain alone, one of the most common pain complaints, has disabled an estimated 7 million Americans and accounts for more than 8 million physician office visits yearly in the United States (M. Clark, Gosnell, & Shapiro, 1977). In fact, as many as 80% of all patients who consult physicians do so for pain-related problems (Bresler, 1979). More than $900 million is spent on over-the-counter analgesic pills and powders and soothing salves, with $100 million spent just on aspirin. To put the figures on aspirin alone in perspective, consider that Americans swallow 20,000 tons of aspirin a year, or 225 tablets for every man, woman, and child (Koenig, 1973)!

To translate these figures to the level of the individual patient, Chapman (1973) has noted that it was not uncommon for patients seen at the University of Washington pain clinic to have experienced as many as

20 to 25 surgical operations, with some patients spending more than $25,000 in health services per year. In a 1978 article, Swerdlow reported that 325 pain clinics had been developed worldwide to handle the health care system's failures. A recent communication from the American Pain Society (1980) indicated that this number has increased to 800 pain clinics in the United States alone!

DIFFERENT TYPES OF PAIN

After the surgery to remove the gallstones, I felt miserable. The pain near the incision was sharp and seemed to spread all over my body. The nurses gave me some pills that took the edge off the pain, and by about 3 days after my operation, the pain was mostly gone.

My pain feels like someone is jabbing my face with a red-hot electric needle. The worst thing about the pain is that it is so unpredictable. I never know what is going to set it off—swallowing, laughing, or talking. Even the smallest thing can set it off, so I try to stay home and go out as little as possible. I don't use makeup, I don't wash my face, and I don't brush my teeth. Sometimes I don't have any pain for days, but I worry about when it might start up again.

The pain feels like a pinched nerve shooting from my shin, through my knee, up to my buttock, and up through the lower end of my back. It is always with me, but sometimes it is worse than other times. If I knew there was no cure for me, I would like to die.

At first I didn't mind the thought of dying, so long as it was not a painful process, but then I began to worry about all those drugs they gave me. The drugs made me groggy and confused, so I couldn't think or really feel like I was alive. At times I didn't take the pills because I wanted to be alert for whatever remained of my life.

I was sitting with my hand in this tank of cold water, wondering how long I could take it and how long the experiment would last. I thought about how I would spend the money I was going to be paid for allowing them to do this to me.

It is important to distinguish between the various types of pain. As the preceding five examples illustrate, not all forms of pain are alike. Pain varies in intensity, quality, duration, and meaning. The sudden onset of pain experienced by the patient suffering from syndromes such as trigeminal neuralgia or causalgia can be contrasted with the progressive pain (and fears such as that of disfigurement or death) experienced with certain types of cancer. The persistence of pain accompanying low back problems can be contrasted with the relatively brief, albeit intense, pain that is a concomitant of abdominal surgery.

We have found it helpful to categorize pain into five different types:

1. *Acute pain*, usually self-limiting and of less than 6 months' duration (e.g., postsurgical pain, dental pain, pain accompanying childbirth).
2. *Chronic, periodic pain* that is acute but intermittent (e.g., migraine headaches, trigeminal neuralgia).
3. *Chronic, intractable, benign pain*, present most of the time, with intensity varying (e.g., low back pain).
4. *Chronic, progressive pain*, often associated with malignancies.
5. *Experimentally induced pain*, with nociceptive stimulation produced in a laboratory setting (e.g., electric shock, radiant heat, muscle ischemia).

Throughout this book we will be discussing each of these five types of pain, how they are assessed, and how they are treated. Let us first consider the concept of pain from a historical perspective.

HISTORICAL PERSPECTIVE

Alleviating pain is not a recent concern. Perhaps the first recorded reference to remedies for pain is included in the Egyptian papyri. In the Ebers papyrus (circa 1550 B.C.), reference is made to the prescription of opium by the god Isis for Ra's headache (Bonica, 1953). In the quest for attenuation of suffering, individuals have submitted themselves to such largely ineffective and often pernicious procedures as purging, puking, poisoning, puncturing, cutting, cupping, blistering, bleeding, leeching, heating, freezing, sweating, trephining, and shocking. The physician's pharmacopoeia has included practically every known organic and inorganic substance. Patients have chewed, imbibed, sucked, or suffered treatment with crocodile dung; teeth of swine; hooves of asses; spermatic fluid of frogs; eunuch fat; fly specks; lozenges of dried vipers; powder of precious stones; oils derived from ants, earthworms, and spiders; bricks; feathers; hair; human perspiration; and moss scraped from the skull of a victim of a violent death (A. Shapiro, 1963).

Consider the treatment that Charles II of England endured at the hands of the best physicians of his day. A pint of blood was extracted from his right arm, and a half-pint from his left shoulder. This was followed by an emetic, two physics, and an enema comprising 15 substances. Next, his head was shaved and a blister raised. Following in rapid succession were more emetics, sneezing powder, bleedings, soothing potions, a plaster of pitch, and pigeon dung was smeared on his feet. Potions containing ten different substances, chiefly herbs, as well as 40 drops of extract of human skull, were swallowed. Finally, application of bezoar stones (gallstones from sheep and goats) was prescribed. Following this extensive treatment, the king died (Haggard, 1929). Whether death was attributable to a medical condition or iatrogenic complications is unclear.

Another example of the medical treatment lavished on the wealthy, in this case George Washington, further illustrates the plethora of treatment techniques. Washington was probably suffering from a throat infection compounded by pneumonia.

> Because he could afford the best care available, he was given a mixture of molasses, vinegar, and butter, and then made to vomit and have diarrhea. But he lapsed. In desperation, his physicians applied irritating poultices to blister his feet and his throat, while draining several pints of blood. Then he died. (Power, 1978, p. 24)

The various treatments administered to and endured by Charles II and George Washington were available only to the rich and powerful, who could afford to pay for physicians and for the costly ingredients of the many preparations employed. Among the peasants and lower classes, treatments for pain often consisted of piercing the painful part of the body with a "vigorous" twig of a tree and then burying the twig deep in the earth. It was assumed that the vigorous twig would absorb the pain from the patient and that burying the twig would prevent anyone from being exposed to the pain. An alternative method was to take the twig after it had lanced the painful part and bake it in gingerbread, which was subsequently pawned off on unsuspecting beggars.

It is also important to consider that, although many of the treatments employed seem rather esoteric today, they proved to be effective in reducing suffering for at least some patients. This point underscores the important contribution of psychological factors to pain and pain alleviation. The "powerful placebo," as Beecher (1955) called it, appears to be an important psychological component of all therapeutic treatments. Until the late 1800s, all medications employed were essentially placebos. The potency of placebos is evident in the description of the siege of Breda in 1625:

> The garrison, being afflicted with scurvy, the Prince of Orange sent the physicians two or three small vials, containing a concoction of camomile, wormwood, and camphor, telling them to pretend that it was a medicine of

the greatest value and extremest variety, which had been procured with very much danger and difficulty from the East; and so strong, that two or three drops would impart a healing virtue to a gallon of water. The soldiers had faith in their commander; they took the medicine with cheerful faces and grew well rapidly. They afterwards thronged about the prince in groups of twenty and thirty at a time, praising his skills, and loading him with protestations of gratitude. (MacKay, 1841/1956, p. 304)

The effect of suggestion and expectancy is no less apparent today. Frank (1975) cited the following dramatic example:

The patient was dying of generalized lymphoma. He had large tumors all over his body, his chest was full of fluid, and he was anemic. He had become resistant to treatment and had been given a prognosis of less than a month. As part of a clinical trial of Krebiozen, a widely touted cancer cure, the drug was given to him because he begged for it and had great hopes for it, although he was not eligible because he was so ill. Two days after the first injection, the tumors had shrunk to half their original size and the chest fluid was gone. He continued to get injections thrice weekly and was discharged in 10 days. After 2 months of practically perfect health, on reading conflicting reports about the efficacy of Krebiozen, he relapsed to his original state. His physician told him to ignore the reports, that the reason for the relapse was that the Krebiozen had deteriorated on standing, and offered him a new double-strength, super-refined batch. This time the injection consisted of distilled water, but the patient's remission was again dramatic, and he was symptom free for two months. Then he read the final AMA report that Krebiozen was worthless. After this, his health declined and he was dead in two days. (p. 57)

(See also Beecher, 1961, and Frank, 1975, for a discussion of placebo effects present even in surgical procedures.) We are reminded of the admonition given to physicians, frequently ascribed to Virchow, to use new treatments before they lose their effectiveness.

Although we may be surprised by the use of such treatments in the past, therapeutic interventions hardly less extraordinary (e.g., acupuncture, biofeedback, transcutaneous electrical stimulation, ultrasound) are frequently employed today in the quest to control pain. Contemporary surgeons have shown great ingenuity in designing operations to relieve intractable pain. Almost every site along the nervous system, from the periphery (sympathectomies and rhizotomies), along the spinal cord (precutaneous cordotomies), to the brain (thalamotomies and prefrontal lobotomies), has been attacked. Although the operations may be brilliantly performed and technically successful, all too often pain recurs following surgery (E. Hilgard & Hilgard, 1975; Melzack, 1973). Not only does the pain tend to return, but new pains may be "unmasked," and other iatrogenic complications such as dysesthesias, "girdle pains," and various sensorimotor losses may occur (Noordenbos, 1959). To date, none of the conventional medical and surgical approaches has resulted in adequate or permanent regulation of pain. The case histories of Charles II and George Washington remind us of the value of skeptical scrutiny of treatment procedures, even if they are endorsed by the most eminent practitioners of the day.

We are too cognizant of the history of various treatment procedures not to appreciate the limitations of the approach that is presented in this volume. We see the cognitive–behavioral approach as a promising way of conceptualizing the assessment and treatment of a variety of health-related problems, including pain, but we do *not* see it as a panacea, a cure for all medical disorders or all pain patients. We have already described some of the ways in which psychological factors play a role along the entire health–disease–illness continuum. We shall describe the literature that suggests the importance of psychological variables in pain, discuss the implications of this literature for assessment and treatment, and then describe the cognitive–behavioral approach to pain in detail. Many of the clinical issues (e.g., resistance, adherence, therapeutic relationship) and techniques (e.g., homework, rational restructuring) that we describe in relation to pain problems are applicable to the various areas of behavioral medicine described in Chapter 3.

THEORIES OF PAIN

Philosophers, religious leaders, health care providers, and lay persons alike have speculated about the nature and cause of pain while seeking effective means of relief. Philosophers, for example, have viewed pain as an emotion (e.g., Aristotle), as the result of physical stimuli impinging upon the body (e.g., Descartes), or even solely as the result of cognitive activity (e.g., Epictetus). Religious leaders, on the other hand, have suggested that pain is imposed by God, as either a test of faith or a form of punishment for original or other sins. How a patient and therapist view pain will determine the strategies employed to alleviate it. This is most clearly illustrated in the late-19th-century model of pain.

Sensory physiologists and psychophysicists of that period provided the first systematic physiological explanation for the pain experience, which still influences current forms of treatment. They conceptualized pain as a function solely of sensory input. Pain varied, they claimed, according to the quality and intensity of the sensory stimulus. Cognitive and affective factors were relegated to a secondary position, since they constituted merely "reactions" to pain. (For a detailed presentation of this sensory position, see Dallenbach, 1939, and Melzack, 1973.) In this view, the amount of pain experienced should be directly proportional to the amount of tissue damage. To put it somewhat simplistically, physical aspects of the stimulus are transmitted from the pain receptors (free nerve endings) along specific peripheral nerve fibers (A-delta and C fibers) to the spinal cord (anterolateral spinothalamic tract), which conducts impulses to the brain (thalamus and higher centers), where these impulses are registered as pain.

This direct-transmission-line model leads to the assumption that pain can be eliminated or reduced by the removal of the pain stimulus, blockage of the "pain pathways" by analgesic agents, severing of the pathways so that impulses never reach the brain, or removal of parts of the brain where pain signals are registered (e.g., thalamus). Blockage or severing of pathways is most often accomplished by surgery, anesthetic nerve blocks, and various pharmacological analgesic agents. Standard medical and surgical interventions have proved reasonably effective with acute forms of pain, but it is estimated that no more than 50% of chronic pain patients have adequate reduction of pain as a function of purely somatic treatment (Toomey, Ghia, Mao, & Gregg, 1977). Physicians have frequently noted, however, the unpredictability of outcome following procedures designed to block or cut pain pathways (J. White & Sweet, 1969). There are frequent recurrences of pain in patients who appear at first to be responsive to treatment. Moreover, patients with apparently identical pain syndromes tend to respond quite differently to identical treatments.

The interest by the medical community in the larger "pain experience" has been prompted further by two recent trends: (1) the increasing dissatisfaction with the results of medically based treatments such as analgesics (particularly narcotics; Halpern, 1974a), nerve blocks (R. Black, 1974), and transcutaneous electrical stimulation (Ebersold, Laws, Stonnington, & Stillwell, 1975), as well as surgery (Stravino, 1970; J. White & Sweet, 1969), and (2) the recognition of complex interactions among pharmacological, physiological, and psychological factors in the perception and elaboration of pain (Bonica, 1974b; Melzack, 1980, S. Snyder, 1977).

Laboratory investigations of the contributions of psychological mediators have underscored the complexity of the pain phenomenon. For example, the literature on predictability and control of pain (e.g., Bandler, Madaras, & Bem, 1969; Bowers, 1968; Staub, Tursky, & Schwartz, 1971) indicates that the subject's perception of control results, in most instances, in higher pain thresholds, higher tolerance, or both. Other investigators (e.g., Bobey & Davidson, 1970; J. Johnson, 1973; Neufeld & Davidson, 1971) have demonstrated that preparatory communications and information that subjects receive prior to the onset of pain affect various pain parameters.

Still other investigators have related pain perception and tolerance to such factors as prior conditioning (e.g., Pavlov, 1927, 1928), early experiences (e.g., Melzack & Scott, 1957), sociocultural background (e.g., B. Wolff & Langley, 1968), the meaning of the situation (e.g., Beecher, 1959), attentional focus (e.g., Blitz & Dinnerstein, 1971), social modeling (e.g., Craig, Best, & Reith, 1974), suggestions and placebos (e.g., McGlashan, Evans, & Orne, 1969), various individual difference measures (e.g., Andrew, 1970; Petrie, 1967), and anxiety regarding the nature and cause of the noxious stimulation (e.g., Hill, Kornetsky, Flanary, & Wilker, 1952a, 1952b). The important influence of such mediators and the relative neglect they have received by many health care providers may explain the apparent inadequacy of the unidimensional sensory model of pain and the treatments predicated on this model.

A pattern theory of pain that contends that pain is produced by spatiotemporal patterns of neuronal impulses (as opposed to stimulation of specific pain receptors) has also proved inadequate (Melzack & Wall, 1965). Pattern theory postulates that the pattern of noxious stimulation is coded by the central nervous system, which results in the perception of pain. The theory proposes that all nerve fiber endings are alike and that the perception of pain is produced by intense stimulation of nonspecific receptors. As Liebeskind and Paul (1977) and Melzack and Dennis (1978) note, the pattern theory ignores evidence of receptor–fiber specialization (A-delta and C fibers). Both the sensory input and pattern theories of pain fail to consider the complex nature of the pain experience.

Recent reviews of the pain literature (e.g., W. Clark & Hunt, 1971; Liebeskind & Paul, 1977; Turk, 1975; Weisenberg, 1977) have provided compelling arguments that pain is *not* simply a function of the amount of tissue damage and that it cannot be defined adequately by specifying parameters of physical stimuli as suggested by simple sensory–physiological theories. Rather, it is suggested that pain be considered a subjective experience defined by an individual, with the amount and quality of the pain determined by such factors as previous experiences, ability to understand the cause and the consequences of the pain, and psychological variables, all in addition to the sensory input. Taken together, the clinical observations and laboratory data suggest that an adequate conceptualization of pain must be *multidimensional* in nature, incorporating cognitive and affective phenomena as well as the physical stimuli and sensory physiology.

Melzack, Wall, and Casey (Melzack & Casey, 1968; Melzack & Wall, 1965, 1970; Wall, 1978) have offered an alternative model to the traditional specificity model of pain, which they label the "gate-control model." Melzack and Dennis (1978) indicated that the gate-control theory proposes the following:

> Neural mechanisms in the dorsal horns of the spinal cord act like a gate which can increase or decrease the flow of nerve impulses from peripheral fibers to the spinal cord cells that project to the brain. Somatic input is, therefore, subjected to the modulating influence of the gate before it evokes pain perception and response. The theory suggests that large-fiber inputs tend to close the gate while smaller-fiber inputs generally open it, and that the gate is profoundly influenced by descending influences from the brain. It further proposes that sensory input is modulated at successive synapses throughout the projection from the spinal cord to the brain areas responsible for pain experience and response. (pp. 2–3)

In other words, the gate-control model views pain perception and response as complex phenomena, resulting from the interaction of sensory–discriminative, motivational–affective, and cognitive–evaluative components. The theory proposes that a neural mechanism in the spinal cord acts like a "gate" that can facilitate or inhibit the flow of nerve impulses from peripheral fibers to the central nervous system. When the amount of information that passes through the gate exceeds a critical level, the neural areas responsible for pain experience and response are activated.

Somatic input is subjected to the modulating influences of cognitive, affective, and behavioral factors before it evokes pain perception. In this manner, a central control mechanism is proposed to account for alterations in pain perception and response produced by psychological factors and psychological control techniques. Psychological factors may mediate pain by altering individuals' appraisals of the threat, their ability to control the quality of noxious sensations, and their emotional arousal. Psychological methods that modulate cognitive and affective factors may thus prevent the development of pain, abolish it entirely, or at least reduce the intensity of noxious sensation. Thus sensory aspects of pain are but one, albeit important, dimension of the pain phenomenon.

Although the posited physiological and anatomical bases for the gate-control theory are speculative and have been criticized (e.g., Kerr, 1975; Liebeskind & Paul, 1977; Nathan, 1976; Weisenberg, 1977), the multidimensional perspective has received considerable support (e.g., E. Hilgard & Hilgard, 1975; Melzack, 1980b; Tursky, 1976; Wall, 1978). As Weisenberg (1977) noted:

> Regardless of the accuracy of the specific wiring diagrams involved, the gate-control theory of pain has been the most influential and important current theory of pain perception. It ties many of the puzzling aspects of pain perception and control. It has had profound influence on pain research and the clinical control of pain. It has generated new interest in pain perception, stimulating a multidisciplinary view of pain for research and treatment. (p. 1012)

Melzack and Wall's multicomponent model of pain has focused attention on the concept that pain is *not* a function of any particular system alone, but rather, that each specialized portion of the entire nervous system contributes to the pain experience. The failure to take this into account can explain the frequent frustration encountered in treating patients with surgery, anesthetic blocks, or other measures designed to block the so-called pain pathways. As Melzack and Casey (1968) suggested:

> The surgical and pharmacological attacks on pain might well profit by redirecting thinking toward the neglected and almost forgotten contribution of motivational and cognitive processes. Pain can be treated not only by trying to cut down sensory input by anesthetic blocks, surgical intervention and the like but also by influencing the motivational and cognitive factors as well. (p. 435)

In short, the gate-control theory of pain suggests that psychology has much to offer in both understanding and treating pain. Recently, an analogous conceptualization of pain was incorporated into the definition of pain proposed by the International Association for the Study of Pain's task force on taxonomy. They define pain as follows:

> An unpleasant sensory *and emotional experience* associated with actual or *potential* tissue damage, or described in terms of such damage. (IASP Subcommittee on Taxonomy, 1979, p. 250, emphasis added)

This definition conveys the multidimensional and subjective nature of pain for various etiologies. This multidimensional perspective on pain is analogous to the multidimensional perspective on health, disease, and illness that characterizes the field of behavioral medicine. The interest in a multidimensional view of pain has led a number of investigators to question how best to manipulate psychological variables in order to augment existing medical treatments. The goals of such multidimensional approaches include eliminating reliance on some of the more drastic medical treatments (e.g., surgery and addictive narcotics), reducing the incidence of recurring pain following treatment, making pain more bearable when it cannot be totally eliminated, and increasing tolerance for unavoidable noxious stimulation (e.g., aversive medical procedures such as debridement of burns; Fagerhaugh, 1974; Wernick, 1982).

In summary, the complexity of the pain phenomenon and the psychological and economic costs of pain should encourage us to search for better ways to achieve pain regulation. The following chapters will outline a cognitive–behavioral intervention strategy that is consistent with this multidimensional view of pain.

CHAPTER 5

PSYCHOLOGICAL VARIABLES AND PAIN

We are more sensible of one little touch of the surgeon's lancet than of twenty wounds with a sword in the heat of fight.—*Michel de Montaigne (cited in Feuerstein & Skjei, 1979)*

This chapter reviews the role that psychological, especially cognitive, factors play in the pain experience. A detailed review of the laboratory and clinical studies indicates the important, complex, and sometimes surprising role of psychological variables in pain regulation. It is apparent that the pain field has been somewhat naive in how it has conceptualized and assessed the impact of cognitive factors on the pain experience. A good deal of emphasis has been placed on the role of coping strategies in pain tolerance. It is not, however, the mere presence of coping strategies that determines the pain experience. The important role of metacognitive processes and "catastrophizing" ideation in the pain experience is noted. The chapter concludes with a description of a multifaceted cognitive-behavioral treatment, stress-inoculation training. The application of this approach to laboratory pain and acute clinical pain is considered.

Montaigne's comment at the opening of the chapter echoes our emphasis upon factors other than the physical aspects of pain, disease, and treatment. This emphasis has a long history. The Stoic philosophers believed that humans could control pain by the "rational repudiation of pain." Aristotle, Descartes, and Spinoza recommended that pain be overcome through "the permeation of reason." More recently, Beecher (1946, 1951, 1959) noted that the personal meaning of a nociceptive event is an important determinant of its painfulness. Objective events (i.e., those observable to others) are not the only, or perhaps even the major, determinants of the amount of pain one feels. As we shall see, how one appraises or interprets the pain also plays an important role.

Beecher's (1946, 1959) research on the pain experienced by soldiers wounded in combat illustrates the role of the appraisal process in the perception of pain. Many soldiers did *not* complain of intense or severe pain despite life-threatening wounds. It was not that they were insensitive to pain, for inept injections resulted in pain expression. But Beecher (1946) was impressed that only one in four injured soldiers reported enough wound-related pain to request analgesics. When questioned later about their reactions to such serious injuries, the soldiers indicated that they viewed their wounds as a "ticket home." They were relieved, sometimes even euphoric, at being able to leave the battlefield. Beecher (1959) summarized:

> The common belief that wounds are inevitably associated with pain, and that the more extensive the wound the worse the pain, was not supported by observations made as carefully as possible in the combat zone. . . . The data in numerical terms and what is known to all thoughtful clinical observers is that there is no simple direct relationship between the wound *per se* and the pain experienced. The pain is in very large part determined by other factors, and of great importance here is the significance of the wound. (p. 165)[1]

So far our discussion of the role of psychological factors in the pain experience has been limited to anecdotal reports and informal clinical observations. Let us now consider the more formal evidence from laboratory studies and studies of acute, clinical pain.

LABORATORY STUDIES: METHODS AND VARIABLES

Much of the information concerning psychological influences on pain has been derived from studies with subjects who voluntarily participate in laboratory research. Typically, these subjects are not initially experiencing pain or any serious disorder, and pain is intentionally induced by the experimenter. In other respects, this research is diverse, and general summaries are difficult. Before examining the results from this literature, we will consider two details: the variety of different pain induction methods that have been used and the types of cognitive manipulations that have been investigated (see B. Wolff, 1978).

---

1. Wall (1979) has taken issue with Beecher's interpretation of the observation of the soldiers wounded in combat. Wall described soldiers from a study conducted in Israel as experiencing guilt, annoyance, and worry rather than relief or euphoria. Wall suggested that absence of pain with an injury occurs during the immediate response to a severe trauma, when attention is necessarily deployed in service of higher biological priorities (escape, eliciting help, etc.). Guilt, annoyance, worry, and distraction are, however, psychological factors that mediate perceptions of pain.

Pain-Induction Procedures

A number of different stimuli have been employed to induce nociception
in the laboratory, including ice water, electric shock, heat, pressure, and
muscle ischemia (depletion of oxygen in muscle, typically in the arm). A
brief description of each of these procedures follows.

   1. Cold-produced nociception is developed by having subjects im-
merse some part of their bodies (usually the hand and part of the arm) in
ice water maintained at a steady temperature (e.g., 2°C). This cold-
pressor task (Kunckle, 1949) produces a rapidly accelerating set of noxious
sensations, which may reach a point of relative numbness in 3–4 minutes.
In most studies employing this procedure, a ceiling of 5 minutes has been
established, with exposure terminated at that point at which local warming
and numbing appear. See Appendix A and Lovallo (1975) for a description of the apparatus employed.

   The cold-pressor task is generally considered to be very painful and
aversive, though just a small proportion of subjects' bodies are involved.
Most persons would pale at the thought of immersing their *whole* bodies
in frigid water. Dreadful though such a procedure might seem in a
laboratory, we are reminded that, each January, members of various
"Polar Bear Clubs" take pleasure in swimming in frigid waters. Even
greater numbers, in fact thousands, of Scandinavians dash straight from
their saunas into tubs of ice cold water or into the snow. The amount of
subjective discomfort induced by nociceptive stimuli obviously, then,
cannot be determined by examining the source of discomfort alone. The
context in which the stimulation occurs and the attitude and previous
experience of the people affected are also very important. We will consider
the implications of these observations in later chapters.

   2. Sometimes experimenters induce pain by exposing subjects to
heat, usually induced by focusing a high-intensity light against a surface
of skin blackened with india ink (radiant heat dolorimetry; Hardy, Wolff,
& Goodell, 1948, 1952). The ceiling tolerance time for this procedure
depends upon the intensity of the light, the distance from the skin, and the
part of the body exposed (e.g., forehead, back, inner surface of the arm).
As in the case of the cold-pressor task, the sensations of discomfort and
pain intensify at a rapid rate, with a ceiling typically reached within 90–120
seconds. Unlike the cold-pressor task, heat dolorimetry can cause considerable localized tissue damage in patients with a high tolerance (Javert
& Hardy, 1950). The earliest systematic use of this procedure and a
description of the apparatus can be found in Hardy *et al.*'s (1952) classic
book. Interestingly, the subjects who participated in the large series of
studies described in that volume were the authors!

3. Pressure pain has become a fairly standardized procedure as employed by Barber and his colleagues (e.g., Forgione & Barber, 1971; D. Scott & Barber, 1977a). They employ the Forgione–Barber strain gauge (1971), which produces a focal pressure to the skin over a bone, typically on the index finger. This procedure produces a continuously building, aching pain. The maximum trial length most frequently employed is 2 minutes. For other methods of producing pressure pain, see Lambert, Libman, and Poser (1960) and Merskey and Spear (1964).

4. Electric shock produces noxious sensations by a nondamaging electric current. Tolerance for shocks is partially a function of such parameters as voltage, current, and duration of the shock. For descriptions of the complexity of this procedure, see R. Martin and Chapman (1979), Price and Tursky (1975), and Tursky (1974).

The shocks are brief and usually delivered in a series varying in amperage. Tolerance is based on magnitude of amperage accepted. The sensations produced by this procedure differ from those previously discussed because of the episodic nature of the shocks versus the constant nature of the other stimuli.

This difference has both advantages and disadvantages. Since electric shock is typically administered by using many brief shocks, it does not very closely resemble most clinical pain for which a patient might seek relief (Nociceptive stimulation produced during the filling of cavities by dentists, however, approximates the stimulation produced by electric shock.) Headache, backache, and postsurgical pain, for example, all involve more prolonged individual occurrences, during which many more cognitive, affective, and behavioral events may influence one's reactions than may occur in the case of electric shock.

On the other hand, it has been proposed that the possibility of delivering many repeated trials of shocks of varying intensity permits more precision of measurement. Signal detection (SDT) methods have been suggested as a way to separate changes in sensory function from changes in subjective bias or attitudes, although there is controversy over the validity of this approach (e.g., see W. Clark, 1974; Lloyd & Appel, 1976; Malow & Dougher, 1979; R. Martin & Chapman, 1979; McBurney, 1975, 1976; McCreery & Bloedel, 1978; Rollman, 1977, 1979).

5. Muscle-ischemic pain is typically produced by the submaximum-effort tourniquet technique (Smith, Egbert, Markowitz, Mosteller, & Beecher, 1966; see Appendix A). This procedure involves the inflation of a blood pressure cuff to a high level (250 mm Hg), followed by a moderate amount of exercise with that arm (i.e., squeezing a hand dynamometer). The intense pressure produced by the inflation of the cuff serves to impede circulation in the lower arm and hand. The exercise serves to deplete the available oxygen already in the arm, producing a steadily intensifying, aching pain. The ceiling for this task is usually 55 minutes; however, the range of tolerance is great, varying from 3.3 minutes to 55 minutes (Smith et al., 1966).

6. Other procedures less frequently employed include injection of hypotonic and hypertonic saline solution and inflation of esophageal balloons to distend the stomach. This list does not exhaust the pain-producing stimuli that have been utilized.

Comparison of the Procedures. There is little agreement in the literature regarding the subjective equivalence of the various pain-producing stimuli or the extent to which they approximate clinical pain (cf. R. Brown, Fader, & Barber, 1973; J. Clark & Bindra, 1956; Davidson & McDougall, 1969; B. Wolff & Jarvik, 1963). An important contrast can be made between the muscle-ischemic procedure, with a maximum tolerance ceiling of 55 minutes, and the other procedures, with ceilings of 5 minutes or less. Muscle ischemia would tend to tax the cognitive coping repertoire, whereas the other procedures may require a limited number of coping strategies for maximal pain tolerance.

The validity of time-limited procedures has been seriously questioned by Beecher (1959) and Zimbardo (1969). Nevertheless, even Beecher, one of the harshest critics of the ecological validity of laboratory-produced pain, concedes that muscle ischemia produced in the laboratory does seem to produce an experience analogous to pathological pain (Smith & Beecher, 1969; Smith et al., 1966). Sternbach (1968) also has asserted that it is possible to produce a response to severe pain in the laboratory that is comparable to pathological pain by creating the slowly mounting, sustained pain produced by muscle ischemia.

W. Clark and Hunt (1971) suggested that, of all the procedures described, muscle ischemia and the cold pressor appear to be the most analogous to clinical pain in the nature of the sensations produced and the length of tolerance. Laboratory studies, nevertheless, must be carefully qualified, since some aspects of the clinical experience are not approximated. Patients, for example, may be concerned about the diagnostic significance of the pain, whether it can ever be controlled, the implications for their lives, and so on. Subjects exposed to laboratory pain-induction procedures experience none of these.

It is the muscle-ischemic and cold-pressor tasks that we have used in our laboratory and clinical research described later, for the pain induced by them seems closer to the quality, duration, and urgency of clinical pain than does that induced by many of the procedures described earlier (Beecher, 1966; W. Clark & Hunt, 1971; Smith et al., 1966). When comparing studies employing different pain-induction procedures, we must keep in mind the differences among procedures and the unknown effects they may have on other aspects of pain.

Cognitive Strategies

The effects of a number of different types of cognitive and other psychological variables on the tolerance to the varied laboratory-induced nociceptive stimuli have been studied. In examining a person's ongoing cognitive experience prior to and during a painful or stressful episode, one can note both cognitions that seem to be attempts to cope with the experience (which are usually referred to as "strategies") and cognitions that seem likely to worsen the experience (which have variously been called "catastrophizing," "negative," or "maladaptive cognitions"). Of course, unrelated or neutral cognitions may also occur.

Let us first take note of some of the classes of strategies that have been used. Cognitive strategies for coping with experimental pain can be divided into two broad subtypes: those that attempt primarily to alter the appraisal of the painful situation and those that attempt primarily to divert attention away from the pain (Genest & Turk, 1979). Turk (1975) further classified the latter attention diversion strategies into categories based on the inclusion of imagery, the ignoring or acknowledging of the intense sensations, and the locus of the attentional focus. Following are descriptions and examples of some of the cognitive strategies people use in dealing with pain.

1. Imaginative inattention involves ignoring the intense stimulation by engaging in a mental image of something that, if real, would be incompatible with the experience of pain. For example, one might imagine a pleasant day at the beach, skiing down a fast run, or attending a party.

2. Imaginative transformation of pain involves interpreting the present sensations as something other than pain or minimizing those sensations as trivial or unreal. Some examples are imagining the affected area's being numbed with Novocain or seeing oneself as a television character such as the Six Million Dollar Man or the Bionic Woman, with mechanical limbs insensitive to pain.

3. Imaginative transformation of context involves picturing the context in which the intense stimulation is received as different from the actual situation. That is, the individual is aware of the intense sensations, but they are pictured as arising in a different context. For example, one might picture oneself as the fictional character James Bond, having been shot in a limb and driving a standard transmission car down a winding road (Knox, 1973), or as an athlete having received an injury in an athletic event, but continuing to participate despite the pain.

Each of these three categories relies to some extent on the production of an image to distract attention. The next three attention-focusing categories do not rely on imagery per se.

4. Focusing attention on physical characteristics of the environment includes watching television, studying the construction of some object, or counting the holes in ceiling tiles. The individual is required to use his or her attention in a directive fashion, and the physical environment is used for centering the focus of attention.

5. Mental distractions involve focusing attention on various thoughts without the production of a vivid image or the mental picturing of any event or circumstance. Some examples are engaging in mental arithmetic, making plans on how to spend the weekend, or singing the words of a song.

6. Somatization involves focusing attention, in a dissociative manner, on the part of the body receiving the intense sensation. This is done by viewing the sensations in an objective, rather than a subjective, manner. For example, one might analyze the sensations in part of the body and compare these to the feeling in another part of the body, or one might reflect on the nature of the sensations as if preparing to write a biology report. Some subjects in our laboratory have reported that they felt the pain in their arm, but that the pain was not "in them," only in their arm, as if there were a barrier between the sensations they felt in their arm and themselves. They seemed able, in some sense, to separate themselves from the pain and to watch the intensity of the pain fluctuate on its own.

D. Scott and Barber (1977a) arrived at a similar categorization of cognitive coping strategies: (1) imagining pleasant events, (2) focusing on other things, (3) dissociating oneself from the pain, (4) imagining the affected area as numb, and (5) concentrating on sensations other than pain.

Treatment Studies

All of the cognitive strategies just described tend to involve some form of distraction. This is not surprising; a widely reported phenomenon is that distraction or withdrawal of attention from a painful stimulus can increase pain tolerance (e.g., Ainslie, 1975; Coger & Werbach, 1975). This distraction has been related to the "right of way of dominant stimuli" (Sherrington, 1906) and to "the law of prior entry to consciousness" (Berlyne, 1951). Barber (1977) has suggested that distraction of attention is the "final common pathway" of all cognitive strategies. But it appears that things are more complicated than these reviews suggest.

Table 5-1 summarizes the research on laboratory studies that have attempted to influence the subject's attentional style by means of cognitive strategies. The table indicates that several different dependent measures (such as pain tolerance, threshold, self-report, and physiological indexes) were examined in relation to a variety of different nociceptive stimuli. The cumulative picture is that of *equivocal results*. It is not clear that the use of any particular cognitive strategy is more effective than a no-treatment control manipultation (group 7 in Table 5-1) in altering the pain experience. A number of studies found differences between an experimental group that received training in some cognitive strategy and a no-treatment control group, whereas other studies did not find such differences. One must interpret the absence of significant differences with caution.

A number of investigators (Barber & Cooper, 1972; Kanfer & Goldfoot, 1966; Turk, 1975) have commented on the fact that individuals come into an aversive situation with well-rehearsed cognitive coping strategies. This point is confirmed by a study conducted by Chaves and Brown (1978) with dental patients and by studies with chronic pain patients (Copp, 1974; Keefe & Rosenstiel, 1980). In these investigations pain patients reported spontaneously employing a wide range of coping strategies to help them endure the noxious sensations they experienced. The reader might take a moment to consider what strategies he or she typically employs to cope with pain. For example, the last time you were at the dental office, or when you underwent a noxious medical procedure or experienced a headache, what sorts of means did you use to help you cope with the pain?

It may be, then, that the subjects in the so-called no-treatment or control groups in the studies summarized in Table 5-1 actually used cognitive strategies, even though they were not instructed to do so. Moreover, a number of reports (Avia & Kanfer, 1980; Barber & Cooper, 1972; D. Scott, 1978; D. Scott & Barber, 1977a; Turk, 1977) provide evidence indicating that some subjects failed to use coping strategies provided by the experimenter. The crucial point is that it is unclear whether subjects adhere to treatment guidelines.

It is extremely important that future research of this sort include manipulation checks to determine the extent to which subjects use the recommended strategies. Similarly, it is important to know whether untreated subjects spontaneously generate and use strategies that approximate those offered to the treatment subjects. These observations have implications not only for research, but also for health promotion and treatment of any medical problem. Patients also have certain expectations

TABLE 5-1. Summary of Laboratory Studies Examining the Efficacy of Cognitive Coping Strategies

Study	Pain stimulus	Dependent variable	Groups[a]										Results
			1	2	3	4	5	6	7	8	9	10	
Neufeld (1970)	Radiant heat	Tolerance	X	X									2 > 1
Neufeld & Davidson (1971)	Radiant heat	Tolerance	X									X[b]	10 > 1
R. Greene & Reyher (1972)	Electric shock	Tolerance	X					X					6 > 1
Strassberg & Klinger (1972)	Electric shock	Tolerance	X						X	X			8 > 1 > 7 (females) 1 = 7 = 8 (males)
Chaves & Barber, (1974b)	Pressure	Self-report	X					X	X	X			1 = 6, 1 > 7 = 8 6 > 7 = 8
Horan & Dellinger (1974)	Cold pressor	Tolerance	X[c]				X		X				1 > 5 = 7
Spanos, Horton, & Chaves (1974)	Cold pressor	Tolerance	X	X					X				2 > 1 > 7
Grimm & Kanfer (1976)	Cold pressor	Tolerance	X	X			X			X		X[d]	1 = 10 > 5 = 8
Beers & Karoly (1977)	Cold pressor	Self-report	X	X			X		X	X		X[e]	1 = 2 = 5 = 7 = 8 = 10
		Tolerance	X	X			X		X	X			2 > 1 = 7 = 8, 10 > 2 = 7 = 8 5 > 7 = 8, 1 = 7 = 8
D. Scott & Barber (1977a)	Cold pressor	Tolerance	X						X				1 > 7
D. Scott & Barber (1977b)	Cold pressor	Tolerance	X	X					X				1 = 2 = 7
		Self-report	X	X					X				1 = 2 = 7
C. Stone, Demchik-Stone, & Horan (1977)	Cold pressor	Tolerance	X[c]			X			X	X	X		1 > 4 = 7 = 8 = 9
		Self-report											1 > 4 = 7 = 8 = 9
Jaremko (1978)	Cold pressor	Threshold	X	X			X		X				2 = 5 > 1 > 7
		Self-report											1 = 2 = 5 = 7
		Electromyogram											1 = 2 = 5 = 7

Study	Stimulus	Measure						Results
D. Scott & Leonard (1978)	Cold pressor	Threshold	X		X	X	X[f]	$10 > 1 = 7 = 8$
								$1 = 8 > 7$
Avia & Kanfer (1980)	Cold pressor	Tolerance			X			$1 = 7$
		Self-report						$1 = 7$
Ladouceur & Carrier (1979)	Cold pressor	Tolerance			X		X[g]	$1 = 7 = 10$
		Self-report						$1 = 7 = 10$
G. Hackett & Horan (1980)	Cold pressor	Threshold/tolerance	X[c]		X	X	X[h]	$7 > 1 = 9 = 10$ (threshold)
		Self-report						$1 = 7 = 9 = 10$ (tolerance)
								$1 = 7 = 9 = 10$ (self-report)
Rosenbaum (1980a)	Cold pressor	Tolerance	X		X			$1 > 7$ (marginally)
Westcott & Horan (1977)	Cold pressor	Tolerance	X[c]		X			$1 > 7$ (females)
								$1 = 7$ (males)
Worthington & Shumate (1981)	Cold pressor	Tolerance	X				X	$1 > 10$
		Self-report						$1 = 10$
Barber & Hahn (1962)	Cold pressor	Self-report	X		X			$2 > 7$
		Skin conductance, heart rate, forearm muscle tension, and respiration						$2 > 7$ (respiration and fore-arm muscle tension)
								$2 = 7$ (skin conductance and heart rate)
Evans & Paul (1970)	Cold pressor	Self-report	X		X	X		$2 > 7 = 9$
		Heart rate and galvanic skin response						
Blitz & Dinnerstein (1971)	Cold pressor	Tolerance	X		X	X		$2 > 7 = 9$
Knox (1973)	Muscle ischemia			X	X			$2 = 6 > 7$
	Cold pressor	Tolerance	X	X	X	X		$2 = 3 = 7$
R. Johnson (1974)	Cold pressor	Self-report	X		X	X		$2 > 7 = 9$ (numbness)
								$2 = 7 = 9$ (warmth)
		Heart rate and galvanic skin response						$2 = 7 = 9$

(Continued)

TABLE 5-1. (Continued)

Study	Pain stimulus	Dependent variable	Groups[a]										Results
			1	2	3	4	5	6	7	8	9	10	
Chaves & Doney (1976)	Pressure	Self-report		X				X				X[i]	2=6>10
R. Stevens (1977)	Cold pressor	Tolerance				X				X	X		4>9>8
		Self-report				X				X	X		4>9>8
D. Scott (1978)[j]	Pressure	Tolerance		X				X	X				2=6=7
		Self-report		X				X	X				2=7>6
J. Brown (1979)	Cold pressor	Tolerance		X					X				2=7
		Self-report		X					X				2>7
Kanfer & Goldfoot (1966)	Cold pressor	Tolerance				X			X			X	4>7=10
		Self-report				X			X			X[k]	4=7=10
Notermans (1966)	Electric shock	Threshold				X			X				4>7
Barber & Cooper (1972)	Pressure	Self-report				X			X				4>7
Kanfer & Seidner (1973)	Cold pressor	Tolerance				X			X				4>7
		Self-report				X			X				4=7
R. Stevens & Heide (1977)	Cold pressor	Tolerance				X				X	X		4=9>8
		Self-report								X	X		?[l]
Shacham & Leventhal (1979)	Cold pressor	Self-report				X		X					6>4
J. Johnson (1973)	Muscle ischemia	Self-report					X		X				5=7
Grimm & Kanfer (1976)	Cold pressor	Tolerance					X		X	X	X		5>7=8=9
		Self-report					X		X	X	X		5=9>7=8
		Heart rate					X		X	X	X		5=9>7=8

Leventhal, Ahles, & Butler (1977)	Cold pressor	Self-report	X X		6 > 5
Shacham (1979)	Cold pressor	Self-report	X	X	5 > 7
Barber & Calverly (1969)	Pressure	Self-report		X X	6 > 7
Spanos, Barber, & Lang (1974)	Pressure	Self-report		X X	6 > 7

[a]Groups: 1 = imaginative inattention; 2 = imaginative transformation of pain; 3 = imaginative transformation of context; 4 = attention diversion—external; 5 = attention diversion—internal; 6 = somatization; 7 = no-treatment control; 8 = placebo control; 9 = relaxation; 10 = miscellaneous.

[b]Neufeld and Davidson (1971) included a group that was provided with accurate sensory information.

[c]Horan and his colleagues (G. Hackett & Horan, 1980; Horan & Dellinger, 1974; C. Stone, Demchik-Stone, & Horan, 1977; Westcott & Horan, 1977) employ a strategy they label "in vivo emotive imagery," in which subjects are told to imagine pleasant scenes described in a tape during the stress exposure.

[d]Grimm and Kanfer (1976) included two additional groups: (1) experimenter motivated and (2) subjects challenged to employ their own strategies.

[e]In addition to the groups listed, Beers and Karoly (1977) included a group that received training in the use of task-irrelevant, rational thinking.

[f]D. Scott and Leonard (1978) included a group that paired category 1 (imaginative inattention) and category 3 (imaginative transformation of context).

[g]Ladouceur and Carrier (1979) included a group in which subjects were asked to keep track of their performance by looking at a watch. In addition, half of each of the three groups were provided with performance criteria of 5 minutes. The other half of each group did not receive performance criteria. The subjects receiving the performance criteria tolerated the cold-pressor task longer than those who did not receive such instructions, regardless of the coping strategy.

[h]G. Hackett and Horan (1980) included a group that received in vivo emotive imagery plus self-instructional training.

[i]Chaves and Doney (1976) included a group instructed to focus upon the sensation.

[j]D. Scott (1978) confounded these strategies because subjects were instructed to listen to tapes describing the strategies during the pain induction.

[k]Kanfer and Goldfoot (1966) included groups told (1) to set goals using a clock on the wall, (2) to verbalize sensation experienced, or (3) to expect severe pain.

[l]R. Stevens and Heide's (1976) self-report results are unclear because subjects engaged in multiple trials and because ratings varied across trials. Also, the study did not account for decreasing number of subjects over time.

and skills upon entering therapy, and these will interact with any treatment suggestions the therapist offers. The therapist will need to tap the patient's expectations about the proposed treatment.

Although one must be cautious in using box-score analyses that collapse across studies without attention to methodological differences, Table 5-1 is informative in providing a qualified picture concerning the usefulness of cognitive strategies in the amelioration of pain. Table 5-2 contains a more specific summary of the results of studies that employed cognitive coping strategies compared to "no-treatment" or placebo control groups. Here the studies are clustered according to coping categories (imaginative inattention, imaginative transformation of pain, etc.).

From Table 5-2 we can note that, in 28 independent studies, it was found that a cognitive strategy group was more effective than a control group; in 16 studies, no differences were found between the two groups. That is, in 64% of the studies, coping strategy training was superior to spontaneously generated coping techniques. Table 5-2 also questions the hypothesis that any particular cognitive control strategy will increase adaptive coping for all subjects, at least in a laboratory pain situation. No one cognitive strategy was uniformly successful.

The studies examined so far have compared a specific coping strategy with a no-treatment or placebo control group. Table 5-3 contains a summary of the results of studies that have compared one cognitive coping strategy with a second cognitive coping strategy. Here the results are rather meager, with little evidence to support the efficacy of any particular category. There is some suggestion that the imagery strategies are more effective than those with no obvious imagery component, but the evidence is not conclusive on this point.

The data reported in Tables 5-2 and 5-3 do not convincingly establish the efficacy of any cognitive coping strategy relative to the strategies that subjects bring to experiments, nor is there sufficient evidence to support the use of any one strategy compared to any other. Since training in specific cognitive skills does *not* uniformly produce improvement across groups of subjects, one cannot assume that a deficit in cognitive coping skills per se accounts for the wide variability in pain tolerance. This does not imply that cognitive skills are unimportant in the coping process. It may be the case that individual differences in cognitions are important (indeed, we have presented some evidence to suggest they are), but that the nature of the differences is not a coping skills deficit per se.

An alternative explanation is that subjects entering a pain study already have general adaptive coping skills in their repertoires that only some of them employ, or they employ them in a role, as compared to an active involvement, manner. Training in coping skills does not necessarily

TABLE 5-2. Comparison of Laboratory Studies Examining Cognitive Coping Strategies with No-Treatment and Placebo Control Groups

Coping category	Dependent variable	More effective than control study	Equal to control study
1. *Imaginative inattention* (i.e., ignoring the intense stimulation by engaging in a mental image, which, if real, would be incompatible with the experience of pain)	Tolerance/ threshold	Strassberg & Klinger (1972) (females) Horan & Dellinger (1974) Spanos, Horton, & Chaves (1974) Grimm & Kanfer (1976) D. Scott & Barber (1977a) C. Stone, Demchik-Stone, & Horan (1977) Jaremko (1978) G. Hackett & Horan (1980) (threshold) Rosenbaum (1980) Worthington & Shumate (1981)	Neufeld & Davidson (1971) Strassberg & Klinger (1972) (males) Beers & Karoly (1977) D. Scott & Barber (1977b) D. Scott & Leonard (1978) Avia & Kanfer (1979) Ladouceur & Carrier (1979) G. Hackett & Horan (1980) (tolerance)
	Self-report	Chaves & Barber (1974) C. Stone, Demchik-Stone, & Horan (1977) Rosenbaum (1980) (marginally)	Beers & Karoly (1977) D. Scott & Barber (1977a) D. Scott & Barber (1977b) Jaremko (1978) G. Hackett & Horan (1980) Worthington & Shumate (1981)
	Physiological measures		Jaremko (1978) (electromyogram)
	Number of unequivocal studies[a]	10	6
2. *Imaginative transformation of pain* (i.e., interpreting the intense stimu-lation as something other than pain or minimizing those sensations as trivial)	Tolerance	Blitz & Dinnerstein (1971) Spanos, Horton, & Chaves (1974) Beers & Karoly (1977) Jaremko (1978) Barber & Hahn (1962) Evans & Paul (1970) J. Brown (1979)	Knox (1973) D. Scott & Barber (1977b) D. Scott (1978) Brown (1979)
	Self-report		Beers & Karoly (1977) D. Scott & Barber (1977b) Jaremko (1978)

(Continued)

TABLE 5-2. (Continued)

Coping category	Dependent variable	More effective than control study	Equal to control study
3. *Imaginative transformation of context* (i.e., acknowledging the intense stimulation, but transforming the situation in which it occurs)	Physiological measures	Barber & Hahn (1962) (respiration and forearm muscle tension)	Barber & Hahn (1962) (skin conductance and heart rate) Jaremko (1978) (electromyogram)
	Number of un-equivocal studies	6	3
	Tolerance Self-report	Shacham (1979) (distress)	Knox (1973)
	Number of un-equivocal studies	1	1
4. *Attention diversion—external* (i.e., focusing attention on physical characteristics of the environment, ignoring the intense sensations)	Tolerance	Grimm & Kanfer (1976) R. Stevens & Heide (1976) Beers & Karoly (1977) R. Stevens (1977)	Horan & Dellinger (1974) Grimm & Kanfer (1976)
	Self-report	Grimm & Kanfer (1976) R. Stevens & Heide (1976) R. Stevens (1977)	J. Johnson (1973) Beers & Karoly (1977) Shacham & Leventhal (1979) (distress)
	Physiological measures	Grimm & Kanfer (1976)	
	Number of un-equivocal studies	2	3
5. *Attention diversion—internal* (i.e., focusing on various thoughts without mental imagery, ignoring the intense sensations)	Tolerance/ threshold	Kanfer & Goldfoot (1966) Notermans (1966) Kanfer & Seidner (1973) Jaremko (1978)	C. Stone, Demchik-Stone, & Horan (1977)

	Unequivocal studies	Equivocal studies
Self-report		Barber & Cooper (1972), Kanfer & Goldfoot (1966), Kanfer & Seidner (1973), C. Stone, Demchik-Stone, & Horan (1977), Jaremko (1978)
Physiological measures		Jaremko (1978) (electromyogram)
Number of unequivocal studies	4	2
6. *Somatization* (i.e., focusing attention on the part of the body receiving intense sensations, but either viewing these in a dissociated manner or attending to sensations other than pain) — Tolerance	Blitz & Dinnerstein (1971), Beers & Karoly (1977)	D. Scott (1978)
Self-report	Barber & Calverly (1969), Chaves & Barber (1974), Spanos, Barber, & Lang (1974), Shacham & Leventhal (1979) (distress)	Beers & Karoly (1977), D. Scott (1978)
Number of unequivocal studies	5	1
Total number of unequivocal studies	28	16
Percentage of total unequivocal studies	64%	37%

[a]Unequivocal studies include studies in which tolerance/threshold, self-report, or physiological measures reveal consistent results. Tolerance scores are the primary measures considered. If subjects tolerate the nociceptive stimulus for a longer period, then "no difference" in self-reports or physiological measures is not taken to be inconsistent; rather, this indirectly supports the effectiveness of the strategy, since subjects are tolerating the stimulation longer, yet do not report the pain as any more painful in self-reports or do not show differences in physiological responsivity despite longer exposure to the intense stimulation.

TABLE 5-3. *Summary of Laboratory Studies Comparing One Cognitive Coping Strategy and Another*

Cognitive coping strategy	Study	Results
Imaginative inattention versus imaginative transformation of pain (1 vs. 2)	Beers & Karoly (1977)	$1 = 2$[a]
	Neufeld (1970)	$2 > 1$
	D. Scott & Barber (1977b)	$1 = 2$
	Spanos, Horton, & Chaves (1974)	$2 > 1$
	Jaremko (1978)	$2 > 1$[b]
Imagination inattention versus attention diversion—internal (1 vs. 5)	Grimm & Kanfer (1976)	$1 > 5$
	Horan & Dellinger (1974)	$1 > 5$
	Jaremko (1978)	$5 > 1$[c]
Imagination inattention versus attention diversion—external (1 vs. 4)	C. Stone, Demchik-Stone, & Horan (1977)	$1 > 4$
Imaginative inattention versus somatization (1 vs. 6)	Chaves & Barber (1974)	$1 = 6$
	R. J. Greene & Reyher (1972)	$6 > 1$
Imaginative transformation of pain versus imaginative transformation of context (2 vs. 3)	Knox (1973)	$2 = 3$
Imaginative transformation of pain versus attention diversion—internal (2 vs. 5)	Jaremko (1978)	$2 = 5$
Imaginative transformation of pain versus somatization (2 vs. 6)	Blitz & Dinnerstein (1971)	$2 = 6$
	Chaves & Doney (1976)	$2 = 6$
	D. Scott (1978)	$2 = 6, 2 > 6$[d]
Attention diversion—external versus somatization (4 vs. 6)	Shacham & Leventhal (1979)	$6 > 4$
Attention diversion—internal versus somatization (5 vs. 6)	Leventhal, Ahles, & Butler (1977)	$6 > 5$

[a]Beers and Karoly (1977) found 2 superior to 1 for tolerance, but found them to be equal on self-report.

[b]Jaremko (1978) found 2 superior to 1 for threshold, but found them to be equal on self-report and electromyographic activity.

[c]Jaremko (1978) found 5 superior to 1 for threshold, but found them to be equal on self-report and electromyographic activity.

[d]D. Scott (1978) found 2 superior to 6 on self-report, but equal on tolerance.

enhance use of such skills. Moreover, training in specific coping skills may even interfere with subjects' preferred modes of coping. This interference was illustrated by one of our laboratory subjects.

Following an initial cold-pressor trial, this woman reported using "dissociative" coping cognitions to tolerate the pain. She said, for example, "This isn't happening to me. I'm somewhere else. It's not my arm; it's *an* arm sitting in the water." At the same time, she reported using other coping strategies very infrequently, if at all. During a treatment intervention, the woman was encouraged to develop an imagery-based coping procedure for a second trial of the cold pressor. During that trial, she did not engage in dissociative cognitions, but attempted to concentrate on an image. In making this change, her performance plummeted. She reported that she lost the sense of control that had characterized her earlier report and that she engaged in "catastrophizing" cognitions (e.g., thinking about how painful the task was). Her tolerance was halved (from 300 seconds to 170 seconds), while her reports of pain intensity rose by about one-third. Even on an individual-case basis, such dramatic changes are intriguing, and we are currently collecting data to examine these events on a group basis.

Such reports indicate the need to conduct a careful assessment of the subject's or patient's coping strategies (Liebeskind & Paul, 1977). Do patients (with pain or other medical problems) have strategies in their repertoires, but do their thoughts and feelings and their low sense of self-efficacy interfere with the implementation of these strategies? If this is the case, treatment might better focus on activation of existing coping skills rather than on skills training. A recent study by Avia and Kanfer (1980) suggests that providing subjects with encouragement to use already-existing coping skills may indeed have potential value. In an investigation using the cold pressor, subjects who were given the set that they could use various means of self-control to handle pain had higher tolerance than subjects who learned the same strategy (e.g., imagining a pleasant trip), but who were not given a self-management set.

Finally, in considering the laboratory studies summarized in Tables 5-1, 5-2, and 5-3, we should keep in mind that a number of procedural and methodological differences contributed to the often equivocal and contradictory results. These included the following:

1. The lack of comparability of the various pain-induction procedures employed (e.g., cold water, heat, pressure) with respect to duration of stimulation, rate of onset, rate of intensification, and subjective interpretation or appraisal.
2. The lack of equivalence of the dependent measures in assessing the efficacy of treatments (e.g., self-report, tolerance, threshold, physiological measures).
3. The explicit and implicit instructions employed in many studies, varying from exhortations to subjects that it is "absolutely crucial for the success of the study that they tolerate the noxious sensation as long as possible" (Knox, 1973) to statements such as "this is not to determine how far you can go" (J. Johnson, 1973; see also Blitz

& Dinnerstein, 1968, 1971; K. Hall & Stride, 1954; B. Wolff, Krasnegor, & Farr, 1965).

4. The range in ceiling effects inherent in each of the laboratory pain-induction procedures employed, with a wide variability among procedures in time of nociceptive exposure.

5. The assumption, in the majority of these studies, that each individual is capable of using information about procedures employed, sensations experienced, or the use of specific coping strategies.

6. Problems in motivation of subjects.

7. The variation in content of information, mode of presentation and who presents the information.

8. The strategies contrasted with each other may not have been perceived as different by subjects (Turk & Wack, 1981; Wack & Turk, 1980).

In summary, the laboratory studies on pain represent a complicated array of findings and two general conclusions. The first conclusion is that psychological and cognitive factors affect performance in pain situations; second, no one form of coping strategy has proved effective in helping individuals improve their tolerance of pain. In fact, the coping strategies that subjects bring into the laboratory may prove as effective as, or more effective than, the coping strategies that the investigator teaches. It is not necessarily the strategy per se, but the subjects' attitudes and sense of confidence about these strategies that may play an important role in the pain situation. We have already emphasized the importance of patients' attitudes and sense of confidence in relation to a diversity of problems incorporated in behavioral medicine (e.g., health promotion, risk behavior, rehabilitation, self-care). It is to the assessment of these cognitions and attitudes that we now turn our attention.

Assessing Cognitions

Research on pain and stress has delineated many of the *physiological* components of such events. Lovallo (1975), for example, has described alterations in blood pressure, heart rate, and other physiological measures that occur during the cold-pressor task. But only recently have attempts been made to capture the flow of the subject's *ideation and affect* during the experience of pain. Some of the possible means of studying these cognitions include asking the person to think aloud during the task, interrupting him or her at various points and asking for a report, or administering a questionnaire after the task is completed (see Meichenbaum & Butler, 1979; Merluzzi et al., 1981).

Certainly there are problems with such cognitive assessment methods (e.g., see Genest & Turk, 1981; Meichenbaum, Burland, Gruson, & Cameron, 1980; Meichenbaum & Butler, 1979; Meichenbaum & Cameron, 1982). For example, it is difficult, if not impossible, to distinguish post hoc rationalizations from actual ongoing thoughts. Further, demand characteristics, availability heuristics, and social desirability influences are formidable (Nisbett & Ross, 1980). And verbalizing thoughts in itself likely changes the thought process. We ought not to delude ourselves into believing that we can ever "capture exactly" a person's cognitive events. Nonetheless, we cautiously proceed. Several sources can provide *convergent information*, which may facilitate the interpretation of self-reports. Moreover, patients' self-reports are likely to influence how they are treated (Gillmore & Hill, 1981) and how they perceive their plight. Let us illustrate some assessments with laboratory pain.

Cognitive Reconstructions

In order to "catch a glimpse" of the subject's cognitions while tolerating the cold-pressor test, we have used such postperformance procedures as self-report diaries, videotape reconstruction, and imagery recall, each with accompanying probing interviews. After the subjects had removed their hands from the water or terminated the muscle-ischemic procedure, either of their own volition or upon instruction from the experimenter at a preestablished ceiling, the subjects were interviewed about the experience.

In one study (Genest, Meichenbaum, & Turk, 1977) female subjects were asked to describe everything they had been feeling and thinking during the immersion, "even if it was brief or random, and even if it seems trivial." To aid the recollection, each woman was shown a videotape of herself made during the cold-pressor task, and she was reminded of the pain ratings she gave at each request point. (Subjective ratings of pain were anchored from 0, representing no pain, to 10, representing severe pain that the subject would like to stop; however, subjects could give ratings higher than 10 if they chose; E. Hilgard, Cooper, Lennox, Morgan, & Voevodsky, 1967.) The women's descriptions were taped and transcribed verbatim. Similarly in Genest's (1978) study, female subjects were interviewed and asked to recall by means of imagery the feelings and thoughts they experienced prior to and during the immediately preceding cold-pressor trial.

These assessment procedures yielded reconstructed chains of cognitions and feelings, with accompanying sequences of pain reports that led to several interesting findings. The subjects naturally clustered into two groups, according to their tolerance times. In each sample we have examined, the distribution tends to be bimodal, with tolerances generally either less than 100 seconds or approximately 300 seconds (the ceiling employed by the experimenters).

Different cognitions were found to be characteristic of the high-tolerance (those who endured the full 5-minute trial) and low-tolerance (those who withdrew early in the trial) subjects. Those in the high-tolerance group seemed to feel that they could use strategies to affect both the *pain* and their *power to persevere* despite the pain, whereas those in the low-tolerance group used strategies with less conviction of their usefulness and with less sense of their own ability to influence their situation other than by removing their hands from the water. The low-tolerance subjects were more likely to catastrophize and to doubt their ability to control the pain. In contrast, the high-tolerance subjects were displaying a sense of self-efficacy and a conviction of the ability to remain in control, and they tended to see the pain as a problem to be solved rather than as an occasion to engage in negative self-referent ideation or catastrophizing thoughts and images. A few brief examples of reconstructions provided by subjects in the study convey the sort of information that can be gleaned from such reports; we also discuss briefly how the reports could be used in clinical situations.

One subject focused on her negative reaction to the pain and the associated physiological changes:

> It's really bugging me now . . . I guess I was just thinking that it was really sore and that I wasn't prepared . . . I was looking at my hand an awful lot. It was swelling and getting white. I was really upset then . . . I was just looking around, trying to keep my mind off my arm, but . . . I wasn't really thinking about anything else except . . . the pain.

Another subject reported as follows:

> I don't think I can do it. I don't think I can use this technique. I'm just not the type of person who is good at this.

This latter subject also focused on the pain and on the desire for it to end. But there is also a complete absence in her protocol of any constructive attempts to handle the sensations in any way. She goes on to add:

> It hurt . . . I was thinking about taking my arm out of the water. It really started to hurt. It really got painful here. I was thinking about taking my arm out of the water and I told myself that I couldn't take it any more. The only thing I remember thinking about was taking my arm out of the water . . . I was saying to myself, "I can't keep it in here any longer."

Although one must be cautious in interpreting such postperformance self-reports, as noted by Nisbett and Wilson (1977), the subjects' verbal reports of their thoughts and feelings are filled with treatment implications, as we will discuss in more detail in Section III. For example, if patients provided such cognitive reconstructions during clinical assessments, the therapist might ask the patient whether his or her attention was similarly occupied when experiencing clinical pain. What is the impact of such thoughts, images, and feelings on the perceived intensity of pain and on the patient's perception of his or her sense of uncontrollability and helplessness? Might a change of attentional focus be helpful, and how could it be accomplished? By raising such concerns, the therapist can use the patient's feelings and thoughts as a basis for conducting a situational analysis and as a way of laying the groundwork for a cognitive–behavioral intervention. We will consider the use of such assessment procedures with pain patients in Chapter 9.

Another example of the potential usefulness of such self-reports was offered by a woman who reported that, when she submerged her hand in the cold water, she imagined that she was at a party and that it was her job to remove the beer from the cold ice chest. She then went on to report that she imagined that she was skiing and that the cold, wet snow went up her sleeve. Finally, she imagined she was letting her arm trail along in the cold water as she sat in a rowboat. In short, this woman reported three imagery-transformation strategies. What surprised us about the woman was that she was able to tolerate the cold-pressor test for only less than 2 minutes and reported high levels of pain intensity.

Thus the mere utilization of such cognitive strategies did not appear sufficient to ensure high pain tolerance and low pain intensity. The postperformance assessment revealed that this woman basically doubted her ability to cope with the pain and shifted from strategy to strategy in a fruitless and somewhat frantic manner, attempting to find anything that would work. This subject highlighted the finding that it is not only the presence or absence of coping skills or cognitive strategies, but also the nature of the beliefs and self-statements about one's coping ability that determines the nature of the pain experience.

An excerpt of the report of a subject who dealt well with cold-pressor immersion illustrates this further. There is an initial shock at the coldness of the water:

> I started thinking, "I wish I hadn't done it." It was worse after a very few seconds and I started to think, "Oh my goodness, it's horrible."

She quickly recovered, however, and changed her approach entirely:

> I sat here and thought, "This isn't happening to me. I'm somewhere else. It's not my arm; it's just *an* arm sitting in the water. I can go on as long as this has to go on." . . . Every time I was ready to give up I thought, "No, it's not killing me because it's not my arm. It's just *an* arm in the water."

Another perspective on the assessment of cognitions is provided by Spanos and his colleagues. In a program of studies centering on hypnosis, these investigators (Spanos & Hewitt, 1980; Spanos, Radtke-Bodorik, Ferguson, & Jones, 1979; Spanos, Stam, & Brazil, in press) have examined the relationships among hypnotic susceptibility, cognitive events, and pain. Using a series of open-ended questions following a cold-pressor immersion, Spanos et al. (1979) were able to categorize subjects' reports into four categories (following the taxonomy of Turk): (1) catastrophizing —focusing on and exaggerating the unpleasant aspects of the situation; (2) imaginal coping—imagining situations inconsistent with the pain situation, such as the experience of being on a warm beach; (3) distraction —focusing attention on nonimagery events other than the pain situation, such as counting backward; and (4) relaxing.

Spanos and his colleagues found a complex interaction between the level of pain reported, the use of strategies, the tendency to catastrophize, and repeated immersion trials on the cold-pressor task. Subjects who were classified as catastrophizers reported significantly more pain than noncatastrophizers. Moreover, Spanos et al. (1979) reported that catastrophizing interacted with the number of coping strategies used by subjects in effecting pain decrements from the first to the second immersion in the cold-pressor task. Subjects classified as catastrophizers showed no increment in pain tolerance from the first to the second immersion, regardless of the number of coping strategies employed. Among noncastastrophizers, however, those who used more than one coping strategy reported a significant reduction in pain from the first to the second immersion, whereas those who used only one or no strategy showed no such reduction.

As Spanos et al. indicated, these findings have a number of important implications. They suggest the important mediating influence of coping cognitions and the role of the subject's attentional style while experiencing pain. The tendency to catastrophize was the single best predictor of reporting pain. Eighty-eight percent of the catastrophizers, but only 39% of the noncatastrophizers, *failed* to report an increment in pain tolerance from the first to the second immersion. Moreover, coping strategies were associated with pain reduction only among noncatastrophizers. More recently, Spanos et al. (in press) found that the higher the percentage of time that experimental subjects engaged in coping imagery while experiencing the cold-pressor task, the less pain they reported, supporting the efficacy of imagery in coping with pain.

These findings are not limited to experimental situations, as is illustrated in a naturalistic descriptive study by Chaves and Brown (1978), who interviewed 75 patients following restorative dental procedures or simple extraction of teeth. The structured interview they employed was designed to determine whether the patients had employed self-generated strategies to control pain and stress. It was found that 44% of the patients spontaneously employed self-generated coping strategies and that 37% engaged in various kinds of "catastrophizing" ideation preceding and during the dental procedures. Catastrophizing took several forms, including negative self-statements regarding their competence, anxiety-arousing thoughts, and extremely aversive images. To illustrate, one patient stated, "How I hated it. I hate having injections. I think, 'Oh no, here we go again.' I hate it with a passion. Just to see that great big needle coming down at you, the next thing you know you start going bananas. I just can't hack it."

Chaves and Brown reported that catastrophizers rated their experience as significantly more stressful than the group that did not engage in such catastrophizing thoughts and images. They went on to speculate that the stress experienced by these patients may be caused, or at least exacerbated, by catastrophizing ideation and that the presence of catastrophizing ideation may be more important than any specific coping techniques. The authors also noted that the noncatastrophizing group reported using a whole host of coping strategies, with no one strategy being used more frequently or proving more effective.

In summary, the studies here indicate (1) there is no evidence that subjects who tolerate intense physical stimuli poorly suffer from a deficiency in the number or type of cognitive coping strategies in their repertoires; (2) no one specific category of coping strategies is consistently shown to be more effective than any other; and (3) what appears to distinguish low- from high-pain-tolerant individuals is their cognitive processes —the "catastrophizing" thoughts and feelings that precede, accompany, and follow the aversive situation—rather than specific elements of the coping strategies per se. Similar conclusions were drawn by Kendall *et al.* (1979) regarding the relationship between thoughts and distress by patients who had undergone cardiac catheterization (see Chapter 3).

So far we have reviewed evidence that psychological, especially cognitive, factors may influence the experience of pain in laboratory and clinical situations. We will now turn to the question of multidimensional training of coping skills to reduce pain.

MULTIFACETED COGNITIVE–BEHAVIORAL TREATMENT

The most extensively examined multidimensional approach is a procedure labeled "stress inoculation" (Genest, 1979; G. Hackett & Horan, 1980; G. Hackett, Horan, Buchanan, & Zumoff, 1979; Horan, Hackett, Buchanan,

Stone, & Demchik-Stone, 1977; Klepac, Hauge, Dowling, & McDonald, 1981; Klepac, Dowling, Hauge, & McDonald, 1980; Meichenbaum, 1977; Meichenbaum & Turk, 1976; Turk, 1975, 1977).

Briefly, the stress-inoculation procedure explicitly teaches patients to regulate pain using such diverse strategies as relaxation, attention diversion, and alteration of attributions, self-labels, appraisals, self-statements, and images. Procedures used in the training are similarly varied, including direct instruction, cooperative development of rationale and intervention procedures, training in utilization of procedures, and cognitive and behavioral rehearsal of the various strategies.

Several aspects of this regimen should be underscored. Patients are provided with an initial conceptualization of pain that emphasizes the contribution of cognitive and affective factors to the pain experience. The implication is that controlling these components should lead to improved self-regulation of pain. The underlying theme is that individuals are not helpless—that they can do something to control the quality and intensity of discomfort experienced. Although patients are provided with information and training in a variety of cognitive and behavioral control strategies, they are treated as collaborators and encouraged to "try on" different strategies in order to establish coping repertoires that best suit them. In other words, in contrast to some treatments, no specific strategy is imposed upon patients or subjects. And finally, patients are provided with graded overt and covert practice to help them consolidate the various skills reviewed and to experience some feelings of self-mastery.

Stress-inoculation training *does not* merely teach a pain patient to have pleasant thoughts or soothing images or to repeat some verbal palliative in order to alter the pain. Much more is involved than verbal persuasion in the manner of Émile Coué ("Every day, in every way, I'm getting better and better") or Norman Vincent Peale (positive thinking). Instead, in a collaborative fashion, the patient is encouraged to generate a variety of coping strategies to deal with the various elements and phases of the pain experience. The details of this treatment approach will be described later; at this point let us briefly summarize some of the preliminary findings using the stress-inoculation procedure.

Both Genest (1979) and Turk (1975, 1977) have reported significant results for groups receiving the stress-inoculation regimen compared to attention-placebo groups matched for treatment credibility and assessment-control groups in laboratory investigations of pain. The control treatments provided subjects with comparable exposure time to credible training materials, procedures, and trainers. Control subjects were encouraged to view pain as partly determined by social (e.g., early learning) and cultural factors and to examine how these variables might play a role in their own experiences of pain. It was suggested that, if the subjects spent some time considering the personal implications of pain and examining anxiety or concerns they had *before* they undertook the posttest, this *work of worrying* would reduce the aversiveness of the actual experience. Turk (1978d) reported that subjects perceived both the stress-inoculation training and the attention-placebo training as equally credible and likely to be effective in reducing perception and experience of pain.

In the Genest and the Turk studies, the pain-producing stimulus employed was muscle ischemia, with dependent measures of tolerance time and self-reports obtained during the pain-induction procedure and retrospectively. The experimental group's mean improvement in tolerance time was more than 80% in one study (from 17 minutes on the pretraining trial to 32 minutes on the posttraining trial; Turk, 1975) and 69% in another investigation (from 17 minutes on the pretraining trial to 27 minutes on the posttraining trial; Turk, 1977), compared to control groups whose improvement ranged from 2.5% to 16%.

In Genest's (1979) bibliotherapy study of stress-inoculation training (a structured format incorporating written and audiotape material and minimal experimenter contact), the mean tolerance-time improvement for the treatment group was 56% (from 16 minutes on the pretraining trial to 25 minutes on the posttraining trial), compared to the control group's 8% improvement (from 17 minutes to 18 minutes). In each of these studies, the stress-inoculation subjects assessed the noxious sensations as no more discomforting or intense than did the control groups, even though they tolerated the noxious stimulation for a significantly greater period of time.

Horan *et al.* (1977) found similar results with a substantially larger number of subjects. Even though the stress-inoculation subjects were tolerating the pain for longer periods of time, they were not perceiving the situation as any more painful. Stress-inoculation training has recently been applied to clinical populations. We will first consider acute pain and in the next chapter consider other forms of pain.

CLINICAL STUDIES: ACUTE PAIN

Numerous combined cognitive and behavioral regimens have been employed with clinical pain populations, including those with postsurgical pain (e.g., Langer, Janis, & Wolfer, 1975), chronic pain (e.g., Gottlieb *et al.*, 1977; Herman, 1978; Herman & Baptiste, 1981; Khatami & Rush, 1978; Levendusky & Pankratz, 1975; Rybstein-Blinchik, 1979; Turk, Kerns, Bowen, & Rennert, 1980; Turner, 1979), dental pain (Klepac *et al.*,

1980), both migraine (e.g., Bakal, Demjen, & Kaganov, 1981; Mitchell & White, 1977) and tension headaches (e.g., Holroyd, Andrasik, & Westbrook, 1977; Holroyd & Andrasik, 1980; Reeves, 1976), and irritable bowel syndrome (e.g., Bowen & Turk, 1979; Harrell & Beiman, 1978). See Turk (1982) and Turk and Genest (1979) for reviews of this literature. Rather than reexamining each of these studies, we will select examples that demonstrate the potential of a cognitive–behavioral treatment approach with different clinical pain populations.

Burns

Studies by Wernick and his colleagues (Wernick, Taylor, & Jaremko, 1978; Wernick, Jaremko, & Taylor, 1981) illustrate the application of stress-inoculation training with burn patients. Following an initial educational phase concerning the nature of stress and pain, a skills acquisition phase included slow, deep breathing; relaxation; autogenic training (relaxing and calming thoughts); and cognitive strategies such as attention diversion and cognitive reappraisal. A cognitive restructuring approach was also employed in order to help burn patients identify dysphoric feelings and specific negative self-statements (e.g., "I can't bear this any longer," "I think I'm going to die," or "I wish they would just let me die and get it over with"). In a collaborative manner, the therapist helped the burn patient react to such negative thoughts as "I think I'm going to die" with coping self-statements such as "This isn't the first time I've had my dressing changed; I'll make it this time, too." Such therapy with the burn patient was followed by rehearsal, in which the patient was asked to imagine such scenes as dressing changes. The patient was guided to use a coping image (imagining the negative self-statements and feelings and then replacing these with coping self-statements).

Following this imagery rehearsal, the application phase of stress-inoculation training was undertaken during the "tanking" (bathing) and changing of dressings. The patient was encouraged to go through the "work of worrying" in preparing a plan of action for coping with the pain that he or she might experience during the next dressing change. During the actual tubbing, the therapist acted as a "coach," providing guidance when necessary. The supports included encouraging the burn patient to relax, to view the tubbing as a series of three phases (physiological arousal, appraisal, and self-evaluation), and to use other coping skills as well. Although Wernick et al. (1981) have reported some encouraging results for this approach for burn patients, the data available must be considered preliminary.

A noteworthy feature of the Wernick *et al.* program is the nature of the *in vivo* application training, in which the therapist extended treatment into the tubbing and dressing-change situations. The transfer of coping skills from a clinical setting to real life is always problematic. It is important to build such transfer into the treatment regimen, as Wernick *et al.* have done.

Postsurgical Recovery

In an examination of postsurgery, Langer *et al.* (1975) provided a group of surgery patients with a cognitive-behavioral treatment designed to reduce stress and augment postsurgical recovery. Patients were trained to reappraise anxiety-provoking cues and events by presentation of a conceptualization of stress and by alteration of negative internal dialogues. Training in the use of attention-diverting, cognitive coping strategies (e.g., distraction of attention, considering positive outcomes of the surgery) was also included, as was sensory and procedural information (namely, what the procedure entailed and what sensation would likely be experienced).

Patients receiving this training were compared to groups receiving (1) only procedural and sensory information, (2) the combined treatment without the preparatory information, and (3) no intervention. The combined-treatment and combined-treatment-minus-preparatory-information groups demonstrated significantly less preoperative and postoperative stress (rated by nurses) than the other two groups. These two cognitive-behavioral groups requested significantly less analgesic medication, and a smaller proportion of the patients in these groups requested sedatives than in either of the other two groups. There were no differences between the information-alone and no-treatment control groups.

Other treatment studies of persons who underwent surgery have been conducted by Egbert, Batit, Welch, and Bartlett (1964); Fortin and Kirouac (1976); J. Johnson, Fuller, Endress, and Rice (1978); and Wolfer and Visintainer (1975). For a review see Turk and Genest (1979). The extent of the training in these studies varied widely (e.g., whereas Langer *et al.*, 1975, provided a brief training, Fortin & Kirouac, 1976, provided a much lengthier, comprehensive approach). For example, Fortin and Kirouac provided herniorrhaphy and cholecystectomy patients with (1) an orientation to the surgical experience and hospital, (2) elementary biological facts related to their surgery, (3) the purpose and techniques of respiratory and muscular exercises, including the routines to follow postsurgically, (4) techniques for changing position in order to minimize postsurgical discomfort (e.g., movement designed to prevent pulling of stitches), and (5) techniques for anticipating and coping with postsurgical nausea, vomiting, pain, dizziness, and weakness (e.g., slow, deep breathing).

Which components of such complex treatments are necessary has not been established, nor have comparisons between various combined techniques been reported. A rule of thumb (we paraphrase Mahoney, 1974a), however, seems appropriate to each of the combined treatments reviewed here and in later chapters: First demonstrate an effect and then conduct component analyses and comparative studies. Investigators should also examine subject-by-treatment interactions to determine the characteristics of subjects who benefit most from the treatment and those of subjects who benefit least.

As we noted earlier, one of our intentions is to evaluate critically the efficacy of cognitive–behavioral treatment programs. The intention is not only to review those studies that support this approach, but also to examine those in which the approach has not proved to be effective.

A recent study by Tan, Melzack, and Poser (1980) examined the efficacy of the stress-inoculation approach as a preventive intervention for the attenuation of acute clinical pain. In this study 36 patients who were to be exposed to a noxious X-ray procedure, knee arthrogram, were assigned to one of three groups: stress-inoculation, attention-placebo, and control. Subjects in the stress-inoculation group were provided with a conceptual scheme of pain based on the Melzack–Wall gate-control theory (Melzack & Wall, 1965), were exposed to a variety of cognitive and behavioral coping techniques (e.g., relaxation, distraction, coping self-statements), and were given a laboratory pain task (pressure pain; Poser, 1962) as a means of rehearsing the coping strategies. The attention-placebo group received procedural information about the arthrogram and a discussion of pain. Both the stress-inoculation and attention-placebo groups received 1 hour of training or information. The control group completed a set of questionnaires and received no additional information or training. The authors reported no significant differences between the groups on subjective pain ratings, radiologist's ratings of patients' pain, or ratings of pain behaviors (e.g., grimaces, sighs, verbalizations).

A number of explanations were offered by the authors to explain the lack of significant results. One possibility offered was that the training may have been too brief. Another possibility is that the intensity of the pain resulting from the knee arthrogram was relatively low (usually rated as mild to discomforting). Thus a floor effect may have been operating. The pain involved with the arthrogram, moreover, usually reaches a peak in about 30 seconds. Patients may not have been able to employ the various coping techniques. In fact, emphasis on training in coping strategies may not have been necessary, since all patients reported using some coping strategies. Regardless of the explanation, it is important to consider nonconfirmatory data such as these in order to enhance our understanding of the applicability and limitations of the stress-inoculation treatment approach or any treatment for that matter. Further studies are required to identify such limitations and to help us modify various components of the treatment approach.

Preparation for Childbirth

We recently came across a newspaper article that provided an interesting comment on prepared childbirth. The article, entitled "South India Agog at Painless Birth" (1974, p. 12), began as follows:

Housewives, newly-wed women and even grandmothers in the south Indian state of Kerala are vigorously participating in a controversy over what newspapers describe as "painless childbirth."

Several women have said that Moslem doctors on the island of Lakshadeep . . . have helped them to deliver their babies without labor pains.

"It took only 15 minutes," 26-year-old Vasuke Menon is quoted saying. "Far from experiencing any labor pain, I brought our third child into the world without being even aware of it."

Mrs. Menon said the doctor who handled her case was popularly known as Baba Sheikh, which means a kind of doctor, holy man, and teacher rolled into one.

Press reports in Kerala say that "at least 200" cases of painless childbirth have been recorded on the island. The doctors are described as experts in ancient Islamic medicine. . . .

Meanwhile, the influential *Times* of India has editorially supported the claim of painless childbirth.

The English-language paper said that "medical authorities have confirmed what they have suspected all along: That labor pains are a myth.

"The pain link has been propagated as one of the human race's ancient myths, a universal malady based upon what is no less than a colossal mass hypnosis."

The *Times* said that the Lakshadeep doctors were only "dehypnotizing" pregnant women of their fear of labor pains.

The article then ended on this pessimistic note:

Family planning officials of the Indian government expressed fear that if painless childbirth gets popular acceptance among women the result may be a baby boom.

We doubt that many prenatal teachers would wish to represent themselves as experts in ancient Islamic medicine, much less as holy men and dehypnotizers, and few now promote a view of even the best birth experience as a completely painless one. Whatever the validity of this newspaper account, the preparation for childbirth is an important area for behavioral medicine. In fact, it appears to be one of the areas that has received the most attention concerning prevention and coping with pain and distress.

Throughout history, attempts to relieve pain related to childbirth have remained controversial, whether the means to alleviate pain was pharmacological or through programs of antenatal training (e.g., "natural childbirth," Dick-Read, 1933; "Lamaze" training, Lamaze, 1958; "psycho-prophylaxis," Velvovsky, Platonov, Ploticher, & Shugom, 1960). A few theologians have argued that attempts to reduce pain during labor and childbirth go against the Creator's wishes, since in the Bible (Genesis 4:3) God is cited as stating, "I will greatly multiply your pain in childbearing. In pain thou shalt bring forth children." Such religious concerns continued to be discussed as late as the 1950s by Pope Pius XII, who wrote an encyclical on the subject giving tacit approval to antenatal training.

When Grantly Dick-Read, perhaps the first to advocate prepared childbirth (*Natural Childbirth*), published his original monograph on the subject in 1933, he was severely criticized for his suggestion that labor and childbirth were not inherently painful (A. Thomas, 1957). His approach was criticized for being "primitive and barbaric" (Reid & Cohen, 1950), "medically unacceptable" (Reid & Cohen, 1950), "likely to create a nega-tive attitude of mothers toward their children" (Fielding & Benjamin, 1962), and "unrelated to neonatal well-being" (Hughey, McElin, & Young, 1978).

At the same time that various approaches to antenatal training have been criticized, they have also been embraced with almost religious fervor and support (e.g., Bing, 1967; Chertok, 1969; Karmel, 1959). In fact, Chertok (1969) suggested that prepared childbirth was one of the most significant advances in modern medicine. Several authors have recently described the interesting history of the controversy between advocates and critics of the approach and between adherents of "different" methods of conducting antenatal training (e.g., N. Beck & Hall, 1978; N. Beck, Geden, & Brouder, 1979).

Investigators have made extensive claims regarding the positive effects of antenatal training (Genest, 1981). For example, studies have reported that training results in the decreased perception of pain (e.g., Bergstrom-Whalen, 1963; Cogan, 1978; Enkin, Smith, Dermer, & Emmet, 1972; Huttel, Mitchell, Fischer, & Meyer, 1972; Klusman, 1975; Norr,

Block, Charles, Meyering, & Meyers, 1977), the increased positive evaluation of the experience (Doering & Entwisle, 1975; Norr *et al.*, 1977), and many other psychological benefits (e.g., Chertok, 1969; Enkin *et al.*, 1972; Huttel *et al.*, 1972; St. Van Eps, 1955; Tanzer, 1967; Yahia & Ulin, 1965).

Other studies have reported that training produced benefits from an obstetric point of view, including the reduced use of analgesic and anesthetic medication (e.g., Flowers, 1962; J. Scott & Rose, 1976; Van Auken & Tomlinson, 1953; Worthington, 1982; see N. Beck & Hall, 1978, and Genest, 1981, for a review); increased cooperativeness on the part of the mother during labor (Chertok, 1969; Huttel *et al.*, 1972); reduction in blood loss and hemorrhaging (Galeazzi & Minella, 1972; Velvovsky *et al.*, 1960); a decreased incidence of significant obstetric interventions, including forceps deliveries, episiotomies, and cesarean sectioning (Flowers, 1962; Van Auken & Tomlinson, 1953); and significant decrease in the length of labor (H. Shapiro & Schmitt, 1973; Van Auken & Tomlinson, 1953; Velvovsky *et al.*, 1960).

Recently, Worthington (1982) has reported that Lamaze-trained pregnant women reported less pain and had a longer tolerance in the cold pressor than women who attended parenting classes that did not teach pain-control methods. Women who managed cold-pressor pain well also requested less medication during labor. (But see the problems in methodology shared by this and other childbirth studies, as will be discussed subsequently.)

Finally, some authors have reported that training produces effects that are beneficial to the child, including increased oxygenation of fetal blood (Petrov-Maskakov, 1972); more rapid initiation of breathing following expulsion (Tupper, 1956); healthier babies, as evident in higher Apgar scores (Apgar, 1953; Enkin *et al.*, 1972); and decrease in the rate of neonatal mortality and sickness (Stahler, Stahler, & Gutanian, 1972).

Many other studies, however, have failed to find results supportive of the data just cited. For example, Huttel *et al.* (1972) found no difference in the duration of labor or in Apgar scores for mothers who had and had not received antenatal training. Davenport-Slack and Boylan (1974) and Cogan, Henneborn, and Klopfer (1976) found no significant effect for antenatal training on mothers' self-reports of pain. And Hughey *et al.* (1978) found no long-term benefits of training on neonatal well-being.

Perhaps the most consistent finding for the effects of antenatal training is that trained mothers received less analgesic and anesthetic medication than untrained mothers. This may be due to motivation on the part of the mother or coach to have a "natural" birth or is perhaps related to self-selection in the groups; moreover, the trained mother may be offered less medication than a nontrained mother (Davenport-Slack, 1974; J. Scott & Rose, 1976). Whatever the reason for the lower drug intake in trained mothers, this result takes on additional significance because obstetricians have become increasingly aware of the harmful effects of drugs on both the progress of labor (e.g., E. Friedman & Sachtleben, 1961) and the condition of the infant at birth (Soule, Copans, Standley, & Duchowny, 1974). Obstetricians concerned with the risks created by drugs have increasingly turned to some form of antenatal training.

One word of caution should be offered. In a comprehensive review of the literature on prepared childbirth, N. Beck and Hall (1978) noted that to date there was an "absence of a single adequately controlled study that allows cause and effect statements regarding antenatal treatment and outcome." The three major concerns regarding these studies raised by N. Beck and Hall are the failure to employ control groups, the non-random assignment of subjects to groups, and the failure to covary such factors as maternal anxiety level, socioeconomic status, reactions toward childbirth, and so on, all known to be related to the childbirth experience (e.g., C. Davis & Merrone, 1962; Klusman, 1975; Zax, Sameroff, & Farnum, 1975).

The failure to incorporate appropriate attention-placebo groups does not permit a determination of the cause of treatment effects. That is, the effects obtained following antenatal training may be attributed to such a nonspecific effect as the attention given by the trainer rather than to any of the specific techniques (e.g., information, relaxation, patterned breathing). These nonspecific effects in themselves, however, may be important components of the training regimen, and their importance should not be overlooked. In addition, the absence of random assignment of subjects to experimental and control groups is often unavoidable in the clinical settings in which these studies are carried out. Unfortunately, self-selection biases may be very important in determining outcome, rendering the implications of the data unclear.

Part of the problem in studying antenatal programs is their complexity. For example, Wright (1964) examined the antenatal preparation literature and identified 33 varieties of training. Common features included in almost all of these are (1) information about labor and birth, (2) muscle relaxation exercises, (3) patterned breathing, and (4) support from attendants during the delivery process (often the father of the child).

Several studies have attempted to identify the factors that may lead to the beneficial effects reported with antenatal training when, in fact, they do occur (e.g., Cogan, 1976; Cogan et al., 1976; Doering & Entwisle, 1975; Doering, Entwisle, & Quinlan, 1980). These studies point to a reduction in anxiety, an increased sense of control, and perceptions of resourcefulness as results of antenatal training (Genest, 1981). In short, the training seems to lead to an alteration of the woman's appraisal of the situation. In Chapters 2 and 3 we emphasized this alteration in appraisals as a common and important factor in many areas of behavioral medicine (e.g., preparation for noxious medical procedures, treatments of stress-related disorders, treating substance abuse and other risk behaviors). In addition, it has been suggested that the support provided by the husband or significant other plays an important role in the woman's coping (e.g., Campbell & Worthington, in press; Genest, 1981).

Given the importance of these processes, one question that might be raised is how to maximize enhancement of women's perceptions of self-efficacy. In addition to the training included in most antenatal courses, a cognitive–behavioral perspective would encourage more explicit attention to the pregnant couple's initial and ongoing thoughts and feelings regarding the course of the pregnancy, the process of childbirth, the potential for control, and the use of some of the strategies taught.

Most antenatal programs emphasize relaxation and patterned breathing *during* contractions, but attend less to what happens *between* contractions. Training women to include positive self-statements (e.g., the positive things to look forward to; Langer *et al.*, 1975) as well as self-statements and images related to the different aspects of labor and childbirth (e.g., preparing for contractions, coping with contractions, feelings at critical moments when the contractions are most intense) may significantly add to treatment efficacy.

The use of a variety of mental distractions between contractions might also be included. For example, Horan (1973) examined the efficacy of *in vivo* emotive imagery (pleasant imagery) during labor and childbirth. In this case study, Horan reported that the imagery procedure was more effective than relaxation. Research of this type is needed in order to examine the effects of coping strategies in antenatal training. We should note that some psychoprophylactic programs do attend to this dimension, encouraging, for example, a focus on feelings of satisfaction and accomplishment following each contraction and on the avoidance of thoughts related to how many are yet to come, possible future unknown events, and so on.

Finally, an inoculation phase of sorts is included in many antenatal training courses. The coach (significant other) is asked to squeeze the woman's knee to simulate the intensity of a contraction, and the woman is told to practice the patterned breathing and muscle relaxation. Sometimes this is extended to having the woman practice the coping responses during the several repetitions and even to an imaginal rehearsal of the whole labor and delivery, from initial signs to the baby's birth (e.g., Campbell & Worthington, 1981).

To date, we are aware of no studies that have attempted to evaluate the stress-inoculation training proposed in antenatal training in comparison with more standard approaches. (See N. Beck & Siegel, 1980, for a more extended discussion of potential modifications of antenatal training employing psychological knowledge regarding pain, anxiety, and stress reduction.) Research along the lines suggested by N. Beck and Hall (1978) is sorely needed, given the increasing enthusiasm for prepared childbirth training.

SUMMARY

In the case of burn patients, postsurgical recovery, and childbirth, as well as in laboratory studies, we have seen the important role of psychological factors in the experience of pain and the potential application of a cognitive–behavioral treatment approach. Many existing training regimens, as in the case of antenatal training, already approximate elements of the stress-inoculation training. These may be further augmented and modified from a cognitive–behavioral perspective. Assessment of individuals' thoughts and feelings about their plight, as well as specific coping strategies, should enhance our understanding of response to pain and provide information that will help in developing comprehensive treatment programs. The potential of the cognitive–behavioral approach is illustrated further in the next chapter, in which we consider the extension of the cognitive–behavioral perspective to other clinical pain populations.

CHAPTER 6

CHRONIC PAIN: PSYCHOLOGICALLY
ORIENTED APPROACHES TO TREATMENT

If we observe the world with which we are concerned here—the *universe* of the patient in chronic pain—we can perceive a similarity to the universe of the nightmare . . . terrible things are being done to him and he does not know if worse will happen; he has no control and is helpless to take effective action; no time-limit is given . . . the patient lives during the waking state in the cosmos of the nightmare.—*Lawrence LeShan (1964)*

This chapter examines the application of a number of psychologically oriented approaches to the treatment of three types of chronic pain: (1) chronic, recurrent pain (e.g., migraine headaches); (2) chronic, intractable, benign pain (e.g., low back pain); and (3) chronic, progressive pain (e.g., pain associated with malignancies). This review reveals some common features that underlie each of the various approaches. Most noticeable is the innovative, but preliminary, nature of much of the work in this area. Second, the approaches have adopted a general, multidimensional perspective on the management of pain. Third, distraction, suggestion, anxiety reduction, and sense of control seem to be incorporated to various degrees in each of the treatment regimens. And fourth, all emphasize the active participation of the patient.

The studies reviewed in the previous chapter focused on the prevention of distress and discomfort in laboratory and acute-pain situations. The focus of this chapter is on chronic pain patients who are already experiencing pain. A variety of psychologically based regimens have been employed with chronic pain patients with a wide diversity of syndromes (e.g., headache, phantom-limb pain, osteoarthritis, low back pain, fibrositis, abdominal pain of unknown etiology, irritable bowel syndrome, peptic ulcers).

119

CHRONIC, RECURRENT PAIN

As noted in Chapter 4, "chronic, recurrent pain" is the phrase we use to describe those pain syndromes that are characterized by intense episodes of pain interspersed with periods of no pain (e.g., migraine headaches, trigeminal neuralgia, myofascial pain dysfunction syndrome). Cognitive and behavioral techniques have been employed for pain management with several types of chronic, recurrent pain. By far the largest amount of attention has been given to the efficacy of psychologically based procedures with migraine headaches, tension headaches, and myofascial pain dysfunction syndrome. In this section we will examine the relative utility of such procedures as biofeedback, relaxation, and comprehensive cognitive–behavioral programs with these three disorders.

Headaches

Headaches are usually classified on the basis of putative etiological factors (Ad Hoc Committee on the Classification of Headache, 1962). Two major classes of headaches are muscle-contraction, or tension headaches and migraine, or vascular headaches. Tension headaches have been attributed to excessive, sustained contraction of the shoulder, neck, and back muscles, whereas migraine headaches have been attributed to a two-step process of prolonged constriction of the intracranial and extracranial arteries, followed by a rebound of dilation associated with the onset of pain. Conventional treatments for muscle-contraction headaches have focused on altering excessive muscle contraction through the use of symptomatic medications (e.g., muscle relaxants, tranquilizers, and analgesics). The medical treatment for migraine headaches also relies on symptomatic treatment (analgesics) and, in addition, prophylactic medications (e.g., propranolol, methysergide).

Parenthetically, the distinction between migraine and muscle-contraction headaches has been questioned (Bakal, 1975; Bakal & Kaganov, 1977; P. Martin & Mathews, 1978; Philips, 1977, 1978; Zeigler, Hassarein, & Hassarein, 1972). These investigators suggest that both types of headaches may be best conceptualized as falling along a continuum of intensity, with excessive muscle contraction present in all headaches. As headaches become more severe, there may be increasing vascular complications. Thus one must be cautious in differentiating between so-called migraine and tension headaches in patients. No matter what the proper diagnosis or cause of the different headache groups, from a cognitive–behavioral perspective the duration and intensity of headaches may be maintained or exacerbated by the patients' thoughts and feelings that precede, accompany, and follow attacks, which, in turn, may increase muscle tension, and so on (Bakal, 1979; Meichenbaum, 1976b).

Recently, relaxation and biofeedback (EMG and temporal artery) have received much attention as treatments that may be beneficial in assisting patients with migraine and muscle-contraction headaches. The relaxation-based biofeedback treatments are designed to modify blood flow in the temporal artery for migraine patients and to reduce excessive muscle tension (usually frontalis muscle tension) for tension headache patients. Although biofeedback has received much popular and professional support, reviews of the existing empirical literature consistently report that there appears to be little advantage to using biofeedback over more conventional relaxation for treating both muscle-contraction and migraine headaches. (See recent reviews by Blanchard, Andrasik, Ahles, Teders, & O'Keefe, 1980; Jessup, Neufeld, & Merskey, 1979; P. Martin, 1980; Neuchterlein & Holroyd, 1980; Turk et al., 1979; Turner & Chapman, 1982; Young & Blanchard, 1980.)

In addition to the physiological etiologies just noted, both migraine and muscle-contraction headaches have been thought to be related to maladaptive responses to psychological stress (Ad Hoc Committee on the Classification of Headache, 1962; Dalessio, 1972; M. Martin, 1966). Muscle-contraction headaches have been most consistently related to patients' responses during stress, whereas migraine headaches have been related to physiological changes occurring during recovery from stress (Cuevas, Hamilton, Katrandies, Safranek, Gannon, & Haynes, 1980; Dalessio, 1972). Traditional psychotherapeutic techniques have been employed to assist headache patients in modifying maladaptive responding to stress (e.g., Dalessio, 1972; Paulley & Haskell, 1975).

Cognitive-Behavioral Treatment of Headaches

More recently, numerous cognitive-behavioral treatment studies have been conducted with headache patients (e.g., Bakal et al., 1981; Holroyd et al., 1977; Knapp & Florin, 1981; Kremsdorf, Kochanowicz, & Costell, 1981; Mitchell & Mitchell, 1971; Mitchell & White, 1976a, 1976b, 1977; Reeves, 1976). These treatments are designed to help headache patients prevent or short-circuit noxious sensations before they crystallize into severe pain. The cognitive-behavioral treatment focus is on the factors that contribute to pain and on those that contribute to dysfunctional physiological processes (e.g., excessive muscle contraction). Some examples will illustrate the potential applicability of cogntive-behavioral treatment approaches to patients with muscle-contraction and migraine headaches.

Holroyd *et al.* (1977) focused on altering the maladaptive cognitive responses assumed to mediate muscle-contraction headaches. Patients were provided with a rationale for treatment that emphasized the function of specifiable maladaptive cognitions in the creation of subsequent disturbing emotional behavioral responses (based on A. Beck, 1976, and Meichenbaum, 1977). Patients were encouraged to attribute their headaches to relatively specific cognitive self-statements and images rather than to external or complex internal dispositions.

Lists of stressful situations were constructed, and patients were taught to focus on (1) the cues that trigger tension and anxiety, (2) how they responded to these (often with anxiety), (3) thoughts prior to and following tension, and (4) the ways in which these cognitions contributed to their headaches. Patients were taught how to interrupt deliberately, at the earliest possible point, the sequence preceding their emotional response and to engage in cognitive control techniques incompatible with further stress and tension (e.g., cognitive reappraisal, attention deployment, fantasy). (See the recent chapter by Holroyd & Andrasik, 1981, for a more detailed description of their treatment regimen.)

This cognitive (stress-coping) training, accomplished in eight biweekly sessions with a 15-week follow-up, was employed with ten patients, who were compared to patients receiving either biofeedback or no specific treatment. At the termination of treatment and at follow-up, only the stress-coping group demonstrated substantial improvement on frequency, duration, and intensity of headaches.

Recently, Holroyd and Andrasik (1980) have reported a 2-year follow-up of the same headache patients. Patients in the stress-coping group reported that they continued to use the coping strategies they had been taught, and daily headache recordings indicated they were still significantly improved. These patients reported more frequent use of (1) problem-solving reattribution ("I identify the source of the stress that is triggering my headache and cope with it by changing my thinking"), (2) self-instruction ("Monitor what I'm saying to myself and talk back to my worries"), and (3) imagery ("Take a break from my worries by immersing myself in a tranquil image").

Moreover, 63% of the patients who received the stress-coping training reported decrements in symptoms other than headaches (e.g. dysphoric affect, psychophysiological symptoms) in contrast to the patients who received biofeedback training, none of whom reported any improvements in symptoms other than headaches. These follow-up data support both the maintenance and the generalization of the effects attributed to the cognitive–behavioral treatment.

A cognitive–behavioral control regimen was also successfully employed by Mitchell and White (1977) with a migraine-headache population. A sequential, "dismantling" strategy separated the effect of the treatment package into four components. Subsets of the inital group of patients received one, two, three, or all four of the components. That is, all patients ($n = 12$) began at the same point, receiving the first component —self-recording of the frequency of migraine episodes—of the treatment package. A subset of the initial group ($n = 9$) returned for the addition of the second component, self-monitoring of antecedent stress cues; a subset of this group ($n = 6$) returned for the presentation of the third component, physical and mental relaxation and self-desensitization; and finally, a subset of these ($n = 3$) returned for the fourth and last phase of the treatment, additional cognitive control strategies (e.g., thought stopping, imaginal modeling, cognitive restructuring). In this manner, the contribution of each phase of the package was assessed.

Patient contact occurred only once per component, with 12 weeks intervening between components. Most of the training was conducted by a series of tapes that the patients heard and used at home. After the 60 weeks of training (with only four personal contacts between the trainer and those patients who received all four components), a 3-month follow-up was conducted.

Mitchell and White (1977) reported that neither the self-recording nor the self-monitoring produced substantial reductions in migraine episodes. Significant reduction in migraine frequency was displayed by the groups receiving three and four components; the group that received all four components, however, showed a significant reduction in migraine attacks at 6 weeks and at a 3-month follow-up relative to the group receiving the three components. These data underscore the utility of the cognitive control strategies in combination with the behavioral strategies.

Demjen and Bakal (1979) used a cognitive–behavioral skills-training procedure for the treatment of chronic headaches. The treatment procedure was found to be equally applicable to both muscle-contraction-headache and migraine-headache patients. In a related study, Bakal et al. (1981) found that chronic headache patients benefited from cognitive–behavioral interventions combined with EMG biofeedback training. Treatment gains were also found to be largely independent of the headache parameters (location of pain, time of onset, or symptoms associated with headache attacks) that often have been used to distinguish migraine from muscle-contraction headaches.

Interestingly, however, Bakal et al. report that headache patients who experienced continuous or near-continuous pain during their waking hours were less responsive to cognitive–behavioral treatment than those for whom headaches were episodic. The patient's headache type by treatment interaction bears careful examination, for it may indicate necessary modifications to a cognitive–behavioral approach. For example, rather than focusing on stressful antecedents of headache episodes, some patients may need to be taught to focus on prodromal signs that may enable them to abort headaches.

To illustrate, Bakal *et al.* (1981) reported on a migraine patient who learned to use attention-diversion skills whenever she experienced a scintillating scotoma (flashing lights), which was a cue for the onset of her headaches. For other patients, persistent feelings of tightness and pressure, primarily in the neck region, were the prodromal cues to use the cognitive–behavioral coping skills. Bakal *et al.* remind us that the conditions that lead to a disorder need not be the same as the conditions that maintain a disorder.

> Headache may begin as a response to psychological stress but with repeated attacks the underlying psychobiological mechanisms may not only become more involved but may also begin to operate in a relatively autonomous fashion. This observation is critical to treatment because it requires a shift in emphasis from dealing with antecedent events to incorporating procedures which modify the sensations, feelings and cognitions that accompany the headache attacks. (p. 3)

Finally, the potential cost-effectiveness of the cognitive–behavioral treatment approach was illustrated in the study by Mitchell and White (1977). In their study, patients were seen in groups by the trainer for a maximum of only four sessions. Most of the training was conducted by means of a series of audiotapes used at home. The usefulness of such automated treatment packages deserves further attention, especially if we consider the ultimate goal of such cognitive–behavioral therapeutic regimens to be their utilization by a variety of health care providers, who are unlikely to expend inordinate amounts of time with a small number of patients.

Hypnosis and the Treatment of Headaches

Hypnosis has received some attention as a means of attenuating pain associated with migraine headaches. The majority of this literature is based on unsystematic reports and case studies. For example, Harding (1967) used hypnosis with 90 patients with intractable migraines. Following hypnotherapy, Harding reports that 38% of the patients had complete relief from migraine symptoms, 32% had moderate relief, and

30% either had no relief or were unavailable for follow-up. Although data such as these are impressive, little in the way of firm conclusions can be drawn because no appropriate control groups were included.

Two studies examining the efficacy of hypnosis for migraine headaches deserve particular attention because they have included comparison groups (J. Anderson, Basker, & Dalton, 1975; Andreychuk & Skriver, 1975). J. Anderson et al. (1975) compared the relative efficacy of hypnotherapy with a prophylactic pharmacological preparation (prochlorperazine). Andreychuk and Skriver (1975) compared hypnosis with two types of biofeedback (electroencephalogram [EEG] alpha enhancement and temperature increase).

J. Anderson et al. treated 23 migraine patients with hypnotherapy and 23 with chemotherapy. Patients in the hypnotherapy group received a minimum of 6 treatment sessions spaced from 10 days to 2 weeks apart. Patients in the chemotherapy group were provided with medication for 12 months. All patients were followed monthly for the 1 year of the study. Patients in the hypnosis group reported significant reduction in the number of migraine attacks during the last 6 months of the study, with 10 of the 23 patients reporting complete remission of migraine symptoms. Patients in the chemotherapy group did not report significant reductions in migraine attacks and only 3 of the 23 patients reported complete remissions. Patients in the hypnosis group had significantly fewer headaches than those in the chemotherapy group during the last 6 months of the study.

Although these results are quite impressive, a number of alternative hypotheses can be put forward to explain the results. First, examination of the treatment provided to the hypnosis group reveals that hypnotic trance induction was *not* included. Rather, suggestions for relaxation and for imagination of swollen vessels dilating were used. Patients in the hypnosis group, moreover, were also instructed to practice self-relaxation and tension- and anxiety-reducing imagery at home during the treatment. The contribution of self-relaxation and suggestions to the treatment is unclear, but such cognitive and behavioral techniques have been employed successfully without hypnosis (e.g., Holroyd et al., 1977).

Additionally, neither the patients nor the health care providers were blind to the treatment assignment, and thus concerns about experimenter bias, placebo effects, and Hawthorne effects must be raised. Finally, patients in the hypnosis group were given substantially more attention by the therapist than patients in the medication group. Thus it is impossible to attribute the successful outcome to hypnotherapy alone.

In a more carefully controlled study, Andreychuk and Skriver (1975) compared the relative efficacy of temperature biofeedback, EEG alpha-enhancement biofeedback, and self-hypnosis in controlling migraine headaches. Each of the three groups received ten, 45-minute sessions. All three groups showed significant reduction in headache activity following the treatment. Unfortunately, no follow-up was conducted. The three groups shared a number of common features that may account for the fact that there were no between-group differences.

All three groups included relaxation, home practice, expectancy of relief, and increased self-control. Moreover, since no follow-up was included, the results may be attributable to regression to the mean. Patients are most likely to seek treatment when they are feeling worse, when headaches are most frequent or most severe (N. Miller, 1974). Since headaches tend to be recurrent, it is possible that reductions in headaches following treatment may result from spontaneous fluctuation toward reduced symptomatology (Turk et al., 1979). The only way to control for such regression effects is to include extended baseline and follow-up assessments. Each of these components (i.e., relaxation, home practice, expectancy of relief, increased self-control, or regression to the mean) may have contributed to the favorable outcome.

Interestingly, Andreychuk and Skriver (1975) assessed the hypnotic susceptibility of each patient and found that the degree of headache improvement in the biofeedback and self-hypnosis groups was strongly related to hypnotizability. These data raise some possibilities regarding the effects of individual differences and the efficacy of both hypnosis and biofeedback. We will consider the treatment approaches of hypnosis and biofeedback in more detail in the next chapter. For now, it is important to appreciate that psychologically based interventions, especially cognitive–behavioral techniques, may prove useful for headache patients. The cognitive–behavioral treatment is designed to help patients to modify and adapt to their environments and to modify their reactions to the environment.

Myofascial Pain Dysfunction Syndrome

Myofascial pain dysfunction syndrome (MPD) is a chronic and fairly common syndrome. It is characterized by recurrent episodes of shooting or radiating, but generally dull, pain that occurs in various locations of the head (especially in the area of the masseter muscle or in the preauricular area) and the neck and that occasionally extends to the back and shoulders (L. Schwartz & Choyes, 1968).

Although some investigators have suggested that MPD contains a psychological component of anxiety and emotional stress associated with muscle tension (e.g., Evaskus & Laskin, 1972; Gessel & Alderman, 1971;

C. Greene, Lerman, & Sutcher, 1969; Reading & Martin, 1976), the condition has generally been treated by dentists using mechanical interventions. These dental interventions have included both reversible procedures (e.g., occlusal splints) and irreversible ones (e.g., occlusal grinding). Evidence suggests that the effects of the conventional dental treatments may be no more than placebo effects (Laskin & Greene, 1972).

Several psychologically based treatments for MPD have been suggested, including psychodynamically oriented psychotherapy (e.g., Lefer, 1966; Marbach & Dworkin, 1975), relaxation (e.g., Gessel & Alderman, 1971), biofeedback (e.g., Carlsson & Gale, 1977; Carlsson, Gale, & Ohman, 1975), and cognitive-behavior modification (e.g., Stenn, Mothersill, & Brooke, 1979; Wepman, 1980). All of these psychologically based treatments consider muscle-tension control a central feature. Unfortunately, no data have been presented to support the position that successfully treated patients actually increased their ability to control muscle tension. With the exception of the Stenn *et al.* study, which we shall discuss next, all of the approaches have relied on self-report measures to support the efficacy of their treatment regimen. No objective dental signs have been reported. Thus neither the cause of the success nor the relative efficacy of any of these treatments can be considered as established.

Stenn *et al.* (1979) examined the relative efficacy of a cognitive–behavioral approach with MPD patients who had previously been treated with conventional dental methods. The 8-week, cognitive–behavioral training consisted of relaxation training and coping skills training (i.e., assertion training, cognitive restructuring, and stress inoculation) with or without the inclusion of masseter-muscle EMG biofeedback.

The results indicated that patients who received either of the two types of treatment, cognitive-behavior modification with or without biofeedback, reported lower ratings of pain, reduced levels of masseter-muscle EMG, and reductions in both subjective and objective dental signs of MPD at the end of training and at a 3-month follow-up. The group that received both the cognitive–behavioral intervention and biofeedback reported lower pain ratings and showed fewer signs of MPD than the treatment group that did not include the biofeedback. There was no difference, however, between the two treatment groups in masseter-muscle-tension readings following treatment or at follow-up. Thus it is apparent that the difference in subjective pain ratings and objective signs of MPD cannot be attributed totally to differences in muscle tension.

The contribution of biofeedback is difficult to discern from this study because the authors did not include a biofeedback-only group. Stenn *et al.* suggested that the increased effectiveness of the combination of biofeedback and cognitive-behavior modification may be attributed to increased expectancies of self-control in the natural environment. Although this hypothesis needs to be examined, this preliminary study does demonstrate the potential of combining a cognitive–behavioral approach with biofeedback for patients suffering from MPD.

Combining a coping-skills-training component with some form of relaxation (either alone or assisted with biofeedback) seems to be an approach with some utility for populations of patients with chronic, recurrent pain. The additive contribution of biofeedback training is unclear. For example, Reeves (1976) reported a case study in which biofeedback successfully augmented the cognitive–behavioral intervention employed with a tension-headache patient. The superiority of the combination of treatments was also noted by N. Anderson, Lawrence, Olson, and Dick (1980), who found cognitive coping training and relaxation more effective in treating tension headaches than either procedure alone. Kremsdorf *et al.* (1981), in two single-case-design experiments, however, reported that biofeedback training did not appear to contribute to the utility of a cognitive skills training treatment used with tension-headache patients. It may be the case that some individuals do benefit from the biofeedback component, and we need to learn more about the characteristics of the patients and the ways in which the training functions to modify headache symptomatology (Holroyd & Andrasik, 1978; Qualls & Sheehan, 1981).

CHRONIC, INTRACTABLE, BENIGN PAIN

The major defining characteristic of chronic, intractable, benign pain is its omnipresence. Although the intensity of pain may vary, patients typically report that it is always present. The devastating consequences of such pain, the large number of patients affected, and the frequently observed psychological concomitants have led to a great many attempts to ameliorate the suffering using a host of psychological techniques.

One of the earliest studies employing a comprehensive, psychologically based program for the management of chronic pain was reported by Draspa more than 20 years ago (1959). Draspa provided patients suffering muscular pain of various etiologies with a treatment regimen that consisted of supportive therapy (reassurance of the innocuous nature of their pain), information related to the causes of excessive muscle contraction, emphasis on the identification of internal and external cues related to muscle tension, and relaxation training. The 112 patients who received this psychologically based training were compared to a matched control group that received standard physical therapy and to a third group that received both the psychological treatment and the physical therapy.

Draspa reported that the combination group achieved significant reductions in reported pain. This study illustrates the potential of combining cognitive and behavioral techniques with conventional medical procedures in reducing chronic pain. Draspa built generalization into his training program by encouraging patients to attend to both internal and external cues of muscular tension and to use relaxation to reduce such tension. This preliminary study received relatively little attention, and there seems to have been about a 15-year hiatus between the publication of the Draspa (1959) study and more recent attempts to employ psychologically based pain-management programs with chronic pain patients.

Much of the impetus for the increased interest in psychological factors in the maintenance and management of chronic pain derived from the pioneering work of Fordyce and his colleagues (e.g., Fordyce, Fowler, & DeLateur, 1968; Fordyce, Fowler, Lehmann, DeLateur, Sand, & Trieschmann, 1973) at the University of Washington. Over the past 10 years, a large number of psychologically oriented chronic-pain-management programs have been developed. We will examine Fordyce's operant conditioning approach in detail in the next chapter. In the remainder of this section, we will briefly describe a number of pain-management programs in order to illustrate the diversity of recent approaches that have been developed for addressing chronic, intractable, benign pain.

Tables 6-1 and 6-2 summarize the range of techniques employed and outcomes reported in a number of studies conducted in comprehensive pain-treatment-clinic programs. These tables include those studies that we have found that have presented the efficacy of comprehensive, psychologically based pain-management programs. Table 6-1 includes a listing of the intervention techniques, the criteria for inclusion of patients, the length of treatment, and the number of patients who in turn applied for, received, and completed treatment and who were included in the follow-up. Table 6-2 describes the specific outcome measures that were used in each study. Despite the large number of such pain-management programs (more than 800), the studies summarized in Tables 6-1 and 6-2 are the only ones that we have found that present any outcome data, no matter how meager. The tables indicate the breadth of interventions and the relative weaknesses of the data base for such interventions.

Illustrative of the treatment research pain is a study by Turner (1979), who examined the utility of the cognitive–behavioral approach with groups of patients having chronic lowback pain. She contrasted three treatments: (1) progressive muscle relaxation, (2) cognitive–behavioral treatment, and (3) an attention control. Each group received five

TABLE 6-1. *Description of Comprehensive Pain-Management Programs*

Study	Intervention techniques[a]	Inclusion/ exclusion criteria[b]	Length of treatment			Patients in study			
			Inpatient	Outpatient	Follow-up	Applied	Accepted	Completed	Followed up
Draspa (1959)	A,C,E,	?	?	—	None	?	100	100	—
Fordyce, Fowler, Lehmann, DeLateur, Sand, & Trieschmann (1973)	B,D,G,H,I	A,B,C,E	$\bar{x} = 7.17$ wk	$\bar{x} = 3.13$ wk	$\bar{x} = 22$ mo	?	?	36	31
Greenhoot & Sternbach (1974); Ignelzi, Sternbach, & Timmermans (1977)	A,C,D	E,G,I	6 wk	—	3 yr	?	?	54	32
Sternbach (1974b)	G,H,K,O	E,G,I	6 wk	—	2-3 yr	?	?	75	?
Heinrich & Fuller (1975)	G,R	B	—	12 sessions	None	?	10	9	—
Shealy & Shealy (1975)	B,D,F,H,M,P	?	?	—	3-6 mo, 1 yr	?	?	?	?
Cairns, Thomas, Mooney, & Pace (1976)	A,B,C,D,G, H,I	A,I	4-6 wk	—	$\bar{x} = 10$ mo	?	175	?	90
Swanson, Floreen, & Swenson (1976); Swanson, Swenson, Maruta, & McPhee (1976); Swanson, Maruta, & Swenson (1979)	A,B,C,D,E, F,H,I	B,E,I,T	3 wk	—	3-6 mo, 1 yr	?	50 (1976) 200 (1979)	27 (1976) 164 (1979)	? (1976) 117 (1979)

Study									
Seres & Newman (1976); Newman, Seres, Yospe, & Garlington (1978)	A,B,C,D,E,F,H,I,K,M	E,F	3 wk	—	3 mo, 18 mo	?	100	100	100
T. Anderson, Cole, Gullickson, Hudgens, & Roberts (1977); Roberts & Reinhardt (1980)	B,C,D,G,H	A,B,C,E,F,G,H	6-8 wk	2-4 wk	6 mo-7 yr	130 (1977) 124 (1980)	60 68	34 34	30 26
Cairns & Pasino (1977)	B,D,G,H	?	?	—	None	?	9	?	—
Gottlieb, Strite, Koller, Hockersmith, Kleeman, & Wagner (1977)	A,B,E,F,G,I, J,N	I	$\bar{x}$ = 6.4 wk	—	1 mo, 6 mo	?	75	50	40
Acharya, Michaelson, & Erickson (1978)	A,B,C,I	?	2 wk	—	12: 5-14 wk; 86: 14-23 wk	?	?	138	98
Alioto & Cox (1978)	A,B,C,F,J,N	?	—	$\bar{x}$ = 8.7 sessions	None	?	48	39	—
Armentrout (1978)	A,B,C,E,F, G,H,J,M,N,R	B,D	6 wk	—	None	62	62	47	—
DeGood, Tung, & Tenicola (1978)	A,C,E,F,J,L, P	B,D,H	—	8 sessions	5-8 wk	102	89	67	?
Hammonds, Brena, & Unikel (1978)	B,D,M	?	?	—	1 mo	?	61	32	—
Herman (1978)	A,C,D,E,F, J,Q,S,T	B,E,I	—	8 sessions	6 mo	?	8-12 per group	approx. 40	20
Khatami & Rush (1978)	C,E,F,J,L,P, S	C,G	—	$\bar{x}$ = 35.8 sessions	6 mo, 1 yr	?	6	5	5
Lack & Bloom (1978)	B,D,E,F,M	I,J	4 wk	—	None	?	47	47	—
Getto, Franks, & Willett (1978-1979)	A,C,I	?	$\bar{x}$ = 12.3 days	?	?	—	12	12	—

(Continued)

TABLE 6-1. (Continued)

Study	Intervention techniques[a]	Inclusion/ exclusion criteria[b]	Length of treatment			Patients in study			
			Inpatient	Outpatient	Follow-up	Applied	Accepted	Completed	Followed up
Morgan, Kremer, & Gaylor (1979)	A,C,D,E,F, J,K,L,N,P, Q,R	?	?	approx. 20 days	8 mo	?	?	197	81
Raft, Toomey, & Gregg (1979)	C,D,E,G,I, K,O	?	2-6 wk	—	6 mo-2.5 yr	?	18	12	?
Rybstein-Blinchik & Grzesiak (1979)	A,B,J,R	B	4 sessions	—	1 mo	?	5	5	5
Cinciripini & Floreen (1980)	B,C,D,E,F, H,I,J,O	A	3 wk	—	None	—	50	50	—
Follick, Zitter, & Kulich (1981)	A,B,C,D,G, H,I,O,S	A,S,C,E,F, G,H	—	10 wk	6 mo	?	8	8	8
Taylor, Zlutnick, Corley, & Flora (1980)	C,E,H	A,G	$\bar{x} = 7.1$ days	$\bar{x} = 3$ sessions	6 mo	7	7	7	6

[a]Specific intervention techniques: A = education and reconceptualization of pain experience; B = physical therapy and exercise program; C = psychotherapy (group, individual, family, marital); D = operant conditioning; E = relaxation training; F = biofeedback as an adjunct to other treatment; G = vocational and recreational rehabilitation; H = systematic medication reduction; I = involvement of significant other(s); J = stress management; K = drug treatment as an adjunct to other treatment; L = home practice of skills; M = physical interventions as an adjunct to other treatment (transcutaneous stimulation, nerve blocks, electrical stimulation, acupuncture, ice rubdowns, facial rhizotomy, massage); N = assertiveness training; O = goal planning; P = self-hypnosis; Q = role playing; R = cognitive coping and problem-solving skills training; S = continuing group therapy or "club"; T = systematic desensitization.

[b]Inclusion and exclusion criteria: A = chronic pain with significant dysfunction; B = no alternative treatments available; C = patient and family actively motivated; D = significant psychosocial component; E = no major personality dysfunction; F = identifiable behavioral goals and reinforcers; G = chemical dependence a second-degree problem or no problem at all; H = no financial issues (insurance, litigation, etc.); I = dysfunction stress-related; J = no assumed malignant process (physical).

TABLE 6-2. Summary of Outcome Measures

Study	Medication				Activity level				Employment		
	Measure	Baseline	Discharge	Follow-up	Measure	Baseline	Discharge	Follow-up	Baseline	Discharge	Follow-up
Fordyce, Fowler, Lehmann, DeLateur, Sand, & Trieschmann (1973)	Converted to standard dosage based on potency of morphine	?	"Significant reduction"	Maintenance of reduction on patients followed	Nonreclining time	59.2 hr/wk	88.9 hr/wk*	94.9 hr/wk*	—	—	—
Greenhoot & Sternbach (1974); Ignelzi, Sternbach, & Timmermans (1977)	Converted to standard dosage based on potency of morphine	Surgical patient = 20; nonsurgical patient = .325	.14* .16*	.05* .16*	Hours active/day	Surgery = 3.5; nonsurgery = 4.0	3.75 6.2*	6.3* 5.0	?	?	27.0%[a]
Heinrich & Fuller (1975)	Mean number drugs	4.17	3.0	—	—	—	—	—	—	—	—
Cairns, Thomas, Mooney, & Pace (1976)	Narcotics	?	0%	58% less than baseline	—	—	—	—	?	?	75%[b]
Seres & Newman (1976); Newman, Seres, Yospe, & Garlington (1978)	Prescription medications	87%	5%	22%	Overall activity rated 1–4	1.09	2.37	2.58	—	—	—
	Converted to standard dosage unit	4.90	.60*	.65*							
Swanson, Floreen, & Swanson (1976); Swanson, Swenson, & McPhee (1976); Swanson, Maruta, & Swenson (1979)	Narcotic	55% of patients	0%	71% maintenance reduction	—		—		?	?	69%[c] (3–6 mo)
	Nonnarcotic	50% of patients	16%								52% (12 mo)
T. Anderson, Cole, Gullickson, Hudgens, & Roberts (1977); Roberts & Reinhardt (1980)	Prescription medication, analgesics	?	67% no analgesics	?	Lying down	?	—	"Significantly less"	?	?	77%
Gottlieb, Strite, Koller, Hockersmith, Kleeman, & Wagner (1977)	—	—	—	—	—	—	—	—	0	81.9%[d]	16.0%[e] (1 mo); 62.0%[f] (6 mo)
Acharya, Michaelson, & Erickson (1978)	—	—	—	—	—	—	—	—	40.1%	72.4%	?
Armentrout (1978)	—	—	—	—	—	—	—	—	?	42.0%[g]	?

(Continued)

TABLE 6-2. (Continued)

Study	Medication				Activity level				Employment		
	Measure	Baseline	Discharge	Follow-up	Measure	Baseline	Discharge	Follow-up	Baseline	Discharge	Follow-up
Hammonds, Brena, & Unikel (1978)	—	—	—	—	Hours exercise/day	Compensation = 3.33; noncompensation = 4.04	8.46 / 8.01	7.58 / 7.20	—	—	—
Lack & Bloom (1978)	?	?	"Significant reduction"	—	—	—	—	—	—	—	—
Getto, Franks, & Willett (1978–1979)	Variety of drugs	100% on medications	"Significant reduction"	—	—	—	—	—	—	—	—
Cinciripini & Floreen (1980)[h]	Self-report of medication reduction	?	68% off all medication	?	0 (= no change)–3(= marked increase)	?	60% marked increase	—	—	—	—
Follick, Zitter, & Kulich (1981)	?	100% on medications	"Significant reduction" in 7 of 8 patients	—	Physical exercise	5 min/day	7 min/day	—	—	—	—
Taylor, Zlutnick, Corley, & Flora (1980)	?	?	?	?	Reclining time	17.73 hr	12.01 hr	11.42 hr	—	—	—
Herman & Baptiste (1981)	Drug intake	?	No significant reduction	?	"Uptime"	?	No significant reduction	?	—	—	28% (21 patients) returned to work 6 mo posttreatment

*Statistically significant reduction.

[a]Returned to work or "regular activities." This is compared to 35% of the control surgical patients.

[b]This percentage is of those selected for vocational training and represents those "in training or working."

[c]"Improved work status." In addition, in the 3- to 6-month follow-up, they show 23.8% working full time, 57.1% working more than at entrance into the program, based on a sample of 21 patients.

[d]This is the percentage of those "with vocational goals," not of the total population.

[e]At 1-month follow-up, 16% employed, 46% in training, 14% "preparing to enter training."

[f]The 62% includes both those working and those in training.

[g]An additional 6% were "preparing for work," and 23% were legitimately retired.

[h]Reduction of verbal pain-related statements from 32% of rating intervals to 4.35%. Nonverbal pain complaints decline from 81.85% during baseline to 26.4% at completion of program.

weekly training sessions. The training provided to the cognitive–behavioral group consisted of relaxation, guided imagery, and positive coping self-statements (for coping with stress and pain).

At the termination of the 5-week treatment, both the relaxation and cognitive–behavioral groups showed substantial reduction in pain (as measured by a visual analogue scale), dysphoric mood, physical dysfunction, and psychosocial dysfunction (as rated by both patients and significant others). The cognitive–behavioral training group differed significantly from the other two groups in the patients' self-reports of ability to tolerate pain and to participate in normal activities.

At the 1-month follow-up, the cognitive–behavioral training group compared to the progressive relaxation group demonstrated further improvements in pain severity, reduction in analgesic medication, anxiety levels, self-reports of ability to tolerate pain, and participation in normal activities. At the 3-month follow-up, there was some relapse noted in the cognitive–behavioral training group. They continued, however, to do much better on all measures in comparison with their baseline scores.

The Turner study provides some preliminary data regarding the efficacy of a cognitive–behavioral approach to the management of chronic, intractable, benign pain. These results should be viewed tentatively, because the follow-up period was rather brief and some regression to the mean might be expected. Another limitation was the exclusive reliance on self-report measures. Finally, Turner herself conducted all of the groups, and thus some experimenter effect may have been operating. A strength of the study is that the two active treatments that were contrasted were rated as equally credible. Most other studies of psychological approaches have not included such comparison groups.

Grzesiak (1977) described the treatment, using relaxation–meditation, of four patients with pain due to spinal cord lesion. First the patients learned muscle relaxation. This was followed by an attention-diverting image, with the patient being instructed to let his or her mind drift gently and effortlessly to a memory or an image that was peaceful and relaxing. The final phase was to have the patient focus attention on the pleasant and relaxing memory or image. Both subjective reports of mood and pain reduction and staff observations of mood suggest the relative utility of the procedures employed. One patient reported that the relaxation procedure "mellowed my pain. . . . Now I can live with it." Again, we must be cautious in interpreting these data, for the same concern as with the Turner study can be raised here.

Rybstein-Blinchik and Grzesiak (1979) described the successful use of a cognitive–behavioral approach with rehabilitation medicine patients with a diversity of chronic pain complaints. The patients were seen for four 1-hour sessions over a 3-week period and were provided with stress-inoculation training. An interesting feature of the intervention was that, during the educational phase, the pain patients were encouraged to omit the use of pain labels for how they felt and to replace them with a cognitive representation such as "I feel numb" or "I feel aroused." An attempt was made to have the patients reinterpret their pain experience as something other than pain. In addition, there was an attempt to teach patients to label their feelings more accurately. Some patients, for example, had been interpreting anxiety or depression as pain.

In another study Rybstein-Blinchik (1979) examined the relative efficacy of several cognitive strategies in reducing pain in 44 rehabilitation patients. The four treatments included reinterpretation of pain, attention diversion, somatization, and control. Treatment lasted for four 1-hour sessions over a 3-week period. Although all cognitive strategies were effective, the reinterpretive group (i.e., the one relabeling pain with other behavioral and affective terms) was somewhat more effective. As Grzesiak (1981) indicated, the chronic pain patient's self-statements change as part of the prolonged experience of chronicity, with the consequence that the patient often loses his or her sense of being a well person.

Varni (1981a, 1981b; Varni, Gilbert, & Dietrich, 1981) recently reported the successful application of self-regulation techniques in several case studies of adult and child hemophiliacs with chronic arthritic pain. Treatment consisted of progressive muscular relaxation, meditative breathing, and guided imagery associated with positive past experiences. Although the treatments were conducted on a case-study basis and more rigorous controlled studies are needed, the impressive long-term changes (up to a 14-month follow-up) indicated that the treatment approach bears careful consideration, especially since an estimated 75% of hemophiliacs are afflicted with chronic arthritic pain.

In a case study of a 65-year-old male with symptoms of chronic abdominal pain, Levendusky and Pankratz (1975) employed a coping-skills-treatment approach. The patient was taught to control pain through a program of relaxation, a cognitive coping strategy (attention diversion), and cognitive relabeling. The authors reported that, following treatment, the patient was able to reduce greatly his extensive intake of analgesic medications. A particularly interesting point to note in this case study is the use of the patient as a collaborator in the development of personally relevant cognitive coping strategies.

Erickson, Acharya, and Michaelson (1978) and Acharya, Michaelson, and Erickson (1980) developed an approach to the management of chronic pian that utilized cognitive restructuring and problem solving during a 2-week inpatient hospitalization. Erickson et al. treated groups of four to six patients by teaching problem-solving skills focusing on the lack of structure in daily life because of inactivity, marital and family conflicts, sexual dysfunctions, uncertain vocational futures, reduced social and leisure activities, and financial complications. Cognitive restructuring was directed toward patients' sense of worthlessness. In addition, patients were also assisted in developing an understanding of the nature of pain and the impact of pain on their lives, as well as being weaned from addictive analgesic agents.

Following discharge from the hospital (5 to 23 months postdischarge), 48% of the patients who had received treatment were no longer actively seeking further medical treatment, while 52% were undergoing only routine follow-ups. Acharya *et al.* (1980) report that, at follow-up, 71% of the treated patients were working in some capacity, in contrast with 41% working prior to treatment. In addition, patients reported substantial improvements in self-ratings of emotional status, attitudes, and personal relationships subsequent to treatment.

Several investigators have developed treatment programs that have combined many of the cognitive and behavioral techniques just described with biofeedback and/or hypnosis (e.g., Hartman & Ainsworth, 1980; Khatami & Rush, 1978; Melzack & Perry, 1975; Sachs, Feuerstein, & Vitale, 1977). We will consider biofeedback and hypnosis from a cognitive–behavioral perspective in the next chapter.

In contrast to the inpatient approach employed in all of the studies reviewed in this section (with the exception of Turner's 1979 study), Khatami and Rush (1978) developed a treatment program for outpatients. The cognitive–behavioral program focused on symptom control (employing biofeedback or relaxation), stimulus control (employing cognitive modification techniques based on A. Beck's 1976 model to modify overt and covert events that might precipitate, exacerbate, or maintain pain), and social-system intervention employing family counseling (to alter the interpersonal reinforcements for pain and for nonpain behaviors; Fordyce, 1976).

Khatami and Rush report that the five patients who were treated with this approach reported significant reductions in ratings of pain, hopelessness, depression, and use of analgesic medications. These improvements were maintained at both 6-month and 1-year follow-ups. The mean number of hour-long, weekly outpatient therapy sessions was 35.8.

Melzack and Perry (1975) reported an interesting experiment comparing the effects of EEG biofeedback and hypnosis in relieving chronic pain. Twenty-four patients who had continuous pain of verified physical origin that was not relieved by surgery or physiotherapy (ten, back pain; four, peripheral nerve injury; three, pain associated with cancer; two, phantom-limb pain; two, pain from earlier injuries; and one, headache pain) participated in their study. Patients were divided into three groups: One group received EEG alpha-enhancement biofeedback; the second group received a modified hypnotic training that focused on increasing energy levels and mental calmness, and on reducing the level of worry prior to patients' becoming upset; and the third group received a combination of both biofeedback and the hypnotic training.

All three groups showed increases in the level of alpha activity, but only the group that received the combined training reported a significant reduction in pain symptoms (36% reduction). The treatment group that received the hypnotic training alone showed a 22% decrease in pain symptoms, whereas the biofeedback-only group evidenced a 10% reduction in pain symptoms. These data suggest that the hypnotic approach was most effective in reducing pain from an unbearable to a bearable level, especially when employed in combination with biofeedback. The evidence for the biofeedback-only treatment was less impressive.

Sachs *et al.* (1977), in a series of case studies, reported the successful utilization of a multidimensional psychological treatment with eight chronic pain patients (pain duration from 8 months to 23 years). The pain-management regimen consisted of four components: (1) relaxation; (2) hypnotic training designed to increase duration of focused attention; (3) self-monitoring designed to provide clear and precise phenomenological descriptions of pain sensation and to identify particular thoughts, feelings, and images associated with deeper levels of relaxation; and (4) cognitive skills training designed to increase the production of thoughts, feelings, and images incompatible with pain. Generalization was built into the training by encouraging the use of self-controlled, pain-incompatible strategies in progressively more real-life situations.

Sachs *et al.* reported that, at a 4-month follow-up, their patients indicated significant reductions in daily pain intensity, the degree to which pain interfered with major life areas (e.g., sleep, social activities), life dissatisfaction, and self-administered pain medications. Again, we must be cautious in interpreting such results, because patients were treated as their own control, with no comparison groups included.

Hartman and Ainsworth (1980) assessed the effects of a stress-inoculation training and EEG alpha-enhancement biofeedback training in a crossover design. Five chronic pain patients received alpha biofeedback in the first block of three training trials, followed by three sessions of stress-inoculation training. For the remaining five pain patients, the order of the two treatment interventions was reversed. Contrary to the investigators' expectations, the stress-inoculation training was significantly more effective than biofeedback in reducing overall pain ratings. Given the small sample size, the limited amount of training, and the short (6-week) follow-up period, it is important to interpret the results cautiously.

Interestingly, the greater effect for stress-inoculation training was significant only when it was presented after alpha biofeedback. This led

Hartman and Ainsworth to suggest that the initial biofeedback may sensitize patients to the process of self-regulation in the cognitive–behavioral techniques. The combination of the two procedures (biofeedback and cognitive–behavioral treatment) seems worthy of further investigation. Finally, Hartman and Ainsworth's concluding observation is worth repeating: "Cognitive and behavioral self-control interventions appear to be much more complex than many investigators have assumed" (p. 42). We will document this repeatedly in Section III of this book, when we discuss the cognitive–behavioral intervention.

Several other therapists have described comprehensive, psychologically based pain interventions that include a wide range of psychological techniques. Herman (1978; Herman & Baptiste, 1981) runs groups of 8 to 12 patients who meet once a week for eight sessions. Her program includes an educational component, a skills-training phase, and an application phase, all similar to the present stress-inoculation regimen. Similarly, Alioto and Cox (1978) developed a stress-management program for pain patients. The 6- to 10-week program included instruction in the psychophysiology of pain (i.e., an educational component), biofeedback, breathing exercises, elements of "self-responsibility" training, and various training regimens, including assertiveness training.

Armentrout (1978) developed a comprehensive treatment requiring an average of 6 weeks' hospitalization that included assertion training, cognitive restructuring, problem solving, self-control, relaxation, vocational counseling, marital counseling, and ongoing outpatient support groups. Bresler's (1978) outpatients with chronic pain receive instruction for 2 hours per week for 7 weeks, focusing on such techniques as stress reduction and relaxation, guided imagery, acupressure, self-massage, exercise therapy, and nutritional supplements.

Heinrich, Cohen, Naliboff, Collins, and Bonebakker (1980) developed a 10-week, 10-session program that included positive goal setting, education about chronic pain, stress-management training, and interpersonal skill training. Finally, Newman, Seres, Yospe, and Garlington (1978) also described a multidisciplinary approach with inpatients, designed to enable them to cope more adequately with their pain rather than get rid of it. Physical, occupational, relaxation, biofeedback, contingency-management, problem-solving, family, and pharmacological modalities are all employed.

Common Characteristics

Some common aspects of the treatment regimens described for chronic, intractable, benign pain are evident. The programs are multifaceted, and they generally adopt a cognitive–behavioral orientation. Each of the programs tends to incorporate, to a greater or lesser extent, distraction, suggestion, anxiety reduction, and an increased sense of self-control. Each of the programs emphasizes the active participation of the patient.

Another characteristic of these programs is their preliminary nature and the absence of careful evaluation. Although several studies have collected follow-up data, each has methodological shortcomings, mainly involving inadequate controls, self-selection biases in follow-up, and the use of questionable dependent measures. We will provide a more detailed evaluation and critique of the more prominent treatment programs (e.g., operant, transactional, and multidimensional) that have appeared in the literature in the next chapter. Despite the limitations of these studies, the investigators deserve much credit for innovative and self-critical attempts to deal with the many problems in conducting clinical research with a challenging population.

CHRONIC, PROGRESSIVE PAIN

There are numerous medical conditions that commonly result in progressive pain (e.g., rheumatoid arthritis, chronic obstructive pulmonary diseases). Cancer is the most common and most feared of the chronic conditions that can result in pain, and it will be considered in detail as exemplifying these, although it is not always associated with pain.

There are a number of physical bases for the presence of pain in cancer, including bone destruction, luminal obstruction, infiltration or compression of nerves, and infiltration or distension of the integument or organ capsule. Additionally, the symptomatic treatments employed with patients with cancer, perhaps more than any other disease, often create a multitude of discomforts, pain, and suffering. It is therefore not surprising that for many people a diagnosis of cancer generates concerns not only about death, but also about the process of dying and, in particular, the presence and intensity of pain.

In our earlier discussion of the psychological contributions to the perception of pain, we indicated that such variables as anxiety, uncertainty, lack of control, the meaning of the situation in which pain arises, and expectancies were important components of the total pain experience. As we emphasized in Chapter 2, ambiguity leads to increased reliance on preexisting attitudes and beliefs in the determination of expectancies and responses. Cancer is, by its very nature, an ambiguous disease. It is of unknown origin, its course is unpredictable and erratic, the likelihood of arresting the disease in uncertain, and the physical sensations created by both the disease and the symptomatic treatments are often vague. Cancer is a particularly frightening disease because the commonly held beliefs about it are overwhelmingly negative. The term "cancer" quickly brings to mind thoughts of death, pain, disfigurement, incapacity, loneliness, helplessness, and hopelessness.

Since cancer patients often withdraw and become introspective, they are likely to become preoccupied with bodily sensations. The beliefs and attitudes of patients regarding cancer may lead them to interpret ambiguous sensations as painful or to overestimate the intensity of the nociceptive stimulation. Such appraisals may result in increased anxiety and even more misinterpretations in a vicious circle of anxiety, misinterpretation, pain, and increased anxiety.

The contribution of psychological factors to perception of pain among cancer patients has been noted in a number of studies. For example, Byron and Yonemoto (1975) found that 77% of patients with advanced cancer obtained complete pain relief for 4 hours or more from placebo medications. It has also been observed that, in the terminal stage of cancer, substantial proportions (from 30% to 50%) of patients do not report pain, even though at autopsy there are no differences in the extent of tissue damage between those who complain of severe pain and those who do not (e.g., Aitken-Swan, 1959; Bonica, 1979; Turnbull, 1971). Despite the demonstrated contributions of psychological factors in chronic, malignant pain, attempts to attenuate pain among cancer patients have relied almost exclusively on surgical and pharmacological regimens as symptomatic or palliative treatments (Turk & Rennert, 1981).

Pharmacological approaches to attenuating pain in cancer patients include the systemic use of various narcotic and nonnarcotic analgesics and psychotropic medications either singly or in combination (e.g., the Brompton mixture, consisting of oral narcotic preparations combined with potent tranquilizers). Various surgical procedures are employed to remove the tumor or to block transmission of pain impulses (e.g., removal of endocrine glands and nerve blocks).

Although the conventional medical and surgical treatments are effective in selected cases, there appears to be a substantial proportion of patients for whom none of the treatments provide adequate relief. For example, Melzack, Ofiesch, and Mount (1976) found that from 10% to 25% of terminally ill cancer patients continued to report experiencing unbearable pain even with the use of the Brompton mixture (perhaps the most potent analgesic preparation).

Another limitation associated with medical treatments is that the effectiveness of various procedures diminishes over time. For example, it has been suggested that, with early tolerance to narcotic analgesics, the patient may not be able to derive adequate relief from pain in the late stages of the disease (Murphy, 1973). Laboratory studies demonstrate that tolerance does occur rapidly and that increasingly larger doses are required in order to obtain the same analgesic effects, with increasing doses eventually reaching the point of "clouding" the cognitive processes and blunting affect (e.g., Houde, 1974; Siegel, 1977). Although others state that tolerance does not present a problem when sufficient narcotics are administered orally on a regular schedule rather than as needed (PRN) (Mount, 1976; Saunders, 1976), tolerance remains a controversial issue. Additionally, procedures involving interruption of pain pathways may produce only temporary relief, with the pain recurring within weeks.

The decision to use a particular medical or surgical procedure requires careful consideration of the associated risks and negative side effects as well as the benefits. For example, complications from the spinothalamic tractotomy, one of the most widely used neurosurgical operations for cancer pain, include weakness or paralysis of the lower extremities or of the bowel and bladder sphincters, abdominal disturbances, girdle pains and paresthesia above the level of anesthesia, orthostatic hypotension, and loss of sexual function (Murphy, 1973).

Side effects of narcotic analgesics include nausea and vomiting, constipation, respiratory depression, and sedation (Black, 1979). Although treatments are available to counteract some of the side effects that accompany heavy doses of narcotics, these medications may have undesirable side effects of their own. For instance, phenothiazines, which are frequently used to control nausea and vomiting, may produce increased sedation and constipation.

The observations concerning the effects of placebos, differential reports of pain in inpatients with the same degree of tissue damage, and the less than completely satisfactory effects of medical and surgical treatments for cancer pain all suggest the importance of psychological variables in pain perception and pain management. That is, psychological approaches to pain management should be included in the health care provider's armamentarium and at the least should be considered as adjuncts of conventional medical regimens.

Cancer patients are often referred to mental health workers to assist the patients in progressing through the so-called stages of dying, described by Kubler-Ross (1969), to eventual acceptance, or to explore the dysphoric affect (e.g., Bloom, 1977; Yalom, 1976). (See Silver & Wortman, 1980, for a critique of the Kubler-Ross stage view of coping.) Although such counseling may be beneficial, it does not directly address the issue of the management of pain in cancer patients.

Several psychologically based approaches have been employed to specifically influence pain perception (e.g., hypnosis: Butler, 1954; Cangello, 1961, 1962; Lea, Ware, & Monroe, 1960; imagery: Simonton, Matthews-Simonton, & Sparks, 1980; McCaffery, Morra, Gross, & Moritz, 1980; biofeedback: Fotopoulos, Graham, & Cook, 1979; relaxation: McCaffery *et al.,* 1980). Although these approaches seem to be of potential utility for at least some cancer patients, carefully controlled investigations are generally unavailable, and thus no firm conclusions can be drawn regarding the efficacy of such techniques in the management of cancer pain.

A more comprehensive approach employing a host of psychologically based techniques is used in the hospice "movement." According to Saunders (1979), hospice personnel endeavor to treat pain in its spiritual, social, and psychological, as well as physical, dimensions. The hospice approach focuses on the patient's entire milieu and makes extensive use of the Brompton mixture. Hospices are concerned primarily with patients in the terminal stages of terminal illness. A distinction, however, should be drawn between the terminal stage of an illness and the earlier phases of a terminal illness. Turk and Rennert (1981) noted:

> Terminal illness is an illness that cannot be cured by means of present day medical technology and generally leads to death within a specified period of time (years or months). During the period of terminal illness, medical treatments may be undertaken in order to prolong life even though the disease cannot be cured. In contrast, the terminal stage of an illness is the time between cessation of medical treatment beyond palliative care, and death (usually weeks or a few months). (p. 169)

In contrast to the hospice approach that focuses on the terminal stage, Turk and Rennert (1981) outlined a cognitive–behavioral treatment approach that might be incorporated with more conventional medical treatments during earlier stages of the terminal illness or used with cancer patients who have good prognosis for long-term survival, despite discomfort associated with cancer treatments. They emphasize the importance of providing patients with information about what to expect both from treatments to arrest the disease and from the disease itself. Turk and Rennert suggest that providing patients with some general information about what to expect should help to reduce the uncertainty and unpredictability that seems to contribute to the distress and suffering of cancer patients.

The program proposed by Turk and Rennert includes enhancement of patients' perceptions of self-control and self-efficacy by including training in the use of relaxation and distraction techniques reported to be of value to cancer patients (McCaffery *et al.,* 1980; Saunders, 1976, 1979; Shawver, 1977; Twycross, 1975, 1979). In the Turk and Rennert model, discussions with patients about the contribution of thoughts and feelings to distress and suffering are also included. The goal of the cognitive–behavioral intervention is to enhance perceptions of control and resourcefulness and to reduce demoralization. The intervention described by Turk and Rennert is prescriptive, but as yet no empirical data are available to support the utility of the approach.

What is quite evident from the discussion to this point is that successful management of chronic, progressive, malignant pain requires awareness of the importance of psychological factors and detailed knowledge of the range of treatment options (Noyes, 1981; Twycross, 1978). To date, the utility of psychologically based interventions is based almost exclusively on anecdotal evidence. The magnitude of the problem of chronic, progressive pain is sufficient to warrant substantially more interest in pain attenuation regimens than currently seems to be the case. This is another area in which workers in behavioral medicine may make a substantial and important contribution to health care.

SUMMARY

In this chapter we have briefly described the range of psychologically based treatment techniques that has been employed with each of the subtypes of chronic pain (recurrent, intractable, progressive). The clinical studies employing multifaceted cognitive–behavioral treatment strategies provide evidence supporting the efficacy of *combined* therapeutic regimens that incorporate both cognitive factors and cognitive and behavioral techniques alone or in conjunction with more conventional medical treatments. Nevertheless, treatments should be viewed in a tentative fashion, given the frequent lack of control groups and single-case and small-group designs. Full-scale clinical trials with appropriate controls are warranted (e.g., Turk & Kerns, in progress), to be followed by systematic dismantling studies. Such treatment outcome and process studies must go hand in hand with continued descriptive and developmental investigations of various pain disorders.

CHAPTER 7

CURRENT PSYCHOLOGICAL TREATMENTS FOR PAIN: A COGNITIVE–BEHAVIORAL PERSPECTIVE

Because pain is such a complex psychological event, often resulting in a pervasive reorganization of one's sense of self, it is stressed that the psychological treatment of pain must involve examining behavioral, interpersonal, and cognitive components in the interest of comprehensive or holistic health care.—*Roy Grzesiak* (*1980*)

In the last chapter we described the encouraging basis for a cognitive–behavioral treatment approach for pain regulation. Recognizing the preliminary nature of these results, we can now consider, from a cognitive–behavioral perspective, several of the most prominent psychologically based treatments for pain.

Prior to our own work on pain, a number of pioneers (e.g., Fordyce, Sternbach) had offered innovative interventions. It is informative to examine these critically, as well as to examine biofeedback treatment and hypnosis from a cognitive–behavioral perspective. Although these treatments were derived from different theoretical models and involve different procedures, we will suggest that the change processes associated with the various interventions may have much in common.

In Chapters 2 and 3 we described the application of a cognitive–behavioral treatment approach to a variety of medical problems. Now we will illustrate how the cognitive–behavioral perspective provides a useful framework for understanding the psychological treatment of patients in pain. Initially we will examine five major treatment strategies for pain disorders. Each approach has usually highlighted its uniqueness, its supposed difference from other procedures. We will note the similarities among an operant approach, a transactional analytic approach, and a comprehensive rehabilitation approach for the treatment of pain patients. We will describe and critically evaluate these respective programs and then compare them from a cognitive–behavioral perspective.

The current state of the art does *not* permit a rank ordering of these three treatment programs, since they vary widely in admission criteria, length of treatment, outcome measures, and length of follow-up (as outlined in Tables 6-1 and 6-2 and as described by Turk & Waldo, 1979). Following an evaluation of these treatment programs, we consider two additional psychologically based interventions for the treatment of pain patients, namely, biofeedback and hypnosis, which were briefly noted in the last chapter.

AN OVERVIEW OF THREE PSYCHOLOGICALLY BASED THERAPIES FOR PAIN

An Operant Approach

Wilbert Fordyce and his colleagues (Fordyce, 1974a, 1974b, 1976; Fordyce, Fowler, & DeLateur, 1968; Fordyce, Fowler, Lehmann, DeLateur, Sand, & Trieschmann, 1973; Fordyce & Steger, 1979) have described the use of operant conditioning in the treatment of chronic pain. Their efforts in developing a psychologically based treatment for pain patients provided an impetus for renewed interest in psychological factors in pain management and for our own work.

Fordyce's operant approach involves manipulating the consequences that are hypothesized to exert control over the continuation of a patient's pain behavior. Treatment goals include reducing maladaptive behaviors, increasing activity level, and descreasing and eventually eliminating analgesic medications. In the well-controlled setting of a pain clinic within a hospital, each of the possible external influences on pain behaviors, such as attention from physicians, nurses, and family members in response to patients' complaints of pain, is used to reduce pain behavior. Verbal and other expressions of pain (e.g., grimacing, moaning, immobilization) by patients are ignored. In addition, environmental control reduces the possibilities for avoiding aversive activities, such as work and activity that is perceived as painful. This treatment regimen avoids indirect reinforcement of avoidant behaviors. Fordyce provides contingent reinforcement of well behaviors, such as physical activity. There is a deliberate attempt to ignore patients' feelings, thoughts, and other cognitive events, since doing so may reinforce pain behavior.

In sum, to influence behavior through operant conditioning, the health professional (1) identifies the behaviors to be produced, increased, maintained, diminished, and eliminated; (2) determines what kinds of reinforcement are likely to be effective for the individual; and (3) regulates the occurrences of reinforcement of the behaviors to be influenced.

In the original case study that illustrated this approach, Fordyce *et al.* (1968) systematically manipulated medication, attention, and rest as positive reinforcements for the "well" behavior of a 37-year-old female with an 18-year history of debilitating back pain. Medication was provided at specific time intervals rather than upon the expression of pain complaints. The attention of staff was contingent upon nonpain behaviors, such as increased walking and activity, and it was withheld upon verbal expression of pain, grimacing, and inactivity. Rest periods were provided as rewards for increased involvement in physical and occupational therapy.

Fordyce and his colleagues have published a study conducted with 36 patients that examines the efficacy of the operant approach to treating chronic pain (Fordyce *et al.*, 1973). This study deserves careful scrutiny. Chronic pain patients referred to the pain clinic at the University of Washington over a 5-year period (1967–1971) were treated by the operant conditioning approach. Patients received from 4 weeks to 12 weeks of inpatient treatment (mean = 7.7 weeks) and from 0 weeks to 24 weeks of outpatient treatment (physical and occupational therapy). In addition to the inpatient and outpatient treatments, the spouses of the patients, whenever possible, received individual counseling in ignoring pain behavior and in reinforcing nonpain behavior (cf. Hudgens, 1979). Thirty-one of the patients were followed for 5 weeks to 175 weeks (mean = 76.17 weeks) following termination of treatment. Fordyce *et al.* (1973) reported that the patients indicated they had significantly less pain at follow-up, less interference with daily activities, a reduction in medication, and a reduction in the amount of time spent reclining because of pain.

A number of methodological concerns may be raised about this study. The length of treatment varied among patients, as did the length of time to follow-up. Before inclusion in the program, patients were screened by a psychiatrist, a psychologist, and a social worker. Screening criteria were not published, nor was there any indication of the number of patients excluded. It is possible that the 36 selected were a biased population, in which case generalization from this group might be questioned. The follow-up data were collected by questionnaire, with patients asked to report retrospectively how much pain they had experienced prior to treatment and at the time of follow-up, as well as how much their condition had interfered with their activities prior to treatment and at follow-up. The reliability of such retrospective reports (some of which were made 3 years following treatment) is problematic. Since no controls were employed, we do not have sufficient grounds to conclude from this study that the results were solely a function of the operant conditioning methods. It is possible that one or more of the occupational or physical therapy procedures or the counseling of the spouses may have contributed to the results.

These concerns make it difficult to draw firm conclusions about the effectiveness of Fordyce's operant treatment. We do not wish to suggest that there is no value in an operant approach to the remediation of chronic pain, but only to indicate that the hypothesis has not been substantiated by this demonstration study. Reports of success with what appear to be some of the most intractable problems, however, deserve attention and more careful investigation. The methodological concerns noted can be raised with the majority of the psychologically based pain-treatment programs described here and in the previous chapters. Perhaps the most important contribution of Fordyce and his colleagues has been the generation of substantial interest in the potential utility of psychologically based pain-treatment programs.

T. Anderson, Cole, Gullickson, Hudgens, and Roberts (1977) reported on the efficacy of the operant model at a different hospital setting (University of Minnesota). The therapeutic strategy was the same as that of the Fordyce group. T. Anderson et al. reported that 74% (25 patients) of the patients completing the program reported "leading normal lives without drugs" when they were contacted from 6 months to 7 years following discharge. Recently, Roberts and Reinhardt (1980) reported on the maintenance of beneficial effects for many of these patients and concluded that, from 1 year to 8 years following treatment, "77% of treated patients were leading normal lives without medication for pain" (p. 151). It should be noted that the T. Anderson et al. (1977) and Roberts and Reinhardt (1980) articles are descriptive reports with no data presented concerning pretreatment or posttreatment subjective pain ratings, objective ratings of occupational activity, or objective ratings of physical activity.

Particularly noteworthy in the Minnesota group's reports is the outline of criteria employed for inclusion or exclusion from treatment:

1. The patient had significant behavior associated with pain that could be identified and probably modified.
2. The patient and family were significantly motivated to undergo the pain-treatment program.
3. Litigation was not pending.
4. All reasonable treatment modalities had been tried and were found unsuccessful or were otherwise ruled out.
5. The patient could perform activities in the program without doing physiological harm.

6. The patient lived with one or more people who were willing to actively participate in the program.
7. A psychotic or severe psychiatric disorder was not present.
8. The staff could identify possible reinforcers that would be effective.
9. Chemical dependency was not a primary problem.

Forty-six percent (60 of 130) of patients referred for the program were accepted for treatment. Unfortunately, no breakdown of the number of patients excluded for any of the criteria is provided. Of the 60 patients accepted for treatment in the program, only 37 (29% of the original 130 patients) chose to enter, with 3 of these dropping out prior to completion. Thus, when T. Anderson *et al.* report that 74% of the patients treated were "leading normal lives," they are actually speaking of only 26 (19%) of the original 130 patients screened over a 7-year period.

Although the syndromes treated usually have been resistant to amelioration by other conventional procedures, we are still concerned about the types and number of patients excluded (see also Kotarba, 1981). Is the subgroup of patients included typical of the more general chronic pain group? This issue needs clarification if for no other reason than to help in screening which patients should be admitted into such an extensive and expensive treatment (8-week inpatient program estimated to cost more than $12,000). Parenthetically, the cost-effectiveness of all multidisciplinary pain clinics has recently been challenged (Kotarba, 1981; Neal, 1978).

In a controlled evaluation of the operant approach, Cairns and Pasino (1977) provided chronic back pain patients with three different treatments to increase daily activity level ($n = 3$ per group). Treatment conditions included:

1. A control treatment in which patients were asked to walk as far as they could over a measured course and then report the distance to the physical therapist. Exercycle riding was also encouraged. Therapists received no specific instructions concerning how to respond to the patients.
2. An experimental treatment that provided the same exercise instructions to patients, but beginning in the ninth session, therapists were instructed to converse with and praise the patients only if their reports of activity increased over previous levels.
3. An additional experimental treatment that similarly requested exercise from patients and then provided daily records of patients' performance by means of a graph displayed over their beds. After 6 days of this, the therapists also began verbal reinforcement for activity (as in condition 2).

Only under verbal reinforcement conditions (i.e. condition 2 and the second phase of condition 3) did the experimental subjects report exercise levels and objectively recorded time out of bed ("uptime") significantly exceeding those of the control group. (Although the graph-alone condition did not differ from the graph-plus-verbal-reinforcement condition, neither did it differ significantly from the baseline or the control-group levels.) Thus it appears that the reported exercise and time out of bed (the latter is less susceptible to recording biases) can be altered by verbal reinforcement in chronic back-pain patients.

Unfortunately, when reinforcement for either walking or biking was not given at the same time at which the other activity *was* reinforced, Cairns and Pasino found that only the reinforced activity increased and that the other activity *decreased*. This suggests little generalization or stability of such reinforcement, at least as it was presented in this program.

Several variants on the Fordyce operant approach have recently appeared in the literature, and these have promising results (Cairns *et al.,* 1976; Follick *et al.,* 1980; Kremer *et al.,* 1980; Seres & Newman, 1976; Sternbach, 1974a; Swanson *et al.,* 1976). (See Tables 6-1 and 6-2 for a summary of these studies.)

Cairns *et al.* (1976) added weekly patient group meetings to the operant approach. These group sessions were designed to identify sources of stress related to pain complaints and to discuss alternatives to a life based on habits of disability. A total of 100 consecutive patients received this treatment intervention. Of these, 90 were assessed from 1 month to 12 months following discharge. The results indicated that 70% of the patients reported significant reductions in pain, with 58% reporting a significant reduction in analgesic medications consumed.

The other variants of operant approaches included a variety of additional therapeutic procedures (e.g., biofeedback, communication skills, assertion training, transcutaneous electrical stimulation). For example, Swanson *et al.* (1976) reported that 54% of an original group of 50 pain patients demonstrated moderate to marked improvement with a combined operant and skills treatment program. At follow-up, 50% of the patients had maintained or increased improvement. These results are mitigated by the fact that one-third of the patients dropped out of treatment before completion of the program. The patients selected for this program received minimal initial screening, which may account for the large dropout rate. Again, it seems critical that efforts be made to examine for whom such approaches are most effective.

In summary, although we have some reservations about the generality and active ingredients of an operant approach to the treatment of pain, it has received extensive attention in the literature (e.g., see "The Pain Clinic: Boon or Boondoggle," 1978; Cameron, 1980; Fordyce, 1976) and merits continued examination.

A Transactional Analytic Approach

Sternbach and his colleagues (Greenhoot & Sternbach, 1974; Sternbach, 1974a, 1974b; Sternbach & Rusk, 1973) have used what they call a "transactional approach" to the treatment of chronic pain. This approach is intended to disrupt patients' "pain games" (e.g., attention seeking, sympathy seeking, avoidance of tasks) as described by Sternbach and his colleagues (Sternbach, 1974b; Sternbach, Murphy, Akeson, & Wolf, 1973). In his first contact with a patient whose pain is disproportionate to medical findings, Sternbach begins with an uncompromising confrontation. In contrast to assuming, as is usually the case in the medical treatment of pain, that (1) a patient really wants to be cured and that (2) given the right treatment, he or she can be cured, Sternbach's approach questions both of these suppositions. Sternbach continues in a forthright manner to challenge patients to give up pain games for more adaptive functioning. It is assumed that patients usually can control their own "pain behavior" if they can be sufficiently motivated and rationally convinced to do so, and if they learn how.

In Sternbach's program, learning how to give up pain games involves patients working with the therapist to develop a set of specific, realistic behavioral goals and steps to achieve these goals. Sternbach has used both individual and group therapy sessions to promote patient progress, to modify behavioral contingencies, and to "*challenge . . . as resistance* any failure in the patient's progress, and . . . [urge] him to be brave and do it, or quit and be doomed" (Sternbach & Rusk, 1973, p. 323, original emphasis). A word of caution: Little attention is given to the fate of those patients who drop out of treatment following such a message. We have some concern about the impact of such a strongly worded message on some patients.

Sternbach (1974b) reported self-report follow-up data on 61 patients examined 6 months after discharge (representing 67% of patients completing his program). The group that was followed up reported significantly less pain than at the time of hospital admission, with some increase following discharge. Activity levels increased following treatment, again with some decrease noted at follow-up. Analgesic medication was significantly reduced at discharge and was maintained at follow-up. These results indicate that treatment effects were maintained reasonably well for at least 6 months, although Sternbach did not consider the large proportion (one-third) of nonresponders to the follow-up questionnaire who might have been treatment failures.

In another study of chronic pain patients, Sternbach and his colleagues reported reduced pain and medication levels and increased activity at a 3-year follow-up (Ignelzi et al., 1977). The changes were maintained at follow-up and did not differ between those patients who had also received surgery ($n = 21$) and those who had not received surgery ($n = 33$) for their pain condition (a decision that was made on medical grounds by the surgeon). In addition to the transactional type of group therapy, patients received physiotherapy, relaxation training, operant conditioning, regulation of analgesics, biofeedback training, transcutaneous electrical stimulation, and vocational rehabilitation. Overall, the total group showed improvements, but interestingly, surgical patients were more likely to have been readmitted for pain problems, and the nonsurgical patients, for other problems. Of course this difference may well be related to the original basis for making the decision for or against surgery.

Given the intractability of many of the pain syndromes manifested by these patients, the results are quite impressive. It is difficult to assess the impact of the various treatment components.

A Comprehensive Rehabilitation Program for Patients with Chronic Low Back Pain

Gottlieb and his colleagues at Casa Colina Rehabilitation Hospital, Pomona, California (Gottlieb et al., 1977), have reported a broad treatment program "aimed at teaching the patient to self-regulate key psychophysiological events contributing to pain" (p. 17). They treated a traditionally refractory population of chronic low-back-pain patients. The patients' complaints of back pain had persisted for 6 months or more; they were unable to work and were supported by Social Security, welfare, or disability payments; and despite previous surgery, they continued to seek medical or surgical relief (Sternbach's, 1974a, "low back losers").

The training developed by Gottlieb et al. (1977) included the following elements:

1. Biofeedback training for teaching self-regulated muscle relaxation.
2. Individual, group, and family psychological counseling aimed primarily at learning "constructive self-control skills for the expression of emotional reactions to stressful anxiety-producing situations" (p. 104).

3. A self-administered medication-reduction program, in consultation with a physician.
4. Patient-participant case conferences.
5. A physical therapy program emphasizing reconditioning and focusing on physical progress rather than pain levels.
6. A vocational counseling program, which also offered assistance in placement.
7. A series of lectures about the relationship between stress and back pain.
8. A therapeutic milieu designed for maximum relaxation, recreation, and socialization.

Obviously, this is quite a comprehensive and expensive inpatient treatment program (mean hospitalization 45 days), but given the refractory nature of the problem, such a "total" program may indeed be required.

The poor prognosis of the low-back-pain patients treated by Gottlieb *et al.* (1977) makes the reported results most encouraging: Following treatment, 79% of the patients demonstrated unimpaired physical functioning levels, and 82% of the 23 patients contacted were employed or in a job training program. Unfortunately, little information is provided concerning the other 49 patients who were treated. Gottlieb *et al.* concluded that a cognitive–social learning view of the low-back-pain patient's problems can lead to success in treating many patients with whom conventional medical and surgical interventions fail. Stressing self-regulation, their program used both behavioral and cognitive components along with more traditional medical interventions. The study is limited by the omission of control groups, but the lack of effective prior medical intervention and the magnitude of the changes support the utility of such combined approaches. The results from this study and a set of case studies by Khatami and Rush (1978) that used a similar combined approach suggest that further examinations should be conducted.

A COGNITIVE–BEHAVIORAL PERSPECTIVE OF PSYCHOLOGICALLY BASED PAIN THERAPY

Let us examine three aspects of the therapies (Fordyce, Sternbach, Gottlieb *et al.*) that have been described: (1) their implicit and explicit conceptualizations of pain and of therapy, (2) the learning of methods of change, and (3) the patient's cognitions concerning change as it occurs.

Conceptualization of Pain and Therapy

Although the three programs that have been described differ in their approach to pain treatment, there are similarities in conceptualization. Each treatment assumes that pain (or pain behavior) can be altered by psychological means, which has crucial implications for patients' views of their problems. Patients are encouraged to change their physiological conceptualizations of pain problems and to become active participants in controlling their lives.

Sternbach and Rusk (1973) noted that pain patients tend to view their problems in purely physical terms, rejecting psychological explanations of symptoms. Patients are therefore likely to approach therapy with a view of their problems that does not render them amenable to change. In fact, pain patients do not usually welcome contact with any *mental* health worker (Sternbach, 1974a). A psychiatrist or psychologist is likely to be viewed as a threat to pain patients' self-esteem, to the veracity of their complaints, and to the legitimacy and dignity of their patient status. "I don't see what good *talking* is going to do me. The problem is this *pain* in my back," argued one of our patients. The patient's concern regarding the health care professionals' view of his pain as being imaginary or "in his head" may not be completely without basis or inappropriate. A recent study (Gillmore & Hill, 1981) found that pain patients with an ambiguous diagnosis (common among chronic pain patients) were viewed by health care workers as not having genuine pain. Moreover, these patients were viewed less favorably than patients for whom definite diagnoses were offered.

The problem at the outset of therapy, then, is to alter the patient's conceptualization so that a psychologically based treatment intervention is feasible. At the same time, the therapist needs to be sensitive to the patient's views and receptive to evidence presented by the patient. Until some *shared conceptualization* of the therapeutic situation is reached, therapist and patient are likely to be working at cross-purposes.

Let us take a closer look at the least professedly cognitive of the treatments we have outlined and note the elements contributing to patients' conceptual shifts. Fordyce (1976) reaches a shared conceptualization primarily by presenting to the patient an operant view of pain behavior. Following a comprehensive medical evaluation, he "orients" selected patients and significant others by means of a didactic presentation of the learning theory basis and procedures of the treatment program. For example, Fordyce offers the following conditioning rationale to pain patients:

If I catch you before dinner and start talking to you about a New York cut, medium rare, you start to salivate. That's not imaginary. You can take the saliva out of your mouth, stick your finger in it, and—sure enough—it's wet. But you can't sit there and decide whether to salivate or not to salivate. You can't turn it on and you can't turn it off. It's a real body process that occurs outside your control. . . . This illustrates how the basic body processes come under the control of a conditioning effect—as true for pain as for any other body function. It's possible that your pain that began with a disc problem is now under the control of a conditioning effect. So that's what I'm going to look for—and the more conditioning I find, the better. There is something we can do about *that*. (Fordyce, cited in "Family Doctor vs. Chronic Pain," 1978, p. 96)

The explanation of conditioning that Fordyce shares with the patient is consistent with the position initially taken by the founders of behavior therapy. Wolpe (1959) and Wolpe and Lazarus (1966) also suggested that a patient about to be treated by behavior therapy be given the principles of conditioning simply and clearly before the "basic psychotherapeutic tools" are applied. Wolpe and Lazarus argued that it is important not only that a patient be conditioned, but that the patient understand the conditioning process and that the therapist "spare no effort" in an attempt to remove the patient's mistaken beliefs. We are arguing that inseparable from the conditioning procedures is the removal of the patient's "mistaken beliefs." (See Fordyce, 1976, Chapter 8, for a detailed account of a patient–spouse orientation session.)

What is important about the rationale that Fordyce offers is not whether it is scientifically valid, but whether it is plausible to the patient. Whereas the pain patient and his or her significant other enter therapy with one view of the presenting pain problem, Fordyce is working to have them shift their view into conditioning terms, so that certain therapeutic steps along reconditioning lines may take place.

Consider, further, the following statements made to patients by Fordyce (1976):

The evaluation process is now complete. The results indicate that we are not going to be able to do much about the physical problem from which your pain originates. There is a real chance, however, that we can help to reduce how much it hurts. (p. 153)

It is possible for you to train your system not to feel the pain so much. (p. 153)

The very best evidence we have about your case indicates both that a specialized treatment approach such as I will describe looks promising as applied to your case *and* that we don't see another way to go that offers a better chance of being helped. (p. 151, original emphasis)

To the extent that your pain is now controlled mainly by learning factors, we can probably help your system to unlearn it and thereby to get rid of the surplus pain. Even if your pain is not now primarily learned, these procedures can probably help you to get along with the problem and have a decrease in the amount of interference from it. (p. 153)

Such communications and others like them, whatever their intentions, do not merely gain patients' cooperation in the program. If they are accepted—and they *are* persuasive communications—they are likely to alter the way in which most patients view their problems: from "pain equals physical disorder" to "pain equals physical disorder and/or learned behavior." Furthermore, patients come to have hope that something may be able to be done about their long-standing problems and to accept that they have key roles to play (e.g., changing the "learned behavior"). In other words, patients shift from a hopeless, passive appraisal to a hopeful, active one that encourages a sense of self-efficacy. In sum, Fordyce's conceptualization of pain conveys that patients may be active contributors to the experience of pain.

Parenthetically, it is worth noting that investigators have seriously questioned the conditioning model offered by Fordyce and others. For example, Brewer (1974) has questioned whether there is indeed evidence for classical and operant conditioning with adult humans, highlighting the role that cognitive factors play even in the salivary response offered by Fordyce. Maltzman (1977) offered these observations:

It now seems apparent that classical conditioning in normal adults, as ordinarily studied in the laboratory, is a consequence of thinking rather than vice versa. . . .

The GSR-OR [orienting reflex] is generated by the participants' covert problem-solving activities. It is not a response elicited by the CS signal as the result of the establishment of an association; it is a consequence of the discovered significance of the CS as a signal for the UCS. (pp. 112–114)

These same observations apply to Fordyce's examples. Our point is not to debate the adequacy or inadequacy of a conditioning model, but to have the reader appreciate that, given our current lack of knowledge, each time we offer our patients a rationale, be it conditioning, transactional, or cognitive–behavioral, we are really encouraging them to view their symptoms, pain, or whatever *as if* they resulted from the factors we suggest. Certain types of interventions naturally follow from each perspective.

This conceptualization aspect of therapy is common to the three approaches (Fordyce, Sternbach, Gottlieb *et al.*) that have been outlined. Each of the therapies involves a *translation* process whereby the patients come to view their problems in different terms, in effect using a different conceptual framework and language. The translation is from the terms of physical medicine, with pain seen as a direct result of tissue damage, to the terms of the particular theoretical approach employed. Fordyce encourages viewing pain as learned, operant behavior; Sternbach, as a means of expression rooted in pain games (Berne, 1964; Sternbach, 1974a); and Gottlieb *et al.* (1977), as having a cognitive–emotional stress component that is susceptible to self-regulation. Common to all three of these particular translations is the notion that pain is not solely a *physical event,* but is a complex, multifaceted, and multidetermined process: a process that the patients influence and *can change.*

This reconceptualization is begun at the outset of therapy, when it is first introduced to patients (as with Fordyce's orientation session). It is not completed here, however, but continues throughout therapy. The questions therapists ask, the homework assignments they offer, and other aspects of the continuing patient–therapist dialogue all contribute to patients' emerging reconceptualizations. The cognitive–behavioral model underscores the importance of this translation process in the treatment of pain patients.

Acquisition and Rehearsal of Skills

Following an initial reconceputalization and planning effort, therapy usually proceeds to a skills-acquisition and rehearsal phase, as described in Chapter 1. In this part of therapy, patients undertake new cognitive and behavioral strategies and strengthen their skills by rehearsing these and other appropriate strategies that may already be within their repertoires.

This time, let us take a brief look at this phase in Sternbach's pain therapy (Greenhoot & Sternbach, 1974; Sternbach, 1974a; Sternbach & Rusk, 1973). As has been noted, these phases are not clearly delimited. The treatment contract that Sternbach and his patients agree upon may be viewed as part of the reconceptualization process, but it also constitutes an initial skills-acquisition step. Once a patient is committed to this therapy, the patient and the therapist work together to formulate (1) a set of specific, behavioral goals of treatment and (2) the steps that will be taken to achieve those goals. Both (1) and (2) involve the acquisition and rehearsal of cognitive and behavioral skills.

Setting Goals

In setting goals, patients are asked how they would live if their pain were removed. Each goal they present is challenged by the therapist. The therapist may argue, for example, that returning to work sounds like a strange goal, for who really likes to work? More money could perhaps be obtained by an increase in pension or disability benefits. Why should the patient really seek work as a primary goal in pain therapy?

> In similar vein we question and challenge each goal, and encourage the patient to come up with a set of goals about which he can get enthusiastic, and which seems realistically attainable rather than goals which he obediently recites in response to assumed expectations of the therapist or "society." . . . Most patients come up with three to five specific behavioral goals they wish to achieve, such as (a) to accomplish a certain amount on a task (job, housework) each day, (b) visit with friends each day, (c) to cultivate a best friend, or (d) to go fishing (or play golf, etc.) at least once a week. (Sternbach & Rusk, 1973, p. 323)

This contracting for goals has an impact on patients' views of their situations and of what consitute realistic means of changing. Setting goals, then, encourages a new cognitive repertoire, or a new set of thinking patterns that come into play when patients attend to their pain. As we noted, the experience of pain is partly determined by ongoing cognitive processes. Through the transactional therapy sessions in which the patients' goals are elicited, challenged, and reformulated, patients come to engage in different cognitions concerning pain: Thoughts, images, and self-statements concerning pain are gradually altered. There is likely to be a shift from hopeless, anxiety-engendering, depressive themes to more realistic, hopeful, resourceful, and positive cognitions. In turn, patients are being influenced to give up self-defeating pain-game behaviors and to begin to engage in self-efficacious behaviors that lead to improvement.

As Frank (1974) and, more recently, Cameron (1978) have suggested, perhaps more important than the specific therapy undertaken are patients' commitments—the belief that therapy will be effective and that change is possible, even likely. Once a conceptualization of the problem and what might be done to help have been agreed upon by both therapist and patient (whether imposed upon the patient or mutually arrived at), the steps of intervention are more or less determined. If, for example, the pain is viewed as an operant, then the contingencies need to be changed; if the problem is considered to be based in pain games and a painful life-style, then the games need to be undermined, and different means of expression and satisfaction substituted; if the problem is viewed as both cognitively *and* behaviorally determined, then multiple interventions are called for. The skills-acquisition and rehearsal phase follows from the conceptualization offered.

Specifying Steps to Achieve Goals

Specifying the steps to attain goals involves developing a series of smaller, discrete goals that lead to the final ones. Again, Sternbach uses transactional techniques in establishing these steps and in motivating patients to carry them out. These "may be no more than writing a letter, or making a phone call, or finding out about the meeting of a singles club, or about a night class" (Sternbach & Rusk, 1973, p. 323).

Sternbach (1978a) advocates diagnostic attention to which of the pain patients' behaviors can be classed as *respondents* and which as *operants,* as does Fordyce (1976). In the therapy setting, however, Sternbach (1974b) encourages patients to make active use of such information themselves. Patients, whether seen individually or in groups, are faced with the challenge of developing a graded set of tasks that will lead them to the goals they have set. Prior attempts at well behavior that failed are examined critically, and new goals are challenged in view of this information.

The specification of behavioral goals is followed up by careful behavioral assessment of success. The data from these assessments are used to motivate further self-directed attempts at change:

> It is an advantage of having specific behavioral goals, and of having daily charts on display at the bedside, that objective signs of improvement become important. What the patient intends, or what he says, is less important. . . . The patient usually protests his good intentions, but we insist that "actions speak louder than words." (Sternbach, 1974b, pp. 105–106)

Whereas Sternbach emphasizes his patients' adoption of new strategies, Fordyce (1976) notes that some desirable behaviors are already within patients' repertoires, but are "not occurring often enough and need to be increased or strengthened" (p. 77).

A behavioral program such as Fordyce's may stress operant techniques to change behaviors (along with reconceptualization and didactic presentations to change cognitions); a game-based program such as Sternbach's may focus on transactional techniques; and a multifaceted, cognitively oriented program such as that of Gottlieb *et al.* may concentrate on a variety of behavioral and cognitive learning techniques. All share the assumption that a change in the amount of pain depends at least partly upon learning new skills and practicing them, or practicing existing ones, or both.

Treatment Generalization and Maintenance

Finally, all therapies are concerned with the generalization and, particularly, the maintenance of therapeutic change. Unfortunately, little long-range follow-up information is available (Ignelzi *et al.*, 1977; Maruta, Swanson, & Swenson, 1979). The Cairns and Pasino (1977) study described earlier demonstrated the need for paying explicit attention to this dimension in treatment. Fordyce (1976) provided an example of the gradual fading of therapeutic intervention but maintenance of contact as patients achieve increasing independence and until they have a stable status in the community and at home. Gottlieb *et al.* (1977) also deliberately encouraged patients' evaluations of themselves by emphasizing the patient's self-regulation throughout the program.

The use of time-limited therapeutic groups may encourage independence from the therapist while enabling patients to provide long-term sources of support for each other. As Davidson (1980) noted, patients will carry treatment effects with them as far as they are given the means to do so, and perhaps the most effective means involve altering their cognitions concerning a problem and how to deal with it and providing the support systems to ensure change.

BIOFEEDBACK TREATMENT: AN OVERVIEW

Another form of treatment for pain patients that has received a good deal of attention is biofeedback. One cannot open a journal or trade magazine or attend a medical or psychological conference without being inundated with promotional materials and endorsements for biofeedback treatment. The approach has been challenged, however. In the last few years, numerous review articles have critically evaluated the usefulness of biofeedback interventions for the treatment of pain disorders. At this point we do not intend to provide another such literature review, but instead we wish to consider the model we have been presenting for biofeedback treatment. The interested reader should see such reviews as Blanchard *et al.* (1980), Jessup *et al.* (1979), Nuechterlein and Holroyd (1980), and Turk *et al.* (1979).

A common theme emerges in these independent reviews, as illustrated in the following passage:

The biofeedback literature for the regulation of pain is reviewed and found wanting on both conceptual and methodological grounds. In particular, studies on the use of biofeedback for the treatment of tension and migraine headaches and chronic pain indicate that biofeedback was not found to be superior to less expensive, less instrument-oriented treatments such as relaxation and coping skills training. (Turk *et al.,* 1979, p. 1322)

Our own impression, as reflected in the Turk *et al.* review, is that biofeedback treatment may be useful with specific pain disorders and with certain patients, but most likely in conjunction with other treatment modalities (e.g., coping skills training, cognitive restructuring) rather than as the sole modality. In coming to these conclusions, one must appreciate the complex nature of biofeedback treatment. In the same way that we have offered an analysis of the components of the treatment programs of Fordyce, Sternbach, and Gottlieb *et al.,* we will offer a similar critique of biofeedback. To appreciate the potential utility and limitations of biofeedback, let us take a closer look at some of the variables involved in biofeedback treatment.

A COGNITIVE-BEHAVIORAL PERSPECTIVE OF BIOFEEDBACK TREATMENT

Cognitive, affective, and social factors play a central role in the biofeedback treatment regimen. This is illustrated in the sequence of a "typical" biofeedback treatment. Although biofeedback treatment varies somewhat, depending on the specific target behavior (e.g., migraine and tension headaches, chronic low back pain, MPD, Raynaud's disease, essential hypertension), there is sufficient similarity across training regimens to permit an examination of the common points at which the patient's cognitions may come into play.

The biofeedback therapy sequence usually involves the patient's initially describing symptoms or reasons for coming to treatment. The therapist then conducts a careful history and performs a situational analysis of the presenting problem (i.e., a discussion of the occurrence of variability in the pain disorder across situations). When the therapist is convinced that the patient is an appropriate candidate for treatment, he or she usually offers an explanation or description of the treatment, providing the patient with a rationale for the use of biofeedback in ameliorating the patient's specific problem(s).

The next phase of biofeedback therapy involves (1) training the patient to develop an increased awareness of the specific physiological response (e.g., muscular tension, hand temperature, heart rate, or blood pressure, depending on the focus of the specific training) and (2) teaching the patient voluntary control of his or her physiological response(s) by means of feedback from various physiological systems. The third phase of the treatment involves employing the newly acquired voluntary controls in the natural environment. It is the training phase of treatment that most experimental and clinical biofeedback studies emphasize, and minimal attention is paid to the initial conceptualization and the final transfer phases of treatment. Let us consider the potential influence of the patient's thoughts and feelings at each of these three phases of biofeedback therapy.

Initial Conceptualization

In biofeedback therapy, as in other forms of therapy, researchers have paid insufficient attention to what happens prior to implementing specific treatment procedures. Therapists usually have subsumed the conceptualization process in therapy under such terms as "nonspecific factors" or have included it in those aspects that go "beyond" therapy (e.g., A. Lazarus, 1972). The events that occur prior to such treatments as biofeedback or other procedures are rarely discussed. The reader is often provided with specific details of how the patient was trained to control some physiological response. The colors of the feedback lights, the nature of the electrode paste, and the sites for placement of electrodes may all be valuable information, but the patient's conceptualization of the problem and treatment expectations are also important, though seldom mentioned.

The patient may come with some physical ailment(s) such as headaches, high blood pressure, or Raynaud's disease. The therapist's attention is usually focused on the physiological responses. But the patient's maladaptive behaviors represent sets of complex responses, including affective, cognitive, and social, as well as physiological, components. Moreover, when the patient seeks assistance, his or her self-perceptions likely include a sense of helplessness or hopelessness and the absence of control. It is important to appreciate that, for one of the consequences of biofeedback treatment may be to change the patient's perceptions, attributions, and appraisals—that is, the patient's internal dialogue about the ability to control physiological responses and about the accompanying cognitions, feelings, and behaviors. Indeed, the improvement following from biofeedback treatment may be mediated in part by such cognitive and affective events.

An appreciation of the "larger" meaning that the physiological disturbance has for the patient will help increase the patient's motivation for treatment. A careful consideration of the internal dialogue that precedes, accompanies, and follows the physiological response, and of the patient's expectations about treatment will result in greater motivation for treatment.

We suggest, then, that biofeedback can be optimized by an initial conceptualization of such phenomenological dimensions. This can be accomplished, for example, by collecting a detailed history; conducting a situational analysis of the patient's problem; giving homework assignments to obtain a reliable baseline assessment of the topography of the maladaptive response(s); examining the interpersonal and intrapersonal meaning of the problem(s); assessing the patient's cognitions and feelings before, during, and after the maladaptive behavior; and evolving a common conceptualization of the problem and of treatment with the patient by means of offering a therapy rationale.

A particular caution concerning the patient's conceptualization of biofeedback therapy was expressed by Turner and Chapman (1982). These authors noted that, although the biofeedback techniques seem to lend scientific credence and respectability to therapy, they can lead to an increased and maladaptive preoccupation with physiology in instances in which psychological factors should be the focus:

> To the extent that preoccupation with a physiology leads to ignoring the complex nature of chronic pain problems, the psychotherapist assumes a position little different from that of physicians using nerve blocks, surgeries, or transcutaneous stimulation. One of the generalizations that can be made about chronic pain patients is that on the whole they tend to deny problems of living and to somatize the stress they experience. The therapist eager to find problems suitable for biofeedback therapy may unwittingly collude in the process of somatization by delivering a physiologically focussed treatment that legitimizes the patient's denial of life problems. In the long run this may support rather than weaken pain chronicity. (Turner & Chapman, 1982, p. 17)

The initiation of biofeedback therapy would, in light of these comments, be ill-advised without paying specific attention to the patient's view of the process. On the other hand, a technical, scientific-appearing undertaking such as this may facilitate the introduction of psychological treatment to patients for whom more verbal approaches might have insufficient face validity.

Training

As mentioned, the focus of biofeedback training is usually on having the patient develop an increased awareness of maladaptive physiological response by means of feedback and then on establishing voluntary control by means of "conscious effort." What role do the patient's thoughts and feelings play during this training phase of treatment?

The biofeedback literature provides little help in answering this question. One finds many suggestions that the patient's thoughts and feelings should be controlled so as not to interfere with biofeedback treatment. Thus, while patients are receiving feedback information about their physiological responses, they are instructed to engage in passive concentration, to master a relaxation of the body, and to attend to the feedback, not letting anything get in the way. An appropriate concern of the biofeedback therapist is to discourage the production of any cognitive and/or somatic, internally generated responses that would interfere with the patient's attention to the feedback.

Do patients actually comply with such instructions? Do some patients instead produce task-irrelevant cognitions while listening to the feedback? What does the patient say to himself or herself and imagine about the meaning of such feedback? We are reminded of G. Schwartz's (1973) patient who was being treated for Raynaud's disease by means of biofeedback. The patient interpreted the reinforcement slides that were used as an occasion to free-associate. One time the slide projector jammed, and the patient viewed the resulting bright white light on the screen as a cue to free-associate about sunny, warm beaches. The patient reported using such "hot thoughts" successfully to control the temperature of his feet outside of the laboratory.

One wonders if the biofeedback therapist could enhance the patient's attentional processes by using *task-appropriate imagery*. Patients could be encouraged to visualize the physiological changes as reflected on a printout or, perhaps more powerfully, to imagine the actual changes the specific bodily area or organ is undergoing. For example, a tension-headache patient could be told the following:

> See in your imagination the muscles of your head, your brow. Good. See the muscles becoming tenser as the feedback beeper goes faster (or louder). Now see the muscles of the head becoming more and more relaxed as the beeps slow down (or become softer). Note the feelings of warmth and calmness you are able to bring forth as you control the feedback, and so forth.

Simonton *et al.* (1980) have described the use of such imagery with cancer patients.

The point is that the biofeedback therapist may be able to employ the patient's cognitive processes as tools to enhance the biofeedback training. This can be accomplished by bringing the patient's behavior under his or her own cognitive control through the use of deliberate self-statements and images. Then, with the development of proficiency, or what Kimble and Perlmutter (1970) call the "automatization of voluntary acts," the patient's cognitions become more incomplete and short-circuited and less intentional, and then completely fade.

In a similar manner, some investigators (Green, Walters, Green, & Murphy, 1969; Sargent, Green, & Walters, 1973) have used relaxation-inducing self-statements (autogenic training) to enhance biofeedback training. Patients were asked to employ such self-instructions or phrases as the following while undergoing biofeedback training:

> I am beginning to feel quite relaxed. . . . My feet feel heavy and re-laxed. . . . They feel comfortable and relaxed . . . warm. . . . My whole body feels quiet, heavy, comfortable and relaxed, etc. (Sargent et al., 1973, p. 131)

Such relaxing self-instructions could be extended to include a variety of coping self-statements and images, which will be considered in Section III.

Transfer of Treatment

The goal of biofeedback training is to have patients develop sets of skills to employ outside of the laboratory or treatment setting. Once again, the patient's thoughts and feelings play a critical role in the success of the transfer stage. To achieve transfer, the patient must first recognize the presence of his or her maladaptive response (e.g., tension headache, back pain) and any accompanying cognitions and feelings he or she is emitting. Prior to therapy, the patient is likely to view his or her target behavior (such as a headache) as a massive, undifferentiated attack and as a sign of further deterioration, both of which engender anxiety and contribute to a maladaptive response cycle.

As a result of biofeedback treatment, the patient is more likely to view his or her headaches differently, noting the tension that precedes a headache (i.e., prodromal signs) and viewing a headache as a series of stages varying in intensity and having time-based or situationally based parameters. The patient becomes aware of how his or her own reactions influence the headache, by exacerbating or easing it. The recognition of such symptoms is a cue—a signal to employ the coping techniques he or she has learned in treatment.

In their report on biofeedback training for tension headaches, Budzynski, Stoyva, Adler, and Mullaney (1973) provided the following description of patients after training:

> They showed an increasing awareness of tension plus they were better able to relax consciously and abort light-to-moderate headaches. . . . The patient now seems to relax automatically in the face of stress and does not have to

make a conscious effort to do so. The headache is now appreciably reduced
or even eliminated. . . . The last stages would seem to indicate that the
ability to relax in the face of stress eventually becomes an overlearned habit
resulting in a change of life style. (p. 404)

The biofeedback therapist can facilitate and help consolidate automatic employment of trained skills with a variety of behavior therapy
tools such as imagery rehearsal, role playing, and modeling films. The
patient can, for example, imagine various scenes in which he or she might
experience the maladaptive response (e.g., headaches) and then visualize
noticing the prodromal tension and using the coping procedures. (This
imagery-rehearsal procedure will be considered in more detail in Chapter
12.) Or patients can be asked to role-play stressful situations (e.g., assertive
situations) that reliably contribute to their symptomatic behavior. The
therapist sometimes can act as patient, modeling how to recognize the
onset of tension and then how to use the coping procedures.

The teaching of coping responses can also effectively be conducted
by means of cognitive-coping modeling films. One could show biofeedback
patients a modeling film of other patients who have undergone biofeedback treatment. In the film a patient (i.e., a trained confederate who is
role-playing a patient) will describe to the therapist how he or she successfully employed the coping procedures in handling various situations, by
recognizing the onset of the symptom (e.g., headache) and how this was a
cue to cope. Consistent with the suggestion that the therapist should
anticipate and subsume the patient's cognitions in therapy, a second
patient model could describe how he or she used the procedures, but
found they did not work; could tell how he or she engaged in an internal
dialogue that included "I knew it would never work. No one can do
anything for my headache. It's useless," and so on; and then could recognize such thoughts and feelings and begin to cope with them—for example,
"Hold on, that's what I always say. I didn't really give the procedures a
chance. I've had these headaches for years, and I've only been in treatment
for a few weeks. Go slowly. Just relax. One step at a time," and so forth.

Such modeling is designed to anticipate and overcome the patient's
negative cognitions in therapy. Then, if the patient emits such cognitions,
they will have a déjà vu flavor (namely, "These are the thoughts and
feelings I saw in the film and that we discussed in treatment. They are the
reminders to cope.").

This brief description of the therapeutic tools available to the biofeedback therapist for use in enhancing the transfer process highlights the
potential role that the patient's cognitions can play in the change process.

A consideration of these procedures may lead to improvement in biofeed-back training.

Recently, several investigators have also noted the role of cognitive and affective factors in biofeedback treatment. Philips (1977) and Nouwen and Solinger (1979) noted that, as a result of biofeedback treatment with tension-headache and chronic low-back-pain patients, changes in muscular tension level did not correlate with improvement in other measures, such as self-report. Philips (1977) reported that pain complaints continued to decrease after treatment, independently of muscular tension level.

A more recent study by Kremsdorf *et al.* (1981) also underscored the usefulness of cognitive skills training as compared to EMG biofeedback in the treatment of tension headaches. In single-case experiments they found that biofeedback training influenced mean frontalis EMG levels, but with no concomitant reductions in headache activity. By comparison, stress-inoculation training resulted in reduction of headache activity. Interestingly, Kremsdorf *et al.* noted the potential value of biofeedback in helping patients identify anxiety-provoking cognitions and as a means of measuring the outcome of cognitive–behavioral interventions. These findings are consistent with those of Holroyd *et al.* (1977), who also found stress-coping training more effective than EMG biofeedback training. In one study Andrasik and Holroyd (1980) found that success in biofeedback training depended more on cognitive strategies generated by the patients than it did on their ability to directly control their EMG activity. As they state:

> Results from the present study . . . indicate that many subjects dealt with their headaches by altering cognitive and behavioral responses to stressful situations . . . It may be less crucial that headache sufferers learn to modify EMG activity than it is that they learn to monitor the insidious onset of headache symptoms and engage in some sort of coping response incompatible with the further exacerbation of symptoms. (p. 584)

It is results such as these that lead us to endorse the conclusion offered by Nouwen and Solinger (1979) that "EMG biofeedback training may be useful in assisting to create a change in attitude toward pain. Future investigators should attempt to address more systematically such cognitive/attitude factors" (p. 110). This observation has been echoed by many other investigators. Although much of the interest of biofeedback investigators is focused on the effects of cognitive acts on physiological responses (the study of alpha enhancement, meditation, etc.), the biofeedback literature could be compared to the verbal conditioning literature prior to the active research on the role of awareness in the conditioning process. The research on awareness (e.g., Dulaney, 1962; Spielberger & De Nike, 1966) questioned whether the experimenter's reinforcement acted in an automatic fashion, and it highlighted the important role of the subject's knowledge of the reinforcement contingencies and his or her motivation to comply. Similar attention to the patient's cognitive and affective processes at each phase of biofeedback training should result in enhanced effectiveness and understanding of the mechanisms that contribute to change.

A COGNITIVE-BEHAVIORAL PERSPECTIVE OF HYPNOSIS

Reports of the utility of hypnosis in alleviating, reducing, or eliminating pain have long been a source of fascination and controversy. We will consider illustrative studies on the uses of hypnosis with laboratory-induced and clinical pain and then look at possible mechanisms underlying hypnosis.

Laboratory-Induced Pain

In laboratory investigations of pain, hypnotically induced analgesia has often been reported effective in reducing pain for subjects who are highly susceptible to hypnosis (E. Hilgard & Hilgard, 1975). One of the more elaborate laboratory studies of pain (Stern, Brown, Ulett, & Sletten, 1977) compared hypnotic analgesia, acupuncture with true loci, acupuncture with false loci, morphine (a moderately strong dose of 10 mg per 70 kg of body weight, intramuscularly), diazepam (10 mg in 2-ml solution, intramuscularly), aspirin (two 5-grain tablets), and a placebo (two white capsules of milk sugar) in their effects on both cold-pressor and muscle-ischemic pain. Hypnotic analgesia with highly susceptible subjects was more effective in reducing both types of pain than any other treatment-by-subject combination.

Less dramatic, but consistent, results are common. E. Hilgard and Morgan (1975), for example, found that two-thirds of their highly susceptible subjects reduced pain by one-third or more in a cold-pressor investigation, and R. Greene and Reyher (1972) reported an average increased tolerance to electric shock of 45%. People who are classified as not very susceptible to hypnosis, on the other hand, experience less effect from hypnotic analgesia. In the Hilgard and Morgan (1975) study, for example, a one-third reduction in pain was experienced by 17% of the medium-susceptible subjects and by 13% of the low-susceptible subjects (compared to the 33% of highly susceptible subjects). As E. Hilgard and Hilgard (1975) summarized:

The relationship is not a perfect correspondence: the most hypnotically responsive subjects are most likely to reduce their pains, but not all of them are successful; and the least hypnotically responsive are less likely to reduce their pains by suggestion, although a few of them can. The relationship can be expressed as a correlation of .50 between measured hypnotic responsiveness and reduction of the pain of ice water. (p. 68)

Clinical Pain

In clinical investigations, case reports, and some experimental studies, there is also evidence for the utility of hypnosis in altering pain (J. Anderson *et al.,* 1975; Andreychuk & Skriver, 1975; Cedercreutz, Lahteenmaki, & Tulikoura, 1976; Crasilneck & Hall, 1973; Daniels, 1977; Finer, 1974; Gottfredson, 1973; G. Graham, 1975; Harding, 1967; Sachs *et al.,* 1977; Stambaugh & House, 1977; Willard, 1974). Not unexpectedly, though, this clinical literature is less clear than the experimental literature (Barber, 1969).

Case studies (e.g., Daniels, 1977; G. Graham, 1975), although sometimes carefully controlled (Stambaugh & House, 1977), have provided an insufficient data base for evaluation. The most common problems in the group studies are the absence of a relevant control group (e.g., Finer, 1974) and the failure to provide an independent evaluation of hypnotic susceptibility (Perry, Gelfand, & Marcovitch, 1979).

Effects and Mechanisms

Despite the problems in the clinical and experimental hypnosis literature, there seems to be sufficient evidence from some well-controlled studies (e.g., McGlashan *et al.,* 1969) to conclude that, at least for subjects who are highly responsive to hypnosis, hypnotic analgesia is effective in pain reduction. The current controversy is less concerned with the existence of hypnosis or hypnotic analgesia than with the mechanisms of hypnotic effects.

There are two predominant trends in the debate. One view considers hypnosis to be an altered state of consciousness brought about by hypnotic induction procedures, which create a dissociation between different levels of consciousness (e.g., Bowers, 1977; Fromm, Brown, Hurt, Oberlander, Boxer, & Pfeifer, 1981; E. Hilgard, 1977). The contrasting perspective does not view hypnotic experiences as entailing separate processes (i.e., a hypnotic trance), but focuses upon the hypnotized subject's disposition to behave differently than he or she would when not hypnotized: in particular, to engage in different cognitive activities and to respond more to perceived demand characteristics of the hypnotic situation (e.g., Barber, 1969; Sarbin & Coe, 1972; Spanos & Chaves, 1970; Stam & Spanos, 1980). We do not need to enter the debate in order to consider hypnotic analgesia from a cognitive–behavioral perspective.

As with biofeedback, cognitive, affective, and social factors play an important role in hypnosis. Attitudes about hypnosis are often colored by erroneous conceptions. The lay person often views the hypnotic situation as coercive, in which an authoritarian hypnotist induces a trance state through the force of his or her "will," with the hypnotized person's having little control. In the case of the use of hypnosis for pain control, the lay person may believe that, after the trance induction, the hypnotist simply suggests away the pain. An aura of mystery and the supernatural often pervades popular portrayals, encouraging such misconceptions.

This image of hypnosis is often based on literary reference to mesmerism (e.g., Svengali in *Trilby*) and stage hypnotists (e.g., a subject comes on the stage, is hypnotized, and then is *made* to bark like a dog or flap around the stage like a chicken). Some misconceptions may be fostered inadvertently by anecdotal reports describing dramatic surgical procedures (e.g., appendectomies, thyroidectomies, cesarean section, open-heart surgery, brain surgery; e.g., see Coppolino, 1965; Lassner, 1964; Marmer, 1969) performed with hypnosis as the sole anesthetic or as an adjunct to more conventional anesthetics. Dramatic accounts of the use of hypnotic analgesia with a variety of severe pain problems also abound (e.g., burns: Crasilneck, Stirman, Wilson, McCranie, & Fogelman, 1955; terminal cancer: Sacerdote, 1966, 1980; trigeminal neuralgia: Sacerdote, 1970; migraine headaches: Basker, 1970).

The greatest amount of attention in anecdotal reports on the use of hypnosis as an anesthetic or analgesic is usually given to the depth of the trance (e.g., light, medium, somnambulistic), the method of approach (e.g., neurophysiological alteration, psychodynamic changes, favorable behavior patterns), methods of induction (e.g., verbal suggestions of relaxation, drowsiness, sleep, eye fixation), deepening techniques (e.g., ego supportive reassurance), and specific suggestive techniques and ideas conveyed to patients (e.g., dissociation, reinterpretation of signals, partial or total amnesia).

A recent emphasis in this literature has been the cognitive events and styles concomitant with hypnotic effects. J. Hilgard (1970) and Spanos and Barber (1974), for example, have noted the role of "a shift in [the highly susceptible subject's] cognitive orientation from an objective or pragmatic perspective to one of involvement in suggestion-related imaginings" (Spanos & Barber, 1974, p. 500) accompanying the onset of hypnosis.

The shift from a more objective or pragmatic perspective carries with it the subject's suspension of critical, analytic processing and an openness to information. Bowers and Kelly (1979) noted that the hypnotic subject neither purposefully complies nor purposefully interferes with the information received. Rather, he or she is uncritically open to new information, becoming absorbed in it (J. Hilgard, 1970; Spanos & Barber, 1974). For a detailed discussion of various techniques and procedures, see Erickson, Hershman, and Secter (1961); Pattie (1956); Sacerdote (1970); or Weitzenhoffer (1957).

Despite the diversity of hypnosuggestive techniques and the range of applications in pain control, a number of common features seem to be incorporated in most reports of hypnotic analgesia and hypnotic anesthesia. To illustrate some of the common features, let us consider a recent description of the use of hypnosis in treating chronic low back pain (Crasilneck, 1979):

> After rapport had been established on the first session, ample time was allotted to deal with any questions concerning the nature of hypnotherapy and its application to the patient's particular difficulty. When it was evident that the patient was comfortable and in accord with the treatment, induction was begun. . . . "Now, to show you the power of your unconscious mind, I give you the suggestion that your eyes are sealed, shut tight—so that even though you try to open them you cannot. . . . Now that we have demonstrated this control of your mind over your body, I want you to relax still more. . . . "Now I give you the suggestion that as you blocked the pain in your finger a few minutes ago, you can block the pain in your back. Nothing is beyond the power of your unconscious mind. You are going to block most of the pain. Most of the pain will come under your control."
>
> Suggestions of this type were repeated until the desired goal was reached for the session. (p. 73)

In addition to the trance induction, a number of important features of hypnotic analgesia are revealed from this excerpt. Before the actual induction began, rapport was established, a convincing rationale for the use of hypnosis was provided, a positive attitude toward hypnosis was established, questions were answered, anxiety was reduced, and a sense of hopefulness was created. During the induction and suggestions, the hypnotist fostered the patient's sense of control and the power of his or her "unconscious mind" over body. Also incorporated into the hypnosuggestions were feelings of relaxation, attentional focusing, and suggestions of pain relief. Following the second of such hypnotic sessions, Crasilneck (1979) taught the patients self-hypnosis and encouraged them to use the self-hypnosis as frequently as necessary.

Following the general presentation of the technique, Crasilneck (1979) provided several case examples that illustrate how he takes into consideration idiosyncratic aspects of different patients' lives and their problems and individually tailors suggestions to be personally relevant and to meet a patient's needs. Crasilneck described the utility of hypnotherapy for a substantial proportion of the low-back-pain patients treated. (The 24 patients treated reported an average of 70% pain relief following six hypnotic sessions; only 4 patients failed to respond to hypnotherapy.)

Unfortunately, no follow-up data are reported, and no control groups were employed, so we have to be very cautious in interpreting these results. We cannot tell from this report whether the trance induction was necessary or what the active ingredients of the treatment were. The Crasilneck account illustrates that a great deal goes on in hypnotherapy in addition to the actual hypnosuggestive techniques employed. In many accounts of hypnosis, relatively little attention is given to factors such as the initial conceptualization provided, the details of the development of rapport, the enhancement of the sense of control, anxiety reduction, relaxation, and so on. Authors tend to make only a passing reference to the establishment of rapport and then provide detailed descriptions of the induction techniques, suggestions, and deepening techniques employed (e.g., Clawson & Swade, 1975; G. Graham, 1975; Wain, 1980).

As in the case of the other psychologically based interventions for pain patients, one can view hypnosis as consisting of three phases: (1) the initial conceptualization and development of rapport, (2) the actual training, and (3) the transfer of training or generalization. In the hypnosis literature, much more attention has been given to the training phase than either of the other two phases. From the cognitive–behavioral perspective, the initial phase and the transfer phase are equally important. A similar analysis of the components in both hypnosis and acupuncture has been offered by Barber and his colleagues, who have arrived at similar conclusions (Barber, 1982; Chaves & Barber, 1974b).

An interesting aspect of the role that cognitive and affective factors play in hypnosis has been offered by Spanos and his colleagues. In several laboratory studies, they have investigated the cognitive and affective processes accompanying hypnotic effects. In investigations of hypnotically induced amnesia, for example, these researchers have developed the position that the amnesia, and, in particular, the disorganized recall that is characteristic of the hypnotic phenomenon, result from the subject's *sustained inattention* to the objects of recall (Spanos & Bodorik, 1977; Spanos, Stam, D'Eon, Pawlak, & Radtke-Bodorik, 1980; Stam & Spanos, 1980).

This inattention is maintained by highly susceptible subjects, but not by low-susceptible subjects, in the face of instruction to do otherwise, that is, to recall actively (Spanos *et al.,* 1980). In a related vein, Spanos and others noted that the occurrence of visual "hallucinations" or vivid images following either waking or the giving of hypnotic instructions partly depended upon the subject's ongoing engagement in imagining an object. In these studies, highly susceptible subjects reported more belief in the reality of their images.

This series of investigations suggests that some hypnotic effects result from very active cognitive processes, even though subjects may be unaware of them or not report them. Similar results have been obtained with hypnotic analgesia. For example, Stam and Spanos (1980) reported that the postexperimental testimony of many hypnotic subjects indicated the use of coping strategies, but when they were queried, these same subjects insisted that they had done nothing to reduce pain. Despite engaging in suggestion-induced coping cognitions, the hypnotic subjects defined their pain reductions as effortless occurrences instead of activities brought about by their own efforts.

Spanos's work suggests that hypnotic responding involves active coping, but that hypnotic subjects make *attributions* of "automatic" and "nonvolitional" control concerning their own behaviors (Stam & Spanos, 1980). Spanos *et al.* (1980) contended that "from our perspective reports of effortless experiencing do not index a quality of behavior" (p. 749), but instead are self-attributions. Whether hypnotic subjects' behaviors *are* volitional is surely not contentious, for as Bowers and Kelly pointed out, "at some level it is surely *the person* who is raising *his* arm, reducing pain, 'seeing' roses that aren't physically present, and so on" (1980, p. 495). Rather, the subjects' self-perceptions of effort are different. Stam and Spanos (1980) note that it is not that hypnotic subjects are "faking" or bearing false witness, but that they are responding to the demand characteristics of the situation, changing their subjective experience accordingly.

The developing attention to cognitive events in hypnosis and the focus on attributional disposition bring hypnosis close to the central concerns of cognitive–behavioral therapy. We hope the result will be an increase in the power of clinical interventions.

SUMMARY

We have examined several major approaches to the treatment of chronic pain, noting how they share common elements. A cognitive–behavioral framework was used as a basis for analyzing these strategies. Similarly, biofeedback and hypnotic interventions were found to have elements in common with the model we have proposed. Although different intervention strategies will continue to stress different methods for achieving change, the cognitive–behavioral perspective may provide a consistent approach to conceptualizing these differences.

COGNITIVE–BEHAVIORAL TREATMENT OF PAIN

CHAPTER 8

PATIENT RESISTANCE, TREATMENT ADHERENCE, AND THERAPIST STYLES[1]

Compliance may currently be one of the greatest challenges facing the health professions.—*Kathy Bloom Cerkoney and Laura Hart (1980)*

This chapter focuses on what have traditionally been called the "non specifics," or the "ambience," of the treatment process. Considered are style and technique designed to increase treatment efficacy and adherence. The chapter underscores the fact that having a set of effective techniques is not sufficient to ensure a favorable outcome. There is a need to prepare patients for interventions and to deal with idiosyncratic reactions to therapy as they occur. The chapter describes some ways to achieve this.

Before we describe specific features of cognitive–behavioral treatment, it is important to raise the issues of patient resistance and treatment adherence. The literature to be reviewed will highlight the serious problems involved in having patients comply with the proposed treatment regimen. No matter how effective a specific set of medical or psychological procedures may be, patients' noncompliance in implementing them defeats the therapeutic process and constitutes a treatment failure. Thus any consideration of the therapy process must take into account possible resistance, premature termination of treatment, and treatment nonadherence.

THE EXTENT OF THE PROBLEM

M. Davis (1968) has estimated that from 15% to 93% of patients usually fail to comply with physicians' orders on health care regimens. Dunbar (1980) reported that only a moderate percentage of patients heed medical

---

1. We are indebted to J. Barnard Gilmore for his help in formulating the ideas for this chapter.

advice: 20% to 50% fail to keep appointments, 20% to 80% make errors in taking medications, and 25% to 60% stop taking their medications before it is therapeutically desirable to do so. In weight-management programs, 20% to 80% of patients drop out of treatment, and 90% to 95% of patients in such programs fail to achieve a desirable weight (Dunbar & Stunkard, 1979). Best and Block (1979) report that up to 75% of people entering a smoking-reduction program resume smoking 6 months after they quit. These statistics underscore the importance of the issues of treatment nonadherence and patient resistance.

Noncompliance can be viewed as one aspect of *resistance,* a difficult and frustrating problem for the physician prescribing medications, the behavior therapist providing specific homework assignments, or the cognitive–behavioral therapist having patients engage in cognitive restructuring. A number of recent reviews, cited in Chapters 2 and 3, indicate the pervasiveness and seriousness of this problem. General practitioners have reported that treatment nonadherence is the single most troublesome factor in their practice (G. Stone, 1979).

The possibility of dire consequences resulting from such nonadherence is illustrated in a study by Vincent (1971), who studied patients being treated for glaucoma. These patients were told that "they must use eye drops three times a day or *they would go blind*" (p. 511, emphasis added). Vincent reported that 58% of the patients did *not* comply at least often enough to create medical complications. When patients were at the point of becoming legally blind in one eye, compliance improved by only 16%, from 42% to 58%. How shall we understand such resistance? Moreover, what can be done to change this behavior?

A second and perhaps more important reason for waving a red flag in this chapter is that, in the course of clinical work, supervision, and giving workshops, we have come to appreciate the very important role of the counselor's or therapist's style in implementing any treatment program, including cognitive–behavioral therapies. We are concerned that the novice therapist, workshop participant, or perhaps even some readers may be so preoccupied with the "how-to" features of the procedures that the manner and style with which the treatment techniques are implemented are ignored.

The social psychological literature on interpersonal relationships in health care underscores our concerns, as reflected in the June 1979 issue of the *Journal of Social Issues,* which was devoted to this topic. Such approaches as equity theory, reactance theory, social power and exchange theories, and attribution theory provide bases for analysis of resistance (e.g., Brehm, 1966; French & Raven, 1959; Thibaut & Kelley, 1959). These analyses highlight the need to view patient resistance from the perspective of a transactional analysis, that is, in terms of the exchanges between patient and therapist that lead to treatment progress and adherence. As Dunbar (1980) noted, the factors that are associated with patient adherence include (1) those having to do with the patient, (2) those having to do with the health care provider, (3) those having to do with the clinic or office environment, and (4) those having to do with the regimen itself.

Given these complexities, exactly how can the therapist prevent resistance or deal with it when it arises? How can the patient be trained or encouraged to anticipate, understand, and alter such resistance and to increase treatment adherence?

INITIAL RESISTANCE

Since most patients who drop out of treatment do so during the initial phase, we will begin with how the therapist can deal with patient resistance from the outset. Therapy, as we have noted, begins wtih the initial contact with the patient. In fact, therapists will likely be more successful if they intervene at an earlier stage by influencing the nature of referrals that are made and the preliminary messages that are provided to the patient.

Referral Agents

The referral stage plays an important role in the patient's initial expectations regarding treatment, which in turn may influence the patient's compliance. Cameron and Shepel (1980) have also noted that the patient's attitude toward the medical practitioner or referring agent may affect the patient's behavior with the new therapist. All too often, physicians who become frustrated with intransigent patients make referrals that implicitly suggest that the patient's problems are "all in his head" (E. Meyer & Mendelson, 1961).

We have received referrals with comments such as "this patient is a crock," "this patient is hysteroid," and "this patient is a dingbat." The causes of the problems of some of the pain patients who were referred to us included "an impoverishment of mental furniture" and "supertemporal disease atrophy" (another way of saying that the patient is stupid).

Although we doubt that any physician would make such comments about patients directly, implicit messages are likely to be perceived by patients and to interfere with attempts to treat patients with psychologically based interventions. This is especially important with pain patients. Pilowsky, Chapman, and Bonica (1977) have presented data suggesting that pain patients were more reluctant to consider their health problems in psychological terms than were other medical patients. Pain patients also were more likely to deny life problems not directly related to disease.

It is important to educate referral agents about psychologically based treatments so that they may view such treatments in a positive way and may transmit this attitude to the patients they refer. As Cameron (1978) noted:

> Psychologists may realize substantial clinical dividends if they invest the time and effort required to cultivate relationships with referring agents by providing information about the nature of the therapy, the rationale underlying it, its limitations, data pertaining to its effectiveness, and prompt feedback in all cases referred. (p. 237)

In treating hospitalized patients, relationships with the ward staff are also important. Often, the attitudes and messages of nursing staff, who spend much more time with patients than do physicians, are critical in influencing patients' expectations and acceptance of treatment (Gillmore & Hill, 1981). Referring agents may be encouraged to provide patients with the perception of free choice rather than coercing them to enter treatment. The manner in which such referrals are offered will affect the patients' internal dialogues (expectations, attributions, etc.), which in turn will influence the success of treatment.

Internal Dialogue

Patients' internal dialogues concerning both their presenting problems and their expectations regarding treatment are an immediate concern for the therapist. Patients often enter treatment feeling helpless, hopeless, and demoralized with regard to their presenting problems. They often feel like victims of their own behaviors, be these physiological symptoms, their accompanying thoughts and feelings, or their response to the reactions of others (Frank, 1974; Strupp, 1970). Moreover, patients often experience what Raimy (1975) has called "phrenophobia," that is, a fear that this problem means that they may be "going crazy." Patients' thoughts about being hopelessly ill, that therapy will be ineffective, and that roads to change are nonexistent or totally blocked provide the potential basis for patients' resistance. The initial phase of therapy (and it is being suggested that this applies to all therapies, psychological and medical) is designed to begin to change patients' internal dialogues concerning their problems and to promote the sense that change is possible.

A central feature of the initial phase of treatment is assessment of the patient. From a cognitive–behavioral perspective, the focus of assessment is on those thoughts and feelings that may contribute to resistance and that may indicate future treatment nonadherence.

ASSESSMENT

The label "resistance" usually reflects a lack of understanding, with a tendency to blame the patient. Once the therapist appreciates the sources of apprehension, fear, beliefs, needs, and so on, that lead to noncompliance, the meaning of "resistance" changes, and dealing with it becomes a part of the therapeutic process. Cognitive–behavioral interventions therefore begin by assessing the phenomenal world of patients in order to understand how they construe their presenting problems.

Insofar as the therapist can accurately and empathically perceive and share patients' experiences, he or she is more likely to be able to understand maladaptive, resistant behavior. As A. Beck *et al.* (1979) indicate, accurate empathy may help the therapist realize that resistant or negativistic patients are people who regard themselves as so incompetent and hopeless that they consider change impossible. The therapist tries to understand the cognitive perspective that contributes to this "paralysis of will."

Before the initial appointment, the experience of sitting in the waiting room will often elicit thoughts and feelings related to initiating treatment. It may be useful, therefore, to begin the assessment of patients' phenomenal experience by asking about the thoughts and feelings they had while sitting in the waiting room. Parenthetically, research on noncompliance to medical treatment has revealed significantly lower adherence with longer waits in the waiting room (Davidson, 1976). One can easily imagine that prolonged waiting can result in rich, counterproductive, negative thinking.

Dunbar (1980) noted that waiting time is related to such factors as the system of patient scheduling, the system used to remind patients of their appointments, the location of the clinic, and the personal manner in which patients are treated. Since these factors are to some extent under the control of the health care provider, they can be modified to enhance the view that the patient is important and respected.

To understand more fully patients' expectations and potential resistance, a number of other inquiries can be made in the initial session. One can ask a patient why he or she wishes therapeutic assistance at the present time. What does the patient think may happen in therapy? On what will the outcome of treatment depend, and how so? Such questioning begins to reveal potential forms of resistance and provides clues as to whether the resistance reflects an attempt to cope, misinformation, fear, or some other source. These sources of resistance can then be dealt with explicitly. Without explicit recognition and attention, such forms of resistance could undermine progress at the initial stages or much later.

In the next chapter we will discuss in more detail some of the clinical tools available for assessing the patient's perspective and for altering it appropriately. We now turn to a source of resistance and nonadherence that is as important as the perspective that the patient brings to therapy— the therapist's characteristics.

THERAPIST CHARACTERISTICS

The therapist's characteristics play an important role in establishing an atmosphere in which the patient may disclose his or her thoughts and feelings. Warmth, accurate understanding, cooperative intentions, and so on, are all helpful in engendering a trusting relationship and play a critical role in preventing or overcoming resistance. Conveying to patients that they are held in high regard as worthwhile persons will help to avoid or reduce resistance.

In conducting cognitive–behavioral interventions with obese patients, Rodin (1979) noted the need to convey a sense of genuine acceptance by reacting positively when the patient mentioned something favorable (e.g., "It is clear that you have a lot going for you"). When something unfavorable is offered, the therapist can respond with a statement such as "It's understandable that you would feel self-critical at times and would want to change." Such statements are designed to convey a sense of worth that will help to mobilize a desire to change.

Dunbar (1980) has also noted the importance of what she calls "approachability," or the ease with which patients will raise concerns with the therapist. Obviously, the warmth and empathy that the therapist conveys to the patient will influence perceived approachability. As Dunbar noted, "hurriedness, interruptions, lack of time for listening, inattentiveness, and not identifying the patient's problems from the patient's own perspective contribute to unwillingness to remain in care" (p. 80). The offering of information and advice in a helpful way, the clarity of the instructions and homework assignments, and the ability not to overwhelm patients with fearful messages of dire consequences that may backfire are important therapist skills that affect patient resistance and treatment adherence.

Dunbar (1980) summarized the treatment elements needed to ensure that patients understand, remember, and implement the treatment regimen. These include:

1. Organizing and presenting information in natural, logical categories, such as diagnosis, treatment, expected outcomes, and so on.
2. Presenting details of the regimen both verbally and in writing, not in just one form or the other.
3. Tailoring the instructions to the patient.
4. Gradually presenting information over time to prevent overloading the patient.
5. Emphasizing the "how-to" component of the regimen rather than the "why."
6. Assessing comprehension and skill by asking the patient to describe what he or she is going to do after the session.
7. Giving the patient a method of assessing his or her own performance of the regimen, perhaps some self-monitoring system.
8. Including the family in the educational process whenever possible.
9. Being aggressive about continued follow-up, to ensure that the patient continues to remember and understand the regimen.

Of these several guidelines, it is particularly worth highlighting item 8, the inclusion of significant others. The importance of involving significant others in the treatment program has been noted by other writers. Baekeland and Lundwall (1975), for example, reviewed 19 studies that examined the relationship between social support and dropout *rate* from treatment. In each case, the lack of significant others' participation or investment was related to a high dropout rate. More recently, Cobb (1979) concluded that the relationship between social support and cooperative patient behavior is "one of the best documented relationships in medical sociology" (p. 168). In Chapters 9 and 10 we discuss some of the ways in which the spouse may be involved in treatment.

BIBLIOTHERAPY

Another means that has been used to reduce resistance and increase adherence is bibliotherapy, that is, providing the patient with written material or cassette audiotapes on aspects of the intervention. The purpose of bibliotherapy is to help consolidate the conceptualization of treatment and to provide information that will form the basis for intervention. A number of cognitive–behavioral therapists (e.g., A. Beck & Greenberg,

1974; Genest, 1979; Mitchell & White, 1977; Novaco, 1978) have written manuals that they use as part of their interventions.

But caution is necessary in the use of such devices. To ensure that the bibliotherapy is indeed read and implemented, a groundwork must be laid for its introduction. The therapist should anticipate and address any possible rejection that the patient may offer. The "set" given to the patient is to read the bibliotherapy material and to see if any of it might fit his or her particular problem. Telling patients that there may indeed be aspects of the material that they may have difficulty accepting or may question often proves helpful. For example, the therapist may say:

> What I would like you to do is read over some materials describing problems similar to yours and what might be done. I have a pamphlet that describes how other patients much like yourself have viewed their problems and what they did about them. As I have mentioned, every person is different, and what I would like you to do is to read this material before our next meeting and note what fits in your case and what does not fit. We will then have an opportunity to discuss your reaction and concerns.

In our experience we have found that one should not provide bibliotherapy material until the second or preferably the third session. It seems necessary to have the patient first collect data from his or her own experience. This prepares the patient for the material covered in the bibliotherapy. It is also important to use written material only as an adjunct to direct contact and to carefully solicit patients' reactions to the content. When patients read and process material on their own, the therapist does not have the opportunity to monitor ongoing acceptance, rejection, understanding, and other reactions. As a result, unless the therapist takes steps to deal with such problems, bibliotherapy materials may be without benefit or may even be detrimental, by producing misunderstandings. If the use of bibliotherapy materials is properly monitored, however, they can provide useful adjuncts to and reinforcements of other therapy methods.

To assist in assessing patients' reactions, the therapist might proceed along these lines:

> As we discuss your reactions to the material you read, it seems to me that a number of different things may be going through your mind. Let me begin by asking you what you felt and thought when you read the booklet.

After this probe, the therapist can voice various hunches about the patient's resistance. These alternatives should be phrased as tentative, reflecting an attempt to make sense of what is going on.

In some cases the patient may be quite resistant, as evident in noncompliance with homework assignments, hesitance in considering certain topics, and so on. In such cases resistance may become the focus of intervention. For example, the therapist might state:

> It is clear that you are quite dissatisfied with your present state of affairs. Yet, as we talk, it seems as if you are reluctant to try to change any of the things in your life that you see as causing—at least in part—your problems. If you really don't want to change things, then someone else saying that you should change obviously isn't going to work. So I think we should take some time to talk about your feelings about what it means to change certain aspects of your life.

Turning explicitly to resistance in such a manner can open the way for the patient to take a different approach—to become a collaborator in attacking a problem that is shared between the patient and therapist—instead of feeling more and more trapped in a defensive stance. The message is that the resistance is not being judged, just that it is there and must be dealt with and that it can be dealt with, with the patient's help. The patient's very consideration of this stance will begin the process of turning him or her from being a "resistant patient" into a more active participant–collaborator in the treatment.

THE ROLE OF AFFECT

The topic of patient resistance is heavily intertwined with the question of the patient's emotions concerning the nature of change. Affect is heavily invested in the patient's expectations and "hidden agendas." The meaning that change has for the patient will influence the nature and degree of resistance. In fact, as one aspect of cognitive–behavioral treatment, the therapist focuses with the patient on the intimate links between thought, behavior, and affect.

Cognitive–behavioral therapies stress that affect (like belief) is *not* under direct voluntary control. To modify affect, one must change thought patterns and behavior. And to change thinking and behavior patterns, it is not sufficient just to reason with or "persuade" one's patients. It is in this respect that cognitive-behavior modification is not merely "talking" therapy or persuasion techniques as some have supposed (cf. Berenson & Carkhuff, 1967; Ledwidge, 1979).

Affect depends in part on what patients believe about their feelings and emotional reactions (or about a specific presenting problem such as

multiple sclerosis, cardiac disease, or pain). These important beliefs—
these personal theories and their connections with presenting problems—
can be modified by careful work that first makes explicit and then
examines the evidence for the truth and the psychological utility of the
beliefs in question. Affect is not out of one's control, as the patient
generally imagines; it is in part controlled by previous affect, through the
mediating links of cognition. The personally interpreted meanings of
previous affective experiences or pain experiences help to determine
succeeding affective or pain experiences. And this key cognitive mediator,
meaning, is the focus of our treatment efforts. Cognitive–behavioral
therapies initially focus upon the interruption of such affect and pain after
they first arise and well before they have expanded into dysfunctional
complexes.

How is such cognitive interruption possible? We have already suggested in Chapter 1 the basic technique of training the patient to use the
scientific model: Identify the working hypothesis, test it empirically,
modify it as necessary, and try out new behaviors that will solve problems
in a world that works according to the model we hold. We try to help the
patient become more scientifically active by modeling a cognitive style
that the patient comes to practice without help, a style that includes such
new cognitions as these: "What are the facts? Let me first rate my pain."
"How are my own reactions contributing to the present level of pain
intensity?" "If I hold these thoughts, what is the evidence for my conclusions?" "Are there other explanations?" "What is the degree of harm to
me if . . . ?" "How serious is . . . ?"

In this context the patient's resistance represents a new occasion for
the patient and therapist to conduct a cognitive–behavioral analysis. If
the set adopted by the therapist and patient is that of a "personal scientist,"
then failures and patient resistance, like anomalous data for the scientist,
provide additional occasions for examining the nature of the patient's
symptoms, cognitions, affect, and behavior, and their interconnections.

PREPARING FOR POSSIBLE SETBACKS

At the outset of therapy, it should be made clear to the patient that
"progress" will almost certainly *not* be linear, but that disappointment
need not spread and that lack of progress itself can be informative. If the
affect or problems experienced by the patient can come to be more
contained and therefore less threatening, then they can be coped with
successfully and used constructively.

It is valuable for the therapist to prepare for resistance by repeated emphasis on the versatility of the therapeutic approach and, by implication, on the resilience of patients as well. A. Beck *et al.* (1979) accomplish this by conveying the following to the patient:

> We have a number of approaches that have been shown to be successful for various problems. We may have to try out several before we find the one that fits you. Thus, if one method is not particularly helpful, it will provide us with valuable information regarding which method is likely to succeed. (p. 132)

There is an element of a paradoxical intention in these instructions, for the therapist conveys to the patient that indeed there may be failures and occasions on which the problem will become more intense, but that such instances are to be expected and are in fact part of the "rocky road" to progress. Thus failures become part of therapy and, as such, are no longer occasions for catastrophizing, but rather occasions for learning.

Cameron (1978) succinctly described several therapy techniques that can be used to mitigate setback in therapy:

> There are a number of things that can be done to prevent over-reaction to slow progress and setbacks. First, the therapist can discuss the time-frame for change with the client at the time interventions are begun. Many clients have unrealistic expectations about how quickly they can change. A person who thinks he is going to change in a month well-ingrained patterns of interaction acquired over a lifetime is almost certainly going to be disheartened by the pace of therapy. Second, structuring therapy so that there are a progressive series of specific intermediate goals rather than a few vague, long-range goals increases the sense of progress. Third, anticipating failures and setbacks may short-circuit over-reaction to them. The therapist can indicate that while these things are normal, people tend to have doubts about whether therapy will work for them or whether they can ever change. In anticipating this negative self-monologue, the therapist can note that it is important for the client to expect this so that when the negative thoughts begin he recognizes them as a normal part of the therapy progress and doesn't take them too seriously. The therapist can wrap up his statement with a suggestion that he has found that simply anticipating these negative thoughts tended to short-circuit them; the client will likely find that when he has such thoughts he will recall this conversation and this will make it possible for him to dismiss the negative self-talk as normal. (p. 246)

Cameron (1978) also suggests that one can and should develop metaphors, aphorisms, and simple demonstrations to illustrate the feasibility of a particular treatment approach. For instance, Cameron and Shepel (1980) described a pain patient, a farmer who took pride in his work. The therapist asked him what he would do if one of his pieces of machinery became rusty. The farmer readily answered that he would carefully sand it down to remove all of the rust before repainting it. The therapist noted that the patient would not deal with the machinery in a superficial way, but that, as the patient had stated, he would "get to the bottom of the problem." The therapist wondered if the same solution might not apply to the patient's problems. The therapist juxtaposed the issue of the patient's taking medication and the work of understanding and dealing with the anxiety exacerbating his pain. The therapist used the "rusty machinery" metaphor as a catalyst in preparing the patient for intervention.

Not all patients are as open to intervention as was this farmer. Sternbach (1974b) reported on a host of pain patients who were resistant to all interventions. Sternbach (1978b) estimated that up to 15% of pain patients are sufficiently angry, demanding, and manipulative to require the negotiation of an explicit treatment contract. Epstein and Wing (1979) reviewed the literature on the use of behavioral contracting with health behaviors. Although such behavioral contracts may be a useful adjunct in some cases, several cautions concerning contracting bear repeating:

> If participation in health habit change programs requires that clients agree to the possibility of significant response costs, such as the loss of money, fewer individuals may be willing to enter the program. It is also possible that the contracts may arouse unnecessary anxiety or lead to unhealthy practices to achieve the contract goals (e.g., taking diet pills to produce weight loss). Contracts may make the client too dependent on the therapist and make long-term habit change more difficult. (Epstein & Wing, 1979, p. 13)

EXPECTATIONS AND PLAUSIBILITY

Another factor that may contribute to patient resistance is the impression that the nature of the intervention is not commensurate with the nature and degree of the patient's problem. The proposed treatment must be perceived as being both credible and acceptable. For example, a patient who has had long-term, severe pain and who has received several major, but unsuccessful, interventions (e.g., surgery, nerve blocks) may view with some skepticism the potential usefulness of relaxation exercises and attention-diverting images: "Do you think those head games will help me?" The proposed intervention may be considered too simple and too low-powered to be helpful.

Several things can be done to create a sense of balance between the patient's perception of the intervention and the patient's perceived problem. One strategy is to illustrate the potency of a particular technique by analogy, by metaphor, and especially by demonstration. For example, a patient with a chronic medical problem may question the utility of distracting imagery (one technique we use with pain patients). Demonstrating the potency of attentional focus by having the patient direct his or her attention to different sensations or external stimuli can be helpful in preparing the patient for the presentation of such techniques for use in relation to his or her pain. We will provide detailed information about the attentional technique in Chapter 10. (See also McCaffery, 1979, Chapter 11.)

Another strategy that has been used is to include technologically more sophisticated interventions, such as biofeedback, in order to enhance the credibility of relaxation training (Cameron & Shepel, 1980). A pain patient, when offered muscular relaxation training, may doubt its potential therapeutic value, especially given a history of multiple medical operations. The status of the relaxation intervention may be enhanced by the use of EMG biofeedback training. The level of technology being brought to bear on the intervention may then appear more commensurate with the patient's perception of the problem.

Cameron (1978) noted that therapeutic adherence may increase if the therapist selects and presents interventions in a way that allows the patient to view them as being sufficiently potent to deal with the problem. Note that the therapeutic efficacy of a treatment procedure such as EMG biofeedback is not the issue at this point. The concern is the fit between the patient's expectations and the plausibility and credibility of the suggested treatment technique. The concern regarding biofeedback raised by Turner and Chapman (1982) in Chapter 7, however, should be taken into consideration.

A patient's beliefs, expectations, self-statements, and images play a paramount role in determining treatment adherence. Since these processes represent the central focus of cognitive–behavioral therapies, we feel that such therapies offer a very promising way of dealing with patient resistance.

HOMEWORK INTERVENTIONS

Cognitive–behavioral therapies make considerable use of homework conducted in the natural environment where the patient must function after therapy is concluded. The homework is a key ingredient in diagnosing and dismantling problem-causing ideas, in strengthening problem-solving ideas, in assessing the sources of new problems and resistance, and in solving those problems that may occur after therapy has ended. Dealing with resistance to homework assignments is an early priority for treatment under cognitive–behavioral therapy. From the very beginning, patients are shown that they will be full collaborators in the therapy process. Patients are made aware that they can contribute very helpful, and sometimes very surprising, data from the homework experiments that are undertaken.

Levy and Carter (1976) contrasted various ways that homework can be assigned. The cognitive–behavioral therapist is particularly concerned that patients develop a sense of efficacy in planning and evaluating experiments and life changes. Consider a patient's probable reactions when he or she has done a homework assignment following each of these three different kinds of directions:

1. "What you are to do is . . ."; "Do the following . . ."; "Do this. . . ."
2. "I would like you to . . ."; "I want you to . . ."; "This is what I am asking you to do. . . ."
3. "So what you have agreed to try is . . ."; "As I understand it, you will . . ."; "So you will take responsibility for. . . ."

The patient's attributions concerning the change process and treatment are likely to be very different under each of these three message styles. The first two sets of directions are presented as demands from the health care provider. No attention is given to the patient's thoughts and feelings concerning the assigned tasks. The third set conveys respect for the patient and commitment by the patient to agreed-upon tasks. This type of directions should enhance the patient's attempts to fulfill homework assignments.

Ideally, the therapist would like to conduct therapy so that the patient comes to suggest the same homework assignments that the therapist has in mind. As noted, our style in achieving this goal is *not* to lecture the patient in a didactic fashion, but to use a Socratic-type dialogue. The involvement of significant others and the gradual introduction of increasingly more demanding homework assignments increase the likelihood of treatment adherence and reduce patient noncompliance. In addition, the effectiveness of what the patient has actually accomplished in homework should be highlighted, so that he or she is fully aware of its contribution to the change process.

The therapist must also ensure that the patient understands the rationale and goal of each assignment. A useful way to assess such understanding is to use a role-reversal procedure in which the patient is asked to explain to the therapist the nature of the homework assignments. Such an explanation, in the patient's own words, is followed by a discussion of the nature of the problems in implementing the homework assignments. The patient may be asked such questions as "How do you feel about this assignment?" "Do you feel it is something useful to tackle?" "Can you foresee some of the possible problems you could have doing it?"

The impact that the patient's "hidden agendas" have on treatment adherence, as well as the impact of the corresponding "agendas" held by others who are significant in the patient's life, must be ascertained. The patient or the significant other may be concerned that complying with homework and treatment plans may result in the loss of workers' compensation or in behaviors that the patient or significant other finds disconcerting. For example, a significant other may sabotage treatment, fearing that the patient's improvement or change may threaten the relationship. Thus both the patient's and the significant other's cognitions, expectations, images, fantasies, and meanings concerning the treatment changes receive a good deal of attention by therapists.

When the homework has not been completed satisfactorily, guilt and discouragement can be reduced first through an appropriate understanding of the reasons (thoughts, emotions, conflicting behaviors) for the patient's inaction and then by appropriate planning for future coping in the face of similar resistance. For example, A. Beck *et al.* (1979) described the following patient reactions: "It is useless to try"; "I can't do it"; "I am too weak to do anything"; "If I try it and it won't work out, I'll only feel worse." Patients usually accept such reasons as valid, whereas the therapist should view these reasons as hypotheses to be tested.

In this light it is interesting to note that an observer of cognitive–behavioral therapy (as reported in A. Beck, *et al.*, 1979) indicated that a noticeable characteristic of cognitive–behavioral therapists is their unwillingness to "give up " in light of repeated patient resistance. Each time the patient reports that he or she "failed" or "can't change," this is *another* occasion for the therapist to have the patient reexamine the data that led to such conclusions. With the therapist's guidance, the patient is encouraged to reexamine the nature of the cognitions and feelings that led to the statements of hopelessness and frustration. Moreover, the therapist is very sensitive to the patient's thoughts and feelings about such failures, and he or she questions and challenges the patient about whether failures mean that the patient "will always" or "must" fail. (Recall the work of Marlatt and Gordon with relapse among alcoholics described in Chapter 3.)

Such consistent analyses and support offered by the therapist provide an important basis for preventing and overcoming patient resistance. When the therapist hears the patient say, "It doesn't work," this is the occasion for the therapist to earn his or her fee by exploring with the patient what he or she is referring to. At first, the therapist may merely reflect, using the patient's own words, but with a tone that turns the patient's phrase, "It doesn't work," into a question, "It doesn't work?" The task for the therapist is to help the patient specify what the "it" is, and the meaning of "doesn't work." What did the patient actually do? When, where, and with whom? How would the patient know if it did work? Does the patient's statement reflect a criterion problem? Is the patient implying that such procedures would never work? These are the key questions that the therapist and patient set out to consider.

The full clinical armamentarium is used to conduct such an interview, so that the tenor of the session is not that of a cross-examination, which could lead to further resistance. Instead, the therapist is attempting to model for the patient a cognitive style that the patient can gradually adopt as his or her own. It is the adoption of this attitudinal set that is viewed as a central objective of cognitive-behavior modification. It is proposed that this set will help patients cope with, reduce, and avoid stress, maladaptive behaviors, and pain.

SUMMARY

As viewed from a cognitive–behavioral perspective, patient resistance and treatment nonadherence are *not* signs of personality defects or of hostility on the part of the patient, but instead are a natural consequence of a maladaptive thinking style, of a set of dysfunctional beliefs, and/or of a set of interpersonal consequences that reinforce resistance. Environmental consequences that follow patient resistance, both within therapy and *in vivo*, are as important as the patient's cognitions and affect. In the remaining chapters, we will discuss adherence, resistance, and therapist style in specific situations as they relate to pain patients.

Any discussion of patient resistance and treatment adherence should end with an *important warning*, one that Davidson (1976) highlighted. It is necessary for us, as health care providers, to ensure the efficacy of a treatment before we start ensuring compliance. Davidson indicated that we tend to view a patient's resistance as "vaguely sinful" and as reflecting something that is wrong with the patient. One must keep in mind the history of various medical and psychological treatments and wonder whether the patient's resistance may sometimes reflect perspicacious wisdom and plain good judgment. Recall our descriptions of the treatment of Charles II and George Washington in Chapter 4. Would they have been better off if they had shown some resistance? It is incumbent upon us to demonstrate the efficacy of our treatment procedures before we bemoan our patients' resistance and treatment nonadherence.

CHAPTER 9

INITIAL PHASE OF
COGNITIVE–BEHAVIORAL TREATMENT:
PART I

I would desire to enforce a principle that I think is not sufficiently and often not at all, considered in practical medicine and surgery. . . . The principle is that, the brain cortex, and especially the mental cortex has to be reckoned with more or less as a factor for good or evil in all diseases of every organ, in all operations, and in all injuries.—*Sir Thomas Clousten* (*1896, cited in Schofield, 1902*)

This and the next four chapters will present in detail a cognitive–behavioral treatment approach. We will use the problem of chronic pain to illustrate the details of the approach. The general orientation and many of the techniques are applicable to many aspects of behavioral medicine (e.g., treatment of various disorders, health promotion, rehabilitation, adherence to therapeutic regimens).

This chapter discusses the initial phase of the cognitive–behavioral intervention. Assessment and treatment are viewed as intimately connected; thus we will consider the assessment procedures in some detail. The reader is referred to the appendixes for specific assessment instruments and procedural guidelines. Finally, although we provide detailed accounts, including some therapist scripts, these are offered as illustrations and are not meant to be employed rigidly. A spontaneous, flexible approach will help to establish an atmosphere of rapport, confidence, and alliance.

We have discussed the various models of pain and a model for cognitive–behavioral interventions and have commented on the role of psychological and, particularly, cognitive variables in pain and its treatment. We now turn to a detailed description of proposed intervention procedures. The approach described is applicable to a broad variety of medical and psychological problems, but we will make specific reference to its use in treating pain problems. A variety of different pain disorders is to be considered, from acute to chronic pain, from pain as the primary symptom (e.g., migraine or tension headaches) to pain as secondary to some other disorder (e.g., cancer).

Although the treatment suggestions presented in the next chapters are quite specific, they are intended neither as proven (although encouraging results have been obtained) nor as rigid prescriptions. There is no substitute for the personal impact of the trained therapist, and there is no easy means of acquiring the sensitivity and judgment that are the fruit of experience. Many practitioners will intuitively or through their own clinical experience be utilizing the methods we describe in the course of their normal contact with patients. We do not wish to suggest that the approach we offer must be formalized in order to be effective. On the contrary, we offer our suggestions as resource material intended for experimentation, revision, and adaptation, and we encourage others to critically evaluate and improve upon our efforts (and to write us about their successes, failures, and suggestions).

Even in the research literature to date, the variability in the application of cognitive–behavioral interventions is notable. Therapy has varied, for example, from involving just one 1-hour session for the treatment of experimentally induced pain to entailing 38 sessions in the clinical treatment of outpatient pain patients (Khatami & Rush, 1978). Therapy has been carried out individually, conjointly with significant others, in groups, by combining both individual and group sessions, and with inpatients and outpatients.

It is our clinical impression, borne out by the data (A. Beck et al., 1979; Genest & Turk, 1979; Herman & Baptiste, 1981; Meichenbaum & Genest, 1977; Rybstein-Blinchik, 1979; Turk, Kerns, Bowen, & Rennert, 1980; Turner, 1979), that group cognitive–behavioral treatment is often as effective as individual therapy. In addition to being more efficient in terms of therapist time, a group approach can capitalize upon group processes such as self-disclosure, the growth of group cohesiveness, group pressure, and public commitment. Group treatment can readily be combined with individual, couple, or family sessions to address idiosyncratic problems.

We will present flexible sequences of procedures, which should be customized to the needs of the particular patient. Some techniques may be recycled at different phases, including the follow-up booster sessions. These procedures are designed to increase the health care provider's repertoire, not to replace other medical or psychological interventions. In studies in which the cognitive–behavioral treatment has been conducted on an inpatient basis with chronic pain patients, such treatment has usually formed one part of the overall therapy regimen, which involves physicians, physiotherapists, occupational therapists, and vocational counselors. Within such a context, it has been impossible to attribute change to the cognitive–behavioral intervention per se. However, with some outpatient groups, such as headache patients, the intervention has been the sole treatment modality (e.g., Bakal *et al.*, 1981; Holroyd *et al.*, 1977).

INITIAL PHASE OF TREATMENT

Table 9-1 details the steps in the initial phase of treatment. The length of this phase obviously will depend upon the overall length of assessment and treatment. The average length of treatment is probably from 12 to 15 sessions, with the initial assessment process completed in 2 or 3 sessions. In some interventions, such as preparing patients for surgery or noxious medical examinations, the total treatment intervention may be limited to only two sessions (e.g., see Kendall, 1982); in such instances, the initial phase may be limited to only a portion of the first session. In contrast, we have had cases in which the initial phase extended over a half-dozen sessions, and the total treatment up to 40 sessions.

Obviously, the full duration of the proposed assessment and treatment will vary with the particular clinical circumstance, but we can describe what we consider a comprehensive cognitive–behavioral treatment for chronic pain patients, an ideal from which circumstances will often force us to deviate. In our judgment, a comprehensive treatment should follow the patient for 1 year to 2 years, with initial assessment and treatment phases of 2 months' duration, followed by a transfer and maintenance phase lasting 3 months to 4 months. This is followed by regular telephone and other contacts (booster sessions where necessary) for 1 to 2 years. Thus our treatment represents a long-term commitment rather than a quick cure. These time estimates may change, depending on whether one is working on an inpatient or an outpatient basis, but the point to be conveyed is the need for a lengthy commitment. Obviously, the practicalities of the situation will determine how much one deviates from this "ideal" treatment plan.

No matter how short or long the intervention, regardless of medical condition, the initial assessment and reconceptualization phases are seen as necessary components. We will discuss each of the elements of this initial phase. The therapist should select those that meet his or her particular style and needs as well as the needs of the patient.

TABLE 9-1. *Steps in the Initial Phase of Treatment*

I. Preparation for treatment
   A. Inform the referral sources about the nature and philosophy of the cognitive–behavioral approach to pain management.
   B. Inform the referral sources about the nature and importance of the message they provide to patients when referring them to the pain-management program.
   C. Provide handout to patients describing the nature of the pain-management program to which they are being referred.
II. Initial contact (may be by phone or during a brief face-to-face encounter)
   A. Obtain a brief description of the patient's pain problem and a history of prior treatment as well as current treatments (e.g., medication, physical therapy).
   B. Elicit information regarding the patient's expectations concerning the program.
   C. Answer questions about the nature of the program and clarify any misconceptions (e.g., the patient's pain is considered to be real).
   D. Arrange appointment with patient and significant other(s). (Spouse, children, employers, or friends may be included, depending upon feasibility and potential sources of support.) Explain that significant others are necessary since pain affects them as well as the patient.
III. Initial assessment sessions (assessment and treatment are not readily separable) Usually two or three sessions are needed to achieve these goals.
   A. Review the nature of the program and clarify misconceptions. Note that the program will be customized to meet the specific needs of the patient, based on age, life circumstances, interests, and pain problem. Note that the therapist will work in collaboration with the patient to establish the goals of the program.
   B. Obtain specific information about the pain. (History of the pain, typography, history of treatments, and current treatments are reviewed.)
   C. Obtain background information about patient's prepain life.
      1. Prior experiences in coping with pain and stress.
      2. How problems are approached (resourceful vs. helpless or passive).
      3. Family structure.
      4. Social supports.
      5. Recreational activities.
      6. Vocational activities.
   D. Conduct separate interview with significant others to obtain clarification of any issues and to determine how the patient's pain affects them (tap their thoughts and feelings) and how they respond to the patient. Then conduct joint spouse–patient interview.
   E. Provide homework assignments. Describe in detail and provide rationale for each task. Patient and significant other should review what they are to do.
      1. Have the patient complete the pain questionnaire that includes part of the Melzack–McGill Pain Questionnaire. This questionnaire is designed to

(Continued)

TABLE 9-1. (*Continued*)

---

    obtain detailed information about the nature of the pain, how it affects different aspects of the patient's life, and how he or she and significant others respond to pain.

  2. Have the significant others complete questionnaires designed to elicit information about how they perceive the patient's pain, how it affects them, and how the significant others respond.

  3. Have the patient complete a diary designed to provide information concerning the time, place, and presence of others during pain episodes, as well as the thoughts and feelings that the patient has preceding, during, and after severe pain episodes. The techniques used or the things the patient does to cope with the pain are also elicited.

  4. Have the significant others complete a diary designed to elicit information regarding the cues the spouse uses to determine that the patient is experiencing pain, what the significant others' thoughts and feelings are when they perceive the patient is in pain, and what they do to assist the patient.

  5. Have the patient complete pain intensity rating cards, to reveal the time course of pain and the fluctuations in pain intensity, as well as the time when medication is used. Significant others may also be asked to complete pain intensity ratings.

IV. Subsequent assessment sessions

  A. Answer questions.

  B. Review homework. The homework data will provide the basis for a situational and performance analysis.

  C. Possibly use imagery reconstructions to identify the nature of the patient's thoughts and feelings during a recent pain episode.

  D. Possibly include a behavioral trial using the cold-pressor and/or the muscle-ischemia task. Videotape reconstruction of thoughts and feelings may be used.

  E. Discuss some of the myths of pain.

  F. Provide a reconceptualization of pain following the gate-control model, emphasizing that thoughts and feelings can exacerbate the pain experienced.

  G. Emphasize the potential for the patient to control pain and discomfort.

  H. Set goals. Negotiate treatment goal with patient and significant others in different areas, such as recreational, vocational. Physical goals will be established in collaboration with the physical therapist and physician.

    1. Explain the use of charts to monitor achievement of goals.

    2. Determine the patient's perception of self-efficacy by completing self-efficacy ratings.

  I. Possibly incorporate additional assessment instruments that assess mood, marital communication, personality style, and so on (e.g., MMPI, Illness Behavior Questionnaire, Beck Depression Inventory).

V. Additional assessment sessions (if required)

TABLE 9-1. (*Continued*)

VI. General points
A. Engender a collaborative working relationship.
B. Use Socratic, rather than didactic, approach.
C. Clarify any potential misconceptions by raising them and discussing them.
D. Use the patient's and significant others' examples to illustrate what is meant by various concepts (e.g., how thoughts can affect pain).

Initial Contact and Background Information

Making the initial appointment with the patient, typically by telephone, often constitutes the beginning of treatment. Preliminary questions on the telephone or in the initial session may concern the source of the referral, the general details of the pain complaint, the general state of health, ongoing treatment (if any), the date of the last physical examination, any additional reasons for contacting a nonmedical pain specialist, and the patient's information and expectations concerning the intervention. One area that should be explored explicitly is the patient's understanding of the purpose of the referral. Any misunderstandings should be clarified.

Liaison with the referring physician(s) or other agent can foster an initial therapeutic alliance with patients (Cameron & Shepel, 1980). Informing referral sources about the therapy approach can assist in this liaison. Appendix B contains an information form we have given to referring agents, which describes the nature of the cognitive–behavioral treatment program. Patients' expectations regarding treatment are often influenced by the referring agents' attitudes, thus underscoring the need for careful consultation. We encourage referral agents to tell patients the reasons for referrals and to convey to patients (1) that their pain is real, (2) that there are currently no medical or surgical treatments available to eliminate their pain, and (3) that they are being referred to a program geared toward alleviating some of their discomfort and toward assisting them to learn how to live a more satisfactory life despite the continued presence of some level of discomfort.

Cameron and Shepel (1980) highlight the fact that, in a hospital setting or in a pain clinic, the timing of a psychological referral and assessment is important. They note that a psychological consultation should occur at the same time at which physical diagnostic tests are conducted, lending further credibility to the comprehensive nature of the workup and treatment plan. If the psychological consultation follows negative results of medical tests, this will influence the patient's interpretation of the referral and may undermine future interventions.

Psychological assessment and treatment may, however, carry little weight with patients until *after* they have received the results of physical assessments, particularly if there is a decision to be made concerning surgery. Maintaining contact with referral agents and providing progress reports concerning referred patients are obvious, though sometimes neglected, aids to maintaining good professional relationships.

Toward a Therapeutic Alliance

From the initial contact, the therapist is engaged in forming an alliance with the patient in order to work jointly on the pain problem. This alliance is as necessary in the assessment process as it is in therapy.

A patient's skepticism concerning psychological interpretations and a consequent unwillingness or inability to contribute relevant information can impede early progress. Most patients will also have some investment in their roles as pain patients, providing further difficulties. Since it is likely that such issues are relevant for all patients, even if they do not voice them, we believe it is appropriate to bring them up and to address each of them. To the extent that we can anticipate problems early and incorporate patients' reservations into the therapeutic alliance, we are less likely to confront resistance in later stages of treatment.

The questions asked by the therapist and the assessment procedures employed do more than solicit information. They are designed to help alter the focus of the patient's attention and to facilitate a translation or reconceptualization of the pain. This translation is the cornerstone of therapy. Moreover, assessment does not cease at some specific time; the emphasis merely shifts gradually to intervention techniques, with continual reassessment and revision of goals and strategies stressed. The cognitive–behavioral approach, then, *involves change from the outset. We do not clearly separate assessment and therapy.*

The initial establishment of a working relationship may be hindered by the common doubts of pain patients about the potential usefulness of seeing a nonmedical person for what is construed *totally* as a medical problem. To deal with resistance to "psychological" inquiries, some preparatory remarks may be offered in the initial session. For example, the therapist may comment to the patient:

> If you have been hurting for a long time, someone has probably suggested that "the pain is all in your imagination," or "it's all in your head." That surely doesn't help, and it simply is not true. You know that you hurt. The pain is real.

Fordyce (1976) has made similar comments to patients:

> We have said that you have more pain than you need to have. That doesn't mean that your pain is unreal or imaginary. Of course your pain is real. It is probably true by now—as it is sooner or later for almost everyone with chronic pain—that someone along the way will have said or, at least hinted, that your problem was psychogenic, imaginary, or all in your head. That is a common misconception about pain and it is nonsense. The proper question is not whether or not the pain is real. Pain is what you feel when you hurt. Of course it is real. The proper question is, what are the factors that influence the pain? (p. 151)

The therapist may continue in this vein:

> At one time we used to think that pain was a simple matter: Something hurt your body and you felt pain. But it's just not that simple. Many different things affect the pain we experience. I would like us to take some time to examine all the things that may be related to your pain so that we can select the best set of procedures to be used to reduce your pain and can help you live a more satisfactory and productive life. We are going to develop a treatment program designed to increase what you can do. If we do that in the right way, you can expect your pain to begin to fade away. But even if your pain doesn't go away completely, you'll be able to do more and to need less medication.
>
> To achieve these goals, it is important for you to understand that I do *not* have any magical techniques or procedures that will immediately take away your pain. Instead, once we both better understand what is going on, we will be able to consider some specific treatment possibilities.

A problem that can arise at this point is that many pain patients have talked about their pain to so many health care providers that they have become rather expert in such descriptions. Some are even angry that they have to go through it again and simply say, "Why don't you see my medical record?" Other patients feel that the therapist does not really care unless they are given an opportunity to tell their story. The therapist has to be clinically sensitive to such potential reactions. It is necessary to establish a relationship that is an *alliance* and is not in any sense competitive or adversary, which the patient has probably experienced all too often.

Information Gathering

The information gathered during the initial interview includes a detailed history of the pain and its role in the patient's life situation. Information regarding use of medication and exercise and vocational, marital, and social histories are also obtained. Because the patient's life did not begin with the onset of pain, the therapist assesses not only the current situation, but also the patient's prepain life, prior experiences in coping with pain and stress, problem-solving style, family structure, social support networks, vocational and recreational activities, and so on (Turk & Kerns, 1980).

Assessment of prepain functioning often provides insights into behavioral, cognitive, and affective responses subsequent to pain onset. In addition, the information assists in the planning of exercises and homework assignments that will be employed throughout the training program and in the development of realistic, personally relevant posttreatment objectives.

The importance of historical information to an appreciation of the context of problems is illustrated by two of our patients. One is a woman who had developed rheumatoid arthritis. Prior to this, she had been particularly close to and quite dependent upon her older sister. She used to spend most of her free time with her sister, shopping, attending church activities, and traveling to historic sites. Unfortunately, about a year before the patient developed arthritis, her sister moved quite a distance away, rendering an important source of support and attention much less available. Part of the treatment plan, then, was to help the patient increase her range of acquaintances and enhance her social support network (cf. Heller, 1979).

Another of our patients, a man suffering from low back pain, had a prepain history of heavy drinking when confronted with a difficult problem. He often avoided directly addressing the problem, but waited and hoped that it would somehow go away. The patient was likely to react similarly to pain, that is, by withdrawing, accompanied by drinking or use of medication. Part of the treatment plan for this patient included discussion and homework assignments to generate alternative coping strategies as well as other problem-solving exercises (e.g., defining problems, evaluating alternatives, anticipating consequences).

Appendix C contains a questionnaire that we have asked our pain patients to complete. Whenever feasible, patients are told on the phone that we will send this questionnaire to them to answer and to bring it to the first session. If patients have minimal facility with English or are hesitant about complying, the questionnaire is incorporated into the first session's interview or is given to them to take home after the initial interview. The pain questionnaire is designed to elicit information about physical aspects of the pain, its etiology, and previous treatment; about patients' thoughts and feelings regarding their capacity to exert some control over pain; and also about other aspects of their lives (e.g., prepain activities).

The questionnaire is also designed to help patients view their pain as episodic, as having a definite beginning, middle, and end. It encourages a view of pain not as life-threatening, but as controllable, fluid, and responsive to the passage of time, life events, and situational factors. Items are constructed so as to maximize their informational content, while stimulating patients to reflect upon and begin reevaluate their pain experience and the factors impinging upon it.

This initial inquiry also serves the purpose of legitimizing the patient's pain as real, and not as "just psychological." Many patients are concerned that seeking help from a psychologist or mental health worker means that their pain will not be taken seriously. This attitude may be fostered by the referral agent, who may be frustrated by the problems posed by patients with chronic pain. Such patients can challenge the health care provider's skills and often fail to benefit from the most concerted therapeutic efforts (e.g., see Sternbach, 1974a; Szasz, 1968). As a result, the physician's attitude and manner of referring (e.g., a last resort, passing along a "difficult" patient) may reflect these frustrations. This is one reason why careful "nurturing" (i.e., educating and support) of the referral agent is so important, as noted previously.

A SITUATIONAL AND COGNITIVE-AFFECTIVE ANALYSIS

From the initial data, we move toward more specific information, which will be used to carry out a situational and cognitive–affective analysis of the presenting problem. The general content of this stage of inquiry is illustrated by a clinical interview outline (Table 9-2) provided by D. Peterson (1968) and by questions suggested by Murphy (1978), among others:

1. What does your pain feel like? How would you describe your pain?
2. When does your pain occur?
3. Is the pain you feel continuous or intermittent?
4. When is your pain worse?
5. What makes your pain worse?
6. What makes you feel better?
7. What does your pain keep you from doing?
8. What do you do less frequently than you used to because of your pain? What do you do more frequently?
9. What have you done to relieve the pain?
10. What effect does medication have on your pain?
11. Why have you come to see me at this time?

TABLE 9-2. *Clinical Interview*[a]

I. Definition of problem behavior
    A. Nature of the problem as defined by client
        "As I understand it, you came here because. . . ." (Discuss reasons for contact as stated by referral agency or other source of information.) "I would like you to tell me more about this. What is the problem as you see it?" (Probe as needed to determine client's view of the problem behavior, i.e., what he or she is doing, or failing to do, that the client or somebody else defines as a problem.)
    B. Severity of the problem
        1. "How serious a problem is this as far as you are concerned?" (Probe to determine client's view of the problem behavior, i.e., what he or she is doing, or failing to do, or somebody else defines as a problem.)
        2. "How often do you (exhibit problem behavior if a disorder of commission, or have occasion to exhibit desired behavior if a problem of omission)?" (The goal is to obtain information regarding frequency of response.)
    C. Generality of the problem
        1. Duration
        "How long has this been going on?"
        2. Extent
        "Where does the problem usually come up?" (Probe to determine situations in which problem behavior occurs, e.g., "Do you feel that way at work? How about at home?")
II. Determinants of problem behavior
    A. Conditions that intensify problem behavior
        "Now I want you to think about the times when (the problem) is worst. What sorts of things are going on then?"
    B. Conditions that alleviate problem behavior
        "What about the times when (the problem) gets better? What sorts of things are going on then?"
    C. Perceived origins
        "What do you think is causing (the problem)?"
    D. Specific antecedents
        "Think back to the last time (the problem) occurred. What was going on at that time?"
        As needed:
        1. Social influences
        "Were any other people around? Who? What were they doing?"
        2. Personal influences
        "What were you thinking about at the time? How did you feel?"
    E. Specific consequences
        "What happened after (the problem occurred)?"
        As needed:
        1. Social consequences
        "What did (significant others identified above) do?"

TABLE 9-2. (*Continued*)

2. Personal consequences
"How did that make you feel?"
F. Suggested changes
"You have thought a lot about (the problem). What do you think might be done to improve the situation?"
G. Suggested leads for further inquiry
"What else do you think I should find out about to help you with this problem?"

[a]From Peterson, D. *The clinical study of social behavior.* Englewood Cliffs, N.J.: Prentice-Hall, Inc., 1968, pp. 121–122. Copyright 1968, Prentice-Hall, Inc. Reprinted by permission.

Another important concern for the therapist is the nature of the patient's emotional state. Intense feelings of depression and anxiety are often evident. The therapist must be sensitive in assessing the presence of suicidal ideation and a depressive state. A number of assessment devices have been used, including self-report measures (e.g., the Beck Depression Inventory or the Zung Depression Questionnaire) and behavioral data drawn from interview data and from reports about *in vivo* behavior. These measures have been described in A. Beck *et al.* (1979).

Lefebvre (1981) has underscored the role of depression in patients with chronic low back pain. Using various measures of cognitive distortions that are evident in depressed patients, Lefebvre found that similar cognitive distortions characterize the thinking style of chronic low-back-pain patients. Although it may be that certain low-back-pain patients become depressed as a reaction to their pain condition, Lefebvre's findings indicate that they still cognitively distort; thus a cognitive therapy component (A. Beck *et al.*, 1979) may be appropriate for low-back-pain patients as well as other pain patients.

Cameron and Shepel (1980) noted that eliciting patients' concerns—the unspoken fears that may impede therapeutic progress—can be particularly difficult with patients who may fear confirmation of their worries, who may fall into a passively helpless state, or who may feel that it is not their place to raise concerns because the medical staff will do whatever is necessary. Cameron and Shepel suggest that merely asking the patient for information may be less helpful in such instances than "normalizing" such fears, as in the following example:

I'd like to know what you think is causing your problem. Many of the people we see have private fears about what's wrong with them. If you have any nagging fears in the back of your mind, even fears you've hesitated to express because you know they're probably groundless, it's important that we know

about them. Many people who come to us have been worrying needlessly for
a long time and find it helpful to be able to bring their concerns out in the
open so they can be discussed. (p. 5)

Although the resolution of such fears is often handled by the diagnosis and treatment, some uncertainty may remain, especially in the cases of
idiopathic pain (pain without clear cause). The impact that such fears
have on the pain experience is a primary concern of the therapist.

An Image-Based Reconstruction

In addition to the situational analysis incorporated in the suggestions of
Murphy and D. Peterson, the therapist is interested in a cognitive–
affective analysis. The therapist may ask patients to share the thoughts
and feelings they have preceding, accompanying, and following a pain
episode or a period when pain is most intense. Patients can be asked to
close their eyes and imagine a recent instance in which the pain and the
accompanying affect were particularly severe. An example:

> Now, what I am going to ask you to do is a bit different. You have been
> answering a number of questions about your pain. In order for both of us to
> understand more fully the nature of your pain, I am going to ask you to sit
> back in the chair and become as relaxed as possible and to consider one of
> the times when your pain was most intense, when you felt most overwhelmed
> by your pain. You described several such examples.
>
> Let's see if we can more fully appreciate what is happening on such
> occasions. Just sit back now, close your eyes, and think about one such
> specific occasion. Do you have one in mind? OK. Now replay the entire
> incident in your mind's eye; sort of run a movie of the entire incident through
> your head, not just when the pain is most intense, but back in time before the
> pain reached that intense point, when you first noticed the sensations. Play
> the scene right through to the end.
>
> I would like you to describe any feelings, thoughts, or images you may
> have had before, during, or after the pain incident, even any passing thoughts
> and feelings, no matter how insignificant you think they may have been. Our
> goal is to come to understand the nature of your pain. Is it clear what I am
> asking you to do?

When patients close their eyes and use imagery, they are likely to attend
to aspects and details of the situation that might otherwise be overlooked
or underemphasized in a direct interview. Patients are directed to the
specifics, the particular thoughts, images, fantasies, and feelings that may
have been experienced in a given situation.

When this assessment is conducted on a group basis, each of the
participants is asked to engage in this imagery, retracing quietly, and then

one member is asked to do it once again aloud while the other members consider whether they have similar thoughts and feelings. Other members of the group may also be asked to replay their scenes. Such assessments may encourage the expression of material that patients are reluctant to share, and the therapist must judge whether the exercise should be delayed until a later session.

One approach is to assess patients initially on an individual basis for several sessions and then decide who will join the group intervention (viz., individual assessment followed by group treatment). Matching of treatment modality (e.g., individual, group, couples) has received little attention. Research is needed to help establish some guidelines for assisting in making such decisions (Turk & Kerns, 1980). At present, the therapist must rely on his or her clinical judgment as well as on available resources in making such decisions.

The following excerpt, from a patient, Sarah, who had suffered migraine headaches, illustrates the potential value of the clinical material obtained from such an imagery procedure:

> For hours and hours! God, will it ever end? How much longer do I have to live this way? I have outlived my capabilities . . . the hours are endless and I am alone. I wish someone could take a sharp scalpel and cut that artery. . . . How long will it be until I am sent to a mental institution? Migraines are not fatal; doctors do *not* care. You live through one, and there is another in a few days. I can't do anything I used to. How am I going to fill the rest of my life? I can't work, can do so little. More and more alone. Isolated.

This patient feels helpless: She views her situation as hopelessly leading to deterioration. She feels victimized by her pain. This material was utilized in our individualized treatment for Sarah. Additional emphasis in treatment was directed toward enhancing her perceptions of control and toward examining the impact of such thoughts and feelings on her experience of pain. We will be more specific about the use of this material in the next section.

Using the Imagery Data

Following the patient's (or patients') description of specific acute episodes, the therapist can empathically assist him or her in considering the impact that such thoughts and feelings might have on the pain experience, in reviewing other situations in which the patient has similar thoughts and feelings (i.e., conduct a situational analysis), and in generating possible means for altering the situation. At this point the intention is more to raise these issues than to find solutions. The line of inquiry can plant a seed of hopefulness in a course of action. The following exchange with the migraine patient, Sarah, illustrates how the imagery-based material can be used.

> *Therapist*: The headaches really seem to be getting you down.
> *Sarah*: Yes, sometimes I don't know what to do with myself.
> *Therapist*: These feelings . . . being alone, helpless—do you have
> them at other times, in other situations?
> *Sarah*: Almost always.
> *Therapist*: Are there times when the feelings become worse?
> *Sarah*: In the evenings when the headaches begin.
> *Therapist*: Tell me about those times.

After Sarah relates this material, and after the therapist has conducted a situational analysis and a historical–chronological analysis of these feelings and thoughts (viz., "When did these feelings begin?" etc.), the therapist may offer the following observation:

> On the one hand, I hear you saying—and correct me if I am wrong—that you are quite depressed and helpless, and on the other hand, you have these headaches. I am wondering how your feelings and thoughts affect your headaches, how these things might go together.

The point of this exchange is to have the therapist, by questions and juxtaposition of data that the patient has presented, raise the possibility that the patient's affective and cognitive reactions contribute to the pain problem. The rather straightforward presentation in this example is not always appropriate. During the initial interaction with the patient, one can evaluate how much the ground must be prepared before posing the relationship between psychological variables and the patient's own pain. The patient usually has a sense that the headaches are causing the dysphoric affect, but the converse—that the patient's affective and cognitive reactions contribute to the headaches—may not have been considered. The therapist's probes are designed to begin the reconceptualization process in which the patient plays an active role in contributing to his or her presenting problems and is not a helpless bystander or victim of the headaches or pain. As this reconceptualization emerges, one implication is that something could be done to change the behaviors, feelings, and thoughts that affect the pain experience.

It is our clinical experience that one should *not lecture the patient*. "Do you see what is happening? Your feelings are contributing to your headaches. It is clear from what you are saying." It is likely that significant others in the patient's life have offered such observations. Instead, the patient may be helped to marshal the data (recall that we are offering an evidential theory of change) that indicate the impact of his or her own behavior, feelings, and thoughts on the pain experience. This does not mean that the therapist should not sometimes offer a timely directive or assertion to the patient, but that the initial assessment phase should help the patient collect data that is persuasive and convincing.

Assisting Cognitive–Affective Productions

Not all patients have equal access to their thoughts and feelings, nor are all equally able to express them. In fact, some reports lead one to doubt that any ideation at all has taken place. Nevertheless, an initial paucity of verbal reports does *not* mean that a cognitive–behavioral treatment is inappropriate; rather, it suggests that the therapist use therapy sessions and homework assignments to help patients become more sensitive to their thoughts and feelings. If no progress occurs through these efforts, then a reassessment of mode of therapy is in order. Some patients, certainly, are not able to make effective use of an approach that makes demands on verbal and intellectual skills. However, it is important to appreciate that, even though some patients may not readily be able to produce these reactions during the initial phase of assessment, they may still be quite responsive to later interventions.

The therapist's sensitivity to patients' internal dialogues about treatment will help in avoiding the problem of therapeutic requests that lead to patients' "negative thinking" or definition of themselves as inappropriate candidates.

In addition to guidance in using the imagery, the therapist may provide some "soft" prompts to reticent or less psychologically minded patients:

> To help you reconstruct the pain incident, why don't you just first describe where you are, what you are doing, who else is present as you begin to experience the pain. . . . Now let's go back and replay that scene one more time, but this time, if possible, share any accompanying thoughts and feelings you might have had.

Therapist prompts may include questions such as the following: What were you thinking about? How were you feeling? Was there anything else going on? Can you tell me more about that?

Even if these prompts and supports do not elicit cognitive and affective material, the therapist can proceed by conveying to the patient that learning to analyze more fully how one feels and thinks in a situation is a skill and that, like any other skill, it must be learned with practice.

The therapist conveys that the patient will begin to become more in tune with such experiences as therapy progresses. Finally, if this therapeutic suggestion is also rejected, or if the patient has not initially offered cognitive and affective material about the pain experience, the therapist can implement the various techniques described.

The Need for Additional Data Sources

The interview and questionnaire-based assessment we have described must be supplemented by more objective behavioral assessment procedures. Self-monitoring and observation, reporting on medication, urinary assays of medication use, "uptime" (i.e., non-pain-related activities), and so on, are other useful sources of data. Significant others, such as the patient's spouse, children, or employees, also play an important role in the assessment process.

Pain Behaviors

Pain behaviors lead an observer to label the individual as being "in pain." One can separate pain behaviors into three categories: *pain complaints*, such as verbalizing the presence of pain, complaining, moaning, grimacing; *impaired functioning*, such as reduction of activities, avoidance of certain activities, impaired interpersonal and sexual relationships; and *somatic interventions*, such as taking medication, seeking treatment. Fordyce (1976) discusses the use of monitoring devices, such as diaries, performance records, graphs, and mechanical counters, that can be used for recording by patients, their spouses and other family members, and treatment staff. It is important to record not only pain behaviors, but also incompatible "uptime" or well behaviors. For example, in one study Brena and Unikel (1976) recorded patients' displays of walking, household chore performance, and participation in active sports. (See Bradley, Prokop, Gentry, Hopson, & Prieto, 1981, for a fuller discussion of assessment alternatives with chronic pain patients.)

Fordyce (1976) has been a prominent advocate of focusing the assessment procedure on pain behaviors, arguing that verbal reports of pain are subjective and unverifiable because they are likely to be subject to distortions and are unrelated to identified physical damage. We agree with Fordyce on the necessity for a careful and thorough assessment of pain behaviors. We would nevertheless argue that pain *behaviors* are also subject to distortions and that their reliability has not been adequately demonstrated (e.g., Block, Kremer, & Gaylor, 1980; Bradley *et al.* 1981; Turk & Kerns, 1980). Pain patients are able to control behavior at low and moderate levels of pain, and thus the behavior may not adequately reflect the actual intensity of the pain being experienced.

Another concern is that, in evaluating overt behavior, the degree of pain becomes confounded with the patient's success in coping. Protective actions taken by patients in an attempt to relieve or avoid pain may be construed as pain behaviors. Such behaviors may be increases in body activity, such as rubbing or supporting a painful area, frequent change in body position, pacing, and so on, or they may be reductions of activity, such as resting an extremity, protecting an area from stimulation, and decreasing body movement. These active attempts to relieve pain may be contrasted with pain behaviors such as grimacing, moaning, or crying, which more directly communicate distress and suffering.

Distinguishing efforts to cope from pain behaviors may be difficult. Pain behavior for one patient may be an attempt to cope by another patient. How pain behaviors are defined, and whether they should be viewed as inappropriate and thus as the focus of change, is a major issue that has not been addressed sufficiently. Although assessment of pain behaviors is important in understanding the pain experience, it is insufficient by itself and should be included within the broader pain assessment, such as we outline. Behavioral assessment alone cannot provide information about various sensory and affective qualities that may be essential for determining etiology, about the choice of treatment employed to reduce pain, or about other such aspects.

Each of the separate pain assessment procedures provides a valuable source of information, but each is inadequate in itself to provide a comprehensive assessment of pain. Together the procedures provide a portrait of the pain experienced by the patient and should facilitate diagnosis and decisions regarding treatment. We will later discuss defining the specific measurable behavioral goals and assessment of treatment progress in terms of achieving these objectives. To establish such joint patient–therapist goals, it is first necessary to develop a better appreciation of the situational impact of the patient's behavior. As Fordyce (1976) has noted, the patterning of a patient's pain in the environmental and social context can offer a great deal of information about the impact of medication, interpersonal interactions, reinforcement schedules, and potential avenues for viable intervention. One way of obtaining this information is through the use of pain intensity ratings.

Pain Intensity Rating Cards

A useful assessment procedure, which involves the patient as a collaborator in the collection of information, is to have the patient monitor pain intensity between sessions. For this purpose, we have used pain intensity rating cards (see Figure 9-1) to provide a 2-week baseline. The format for these cards follows the guidelines offered by Budzynski *et al.* (1973).

The cards contain the hours of the day and a 6-point scale of pain intensity, with 0 equal to no pain, and 5 equal to excruciating, severe, incapacitating pain. Patients are asked to rate the intensity of the pain they experience during each waking hour. It should be noted that the adjectives (excruciating, horrible, distressing, discomforting, and mild) used on the pain intensity scale have been chosen very carefully. Melzack (1975a) has demonstrated that these five adjectives or anchor points constitute an equal-interval scale. This provides an important quantitative basis for evaluating changes in self-reports of pain before and after treatment. Space is provided for recording the times medication is taken, as well as the thoughts and feelings that accompany intense pain.

The following is an example of a patient's introduction to this procedure by the therapist:

I would like you to keep an hourly record of your pain. Here are seven cards [if a 2-week period is used between initial sessions, then 14 cards are given], one for each of the days before our next session. The record keeping is quite easy and straightforward. It consists of rating your pain each hour on a 3-inch by 5-inch card. On the card you will see, first, that the hours of the day are indicated on the top, going from 6 A.M. to 5 A.M., so that each card covers the full 24 hours of 1 day.

Second, as you will notice, under each hour of the day are listed the numbers 0 to 5. These refer to the severity of your pain:

5 indicates intense, incapacitating pain. The pain is so severe that you can do almost nothing. You consider the pain *excruciating*.

4 represents a very severe pain attack that makes concentration difficult, but you can do some tasks or something that is undemanding. You consider the pain *horrible*.

3 is painful, but you are able to continue at your job or whatever you were doing. You consider the pain *distressing*.

2 represents a pain level that can be ignored at times. You consider the pain *discomforting*.

1 represents a very low level of pain that enters awareness only at times when attention is devoted to it. You consider the pain *mild*.

0 represents *no pain*.

These ratings are summarized on the back of each card.

I would like you to rate your pain each waking hour of the day. That is, at the end of each hour, think back over the last hour and rate your pain on the 0-to-5 scale. Rate the intensity of the pain you experienced. Was the pain excruciating? If so, circle the number 5 under the hour you are rating. Was the pain horrible, but could you occupy yourself with undemanding tasks? Then circle the number 4. You can similarly use the ratings of 0, 1, 2, and 3 to describe how the pain affects you. On the back of the card is a key to the severity-of-pain scale. What rating would you give to your pain right now? Look at the card and decide on a rating. This is what I would like you to do each hour that you are awake. After you do it several times, you will see that it takes very little time to make such ratings.

You should only rate yourself for the waking hours. If you do wake up, you can indicate this on the back of the card, where comments are asked for. Under the comments section, indicate whether you got up because of the pain and the intensity of the pain. In addition, please feel free to make any additional comments about the kinds of pain you are having—for example, are they of the dull, aching type, or do they quickly come and go?

I would also like you to indicate each time you take medication to reduce your pain by simply marking an $\times$ over the rating for that hour. For example, if you take some medicine at 2 P.M., and if you have rated your pain a 4, mark the 4 with an $\times$. In the space provided on the back of the card, write the name and the amount of medication you took and also the time you took each dose. [The therapist ensures that the patient understands how to use the pain rating cards.]

It is important for you to keep the rating card with you and to get in the habit of rating yourself each waking hour. You should *not* fill out in the evening the ratings for a whole day. Rather, rate each and every hour. If you somehow forget the card, then jot down your hourly ratings on a piece of paper and copy them onto the card later. This information will be most valuable for our understanding of the nature of your pain. If you forget to rate your pain, don't try to fill in the previous hours' ratings; just continue the ratings.

Finally, be sure to put your name on each card, as well as the date (e.g., Thursday, December 10, or whatever day and month it is). You should begin your ratings from whenever you wake up tomorrow and continue them for the next 7 days [14 days].

The therapist then reviews the cards with the patient and engages him or her in a discussion to check that the patient understands what is expected, why the homework assignment is being given, what kinds of problems may be expected in implementing the self-monitoring, and possible solutions to these problems. *A homework assignment is never given without the therapist's providing a rationale and checking with the patient about his or her comprehension and discussing the possible problems with its implementation.*

Typical problems that emerge during use of the pain intensity ratings include (1) possible confusion about the nature of the 6-point scale and

Front

Name: _____ Date: _____

Note: Key and space for comments on back.

Time

	a.m.						p.m.												a.m.					
	6	7	8	9	10	11	12	1	2	3	4	5	6	7	8	9	10	11	12	1	2	3	4	5
Level of pain	5	5	5	5	5	5	5	5	5	5	5	5	5	5	5	5	5	5	5	5	5	5	5	5
	4	4	4	4	4	4	4	4	4	4	4	4	4	4	4	4	4	4	4	4	4	4	4	4
	3	3	3	3	3	3	3	3	3	3	3	3	3	3	3	3	3	3	3	3	3	3	3	3
	2	2	2	2	2	2	2	2	2	2	2	2	2	2	2	2	2	2	2	2	2	2	2	2
	1	1	1	1	1	1	1	1	1	1	1	1	1	1	1	1	1	1	1	1	1	1	1	1
	0	0	0	0	0	0	0	0	0	0	0	0	0	0	0	0	0	0	0	0	0	0	0	0

Circle your level of pain each hour you are awake.
Put an × through the times you take pain medication.

Back

5 = excruciating, incapacitating, intense, severe
4 = horrible; pain severe, but undemanding tasks possible; concentration difficult
3 = distressing; painful, but able to continue job
2 = discomforting; pain can be ignored at times
1 = mild; low-level pain only when attended to
0 = none; no pain

Comments:

Example (front)

Name: Mary Jones   Date: 12/10/81

Note: Key and space for comments on back.

Time

	a.m.						p.m.												a.m.					
	6	7	8	9	10	11	12	1	2	3	4	5	6	7	8	9	10	11	12	1	2	3	4	5
Level of pain	5	5	5	5	5	5	5	5	5	5	5	5	5	5	(⊗)	(5)	5	5	5	5	5	5	5	5
	4	4	4	4	4	4	(4)	(⊗)	4	4	4	4	4	(4)	4	4	4	4	4	4	4	(⊗)	4	4
	3	3	3	3	3	(3)	3	3	(3)	3	3	3	3	3	3	3	(3)	3	3	3	3	3	3	3
	2	2	2	2	2	2	2	2	2	2	2	2	(2)	2	2	2	2	(2)	2	2	2	2	2	2
	1	1	(1)	1	(1)	1	1	1	1	(1)	1	1	1	1	1	1	1	1	1	1	1	1	1	1
	0	0	0	(0)	0	0	0	0	0	0	(0)	(0)	0	0	0	0	0	0	0	0	0	0	0	0

Circle your level of pain each hour you are awake.
Put an × through the times you take pain medication.

FIGURE 9-1. (*Continued*)

Example (back)
5 = excruciating, incapacitating, intense, severe
4 = horrible; pain severe, but undemanding tasks possible; concentration difficult
3 = distressing; painful, but able to continue job
2 = discomforting; pain can be ignored at times
1 = mild; low-level pain only when attended to
0 = none; no pain

Comments:
1 p.m. took 2 Tylenol.
8 p.m. took 2 Darvon.
3 a.m. took 2 Darvon and 1 Tylenol.
Awoke briefly at 3:15 a.m. Lots of pain, which lasted 15 minutes. I put a heating pad on my shoulder.

FIGURE 9-1. *Pain intensity rating card.*

when one should use the extreme points; (2) how one remembers to use the cards; (3) what the patient should do when someone else sees him or her making a rating; (4) forgetting to fill out the cards for one or more periods and using this as evidence of being incapacitated or unsuited for this treatment; and (5) what to do if the patient reports that he or she is in such a mood that everything seems to be a chore, including keeping track of the ratings and filling out the other questionnaires and the diary. If patients do not exert the effort needed to undertake these assessment techniques, then it is unlikely that they will manifest sufficient motivation to implement the more demanding exercises and activities given later. The therapist can anticipate whether an unmotivated state is likely and can bring this up during the discussion. For example:

> I am not sure this will apply in your case, but some patients who have participated in our program began by conscientiously recording the information, even enjoying becoming their own Sherlock Holmes in figuring out the nature of their pain. But for a small group, the person's pain and his or her mood seemed to make this effort at recording feel like a real chore, a burden. It was becoming too much and some sense of—how shall I describe it?— helplessness, hopelessness set in. Has this been the case in your own situation?

If the patient reports such problems, then the therapist and patient discuss what thoughts, feelings, and circumstances are contributing to this state and what can be done about it. As we noted in the previous chapter, noncompliance is seen as the occasion to engage in problem solving, not the occasion to catastrophize.

One way to determine the presence of problems such as these is to have the patient describe to the therapist how the cards are to be employed and what the patient's task is to be, following the therapist's initial discussion of the rating procedure. The therapist can even ask the patient to tell how he or she would describe the use of the ratings to another patient. In this manner, the therapist can clarify any obvious misunderstandings. The therapist can also suggest potential difficulties to the patient and ask the patient to generate ways that these difficulties could be handled. A Socratic manner permits the therapist to help generate personally relevant approaches rather than simply offer suggestions. For example, the therapist might say:

> Now that you seem to have a good handle on how to use the rating cards and on what you are supposed to do, I'm wondering what you might do if someone sees you pulling a card out of your pocket and marking on it, and then asks you what you are doing? What might you say?

If patients have difficulty responding to this question, the therapist may offer several alternatives and ask whether these suggested responses would be useful and whether the patient would be likely to make such responses. The alternatives suggested by the therapist might include something as simple as "I'm just trying to gather some information related to my back pain (headaches, etc.)" or "This is information I need to collect to help develop a management program for my pain problem."

The therapist might also note that some patients have reported that they forgot to complete the cards for several hours. The therapist can ask what the patient might do should this happen to him or her. The important point to convey is that, even if patients forget to complete the ratings for some period, they should begin to record the pain intensity as soon as they realize the oversight and should *not* give up the task completely because of such a lapse in memory. The patient should *not* go back and fill in prior missed ratings because of the low reliability of retrospective reports.

The therapist and patient can consider memory aids for filling out cards. Some possibilities are placing a piece of colored tape on a watch face as a reminder or placing reminders at strategic points, such as on the television or refrigerator. Engaging the patient in developing such reminders should enhance the therapeutic relationship, engender patient participation and responsibility, and short-circuit potential problems before they arise.

There is a need to obtain baseline data for at least a week, and preferably 2 weeks, in order to determine if there are any patterns in the pain intensity reports, such as variations tied to specific days or times of day, activities, or medication. For some patients a 2-week period may be used between contacts. However, if the pain is very severe, if there is intense affect such as severe depression or suicidal ideation, or if there is some concern about the patient's compliance with monitoring over a 2-

week period without further contact, an appointment may be scheduled sooner. A telephone contact may also be useful. Completion of such homework assignments provides a useful indication of future compliance problems. Failure to comply may lead to a discussion of reasons and an emphasis on the importance of this material in the development of the best therapeutic regimen.

A Note on Reliability

The therapist should not, of course, assume that completed rating cards reflect a patient's reliable compliance with the pain reporting procedure. An investigation by Collins and Thompson (1979) of the reliability of self-reports of headache pain suggests the need for caution in collecting and using such data. Through relatively unobtrusive detection techniques, these authors were able to detect 50 of 124 subjects (40%) as having been noncompliant at least once in making ratings of their headaches *four times a day* for 8 weeks. The mean number of detected instances of failure to rate for each subject was 2.42, with a range of from 1 to 8. Most of the detections indicated that subjects had filled out a whole day's ratings retrospectively (a day or more later); some ratings were even made ahead of time. The findings are particularly significant when one considers that the procedures for data collection used in the study were ones that the authors believed would, on the basis of the available information, "facilitate reliable responding and accurate headache information while placing a minimum of demand on subjects" (p. 77).

Often, the procedures used clinically may place considerable demands upon patients (such as making hourly ratings). Noncompliance can have an impact on the patient's data and on the assessment process in general. Further, the data for the Collins and Thompson study are likely to be conservative estimates of noncompliance, since several sorts of noncompliance were not detectable by their procedures. For example, headaches are infrequent events, and thus it is quite easy to forget to complete pain intensity ratings. However, chronic, intractable pain is present at least at some level most of the time and is less likely to be forgotten. We would like to see the Collins and Thompson study replicated with other forms of pain and with different populations.

To maximize compliance with pain ratings (or ratings of other, similar variables), one may attempt to keep the demands of the method to a minimum while attempting to provide some memory aid. The use of small rating cards such as we have suggested is one means of accomplishing this. The cards are small enough to be convenient to carry, yet their constant presence can help to remind the patient to make ratings.

We have had patients mail in cards daily, and in some cases have reduced the number of ratings from hourly to only several times a day (e.g., upon waking, at meals, and at bedtime). Research is needed to examine the efficacy of these procedures.

Two other examples further illustrate the difficulty in obtaining reliable data. Taylor, Zlutnick, Corley, and Flora (1980) recently found that all nine patients who had completed a pain treatment program reported substantial reductions in consumption of analgesic medication at a 3-month follow-up. An analysis of analgesic levels in the patients' urine revealed that eight of the nine patients had in fact continued to take large quantities of analgesics despite their reports to the contrary.

If lapses in patients' self-reports are not enough to contend with, consider the demand characteristics of the assessment procedures. Harris and Monaco (1978) commented that the kinds of questions we ask patients influence the nature of the answers. Harris and Monaco cite a study by Loftus (1975), who asked subjects (who were not headache patients) either (1) Do you get headaches *frequently*, and if so, how often? or (2) Do you get headaches *occasionally*, and if so, how often? Subjects questioned with (1) reported a mean of 2.2 headaches per week, whereas those questioned with (2) reported only .7 headaches per week. These findings call for caution in the interpretation of self-report data. Undaunted, the therapist nonetheless proceeds with caution, using self-report data (e.g., pain intensity ratings) for clinical purposes. Perhaps it is comforting, though dismaying, to realize that behavioral and physiological measures have their own reliability and validity problems. There is *no* easy or right way to measure the subjective experience of pain. Convergent measures are clearly indicated (cf. Meichenbaum & Butler, 1979).

Clinical Use of Ratings

The pain intensity rating cards are designed both to collect data and to ensure that patients and their significant others (family, spouse, boss, etc.) are aware of the relative fluctuations in pain. Patients rarely experience the most intense pain (ratings of 5) over extended periods. Instead, the intensity of the pain ebbs and flows. In our experience, no patient has ever reported the intensity to be at level 5 every waking hour over a 2-week baseline period. Patients often find this fact to be quite surprising in view of their earlier descriptions of the pain.

Family and significant others may also benefit from information obtained from the pain intensity ratings. The wife of one patient believed that her husband was experiencing incapacitating and severe pain every waking hour of his life. This belief contributed to her preventing him from participating in any but the simplest chores around the house. Their social life had deteriorated, and the couple had grown increasingly depressed over the course of 4 years. Upon hearing that her husband experienced only moderate pain most of the time, that he indeed felt capable of various tasks, and that he actually resented his wife's efforts at pampering him, she was helped to alter her behavior. Misunderstandings of this sort do not always have such dramatic consequences, but it is best to monitor the family's involvement in the situation. We will have more to say about the involvement of significant others in the asessment process in the next chapter.

The rating cards also provide an opportunity to determine whether the pain intensity follows any particular pattern either at various times of the day or on specific days. For some patients pain is typically severest during the evening, when they are tired and have little in which to involve themselves. Is this pattern ever broken? If so, what breaks it? Have there perhaps been occasions on which patients have been totally occupied by something during a typically "bad" time, and afterwards noted that they "missed" the pain that evening? Does the pain vary in any particular manner? In the case of one young woman who had arm and shoulder pain resulting from a fall several years earlier, the pain was severest on Wednesdays and Fridays. We were able to establish that she was involved in team teaching on Tuesdays and Thursdays and that she was having a great deal of conflict with her teaching partner.

The therapist may assist patients in achieving such "insight" into the possible connection between certain situational events, such as conflict, and the variability in pain. As noted, the approach we favor uses clinically sensitive questions and the juxtaposition of bits of data (such as the information obtained from the situational analysis and the pain intensity ratings) to have patients entertain the notion that the pain they experience is indeed complex and subject to a variety of influences. This assessment process helps patients to collect the data that will lead to their own alteration of their conceptualization of pain. This reconceptualization will provide the basis for the treatment rationale to be offered. The therapist might use the following approach to help patients achieve insight:

> You have done a fine job completing these pain rating cards. Let's look at them together. I wonder if you have noted anything special about what you have recorded. [Patients often fail to see any patterns, so the therapist might proceed.] As I look at these, several things seem apparent. For example, you noted that you took your pain medication at different times, but sometimes you took the medication when you rated your pain as 5 (severe, excruciating), and other times as 3 (distressing, yet you were able to complete tasks you

were working on). At still other times when you rated the pain as 5, you did not taken any medication. What determines when you will take medication, and when you won't?

Or the therapist might say:

Some patients have indicated that they have started taking medication at certain times more out of habit than because of the pain, and other patients have told us that they take medication when they are feeling depressed rather than when the pain is severest. How would you describe your taking medication?

Another tactic might include the following:

Something else I can see from your ratings is that your pain seems to be rated as severest between 5 P.M. and 6 P.M. Is there anything special going on in your house at this time of day?

Or consider the way Fordyce (1976) queries patients about what happens when they awaken during the night with pain. Fordyce asks, "If I were there when you awakened, what would I see and hear?" (p. 126). Similarly, with regard to tapping daytime interpersonal behaviors, Fordyce asks, "If I were in your living room when you were present experiencing pain, what would I see you do and what would I see those around you do and hear you say?" (p. 127). We have found that such questions help solicit needed behavioral data.

Many patients have been able to report that certain events consistently occur simultaneously with increases in pain. One patient noted that the pain always seemed to be worse around the time her husband came home from work. When the therapist asked her what she thought might be the cause of this, she reported that she always described her day and the amount of suffering she had endured to her husband at this time. The therapist followed this up by asking what impact such complaining might have on others as well as on her own pain. The patient admitted that perhaps her talking about her pain made her focus on it more and that attending to the pain made it worse. The patient also acknowledged that her husband's typical response was sympathy and concern and that she liked the extra attention he gave when she described a particularly bad day. At this point the therapist raised the possibility that the patient's talking about pain and the extra attention might be related to the regular occurrence of the more intense pain recorded at this time of the day.

The therapist continued by noting that the patient had rated the pain as being particularly severe during one afternoon and evening: "I'm wondering what was going on last Wednesday when your pain was particularly severe. What was different about Wednesday?" The patient recalled that she had had a fight with her mother-in-law that morning. The therapist questioned the patient about any relationship between the fight and the pain intensity. The therapist also asked what the patient's thoughts and feelings had been prior to, during, and following the acute pain episode. The patient acknowledged that she had been angry and had felt that she was not receiving any support from her mother-in-law, who was always critical of her. The therapist continued by asking whether the patient had recorded any other conflicts in her pain diary (to be described later) and whether there was any relationship between pain and conflicts or stress. Examination of the pain records revealed that this was the case, and the patient was able to note this relationship.

The pain rating cards and accompanying notes are particularly useful in making many points about the relationship between pain and the responses of others, the use of medication, and conflict and stress. Repeated pain intensity ratings also prove useful in assessing patients' medication regimens. Rather than the patient's taking medication at regular time intervals (e.g., three times a day) or PRN, it is possible to help him or her to plan and implement medication times based upon periods preceding the most intense pain. In this way, use of medication may become increasingly situation-dependent rather than being pain-focused. This helps to convey further a sense of control through predictability; peaks and troughs of pain, once recognized, are amenable to self-management strategies. Peaks may be modified in a variety of ways. Troughs may be put to better, more satisfying use with more effective use of analgesic medication. This will help to reduce a mindless dependence on analgesics and to contribute to withdrawal from medication, often a goal of treatment.

The pain ratings can also be used in planning the use of other coping skills such as relaxation, controlled breathing exercises, and attention-diversion techniques. The cognitive and behavioral coping skills may be substituted for medication. For example, if the ratings revealed that the patient's pain was severest at 10:00 A.M., the patient might program relaxation exercises at 9:30 A.M. Other such examples will be given in later chapters.

When treatment is conducted on a group basis, the pain intensity records may be used as a basis for group discussion. The therapist can encourage members to share with each other their respective pain records and then begin to speculate on reasons for the changes in pain levels. In this way, the group members themselves can begin to suggest some of the complex relationships among behavior, cognitions, affect, environmental events, and pain, which will form the basis for later interventions. The therapist can guide the members of the group in conducting detailed situational analyses of their pain in which they attempt to identify environmental events that influence pain intensity or pain *intrusiveness*.

Throughout this discussion, the therapist can encourage group members to view the formulation of their problems and strategy planning as cooperative efforts, not as interpretations and techniques rigidly imposed on them by the therapist. In this view, Cameron (1978) noted the following:

> The client is likely to be resistant to attempts to educate him if he believes that the therapist is mechanically imposing a prefabricated conceptualization upon his problem. . . . While it is undoubtedly advantageous for a therapist to be enthusiastic with clients, clients need to believe that they can honestly report lack of understanding, misgivings, or lack of progress. (p. 243)

Pain Diary

A pain diary (see Figure 9-2) is another means by which to have the patient collect data that can be used to contribute to a reconceptualization. This diary, which should be kept on a daily basis, can be used in combination with the pain intensity ratings. The therapist may introduce the diary in the following manner:

> Since each patient is different, and since it is important for both of us to understand your pain in as much detail as possible so we can choose the correct treatment program, I would like you to keep a daily diary of your pain behavior. Have you ever kept a diary before? . . . Well, the diary I am going to ask you to keep is very simple. It involves answering a few questions about your pain each day. It does not take much time. Other patients like yourself have indicated that the diary information proved quite revealing and helpful. Let me explain what is involved.

The pain diary is then given to the patient, who is asked to keep it for one or two weeks prior to beginning the pain-management program. The diary should be kept on a daily basis. The diary may be employed at treatment termination and follow-up as well. The therapist then gives the following instructions to the patient:

To help us learn more about the nature of your pain, it is important that you keep careful records. This diary is designed to provide detailed information about periods when your pain is severest, periods when your pain is least severe, and the use and effectiveness of your pain medication. This information will help us develop the most effective treatment for your pain.

There are two things I would like you to do between now and your next appointment. These are in addition to your completion of the pain intensity ratings.

1. On the sheets provided, note the time, the place, and who is present every time your pain rises to its *highest level* (the highest level you rate the pain on the pain intensity rating cards). We would like you to describe what you think might have led to the increase in pain (e.g., physical activity, a change in the weather, an argument). You should also try to list any thoughts or feelings you had that were related to the pain at that time (e.g., "Here it goes again," "I can't take it," "I feel so helpless," "Nobody understands"). Next, I would like you to note what you tried to do to relieve the pain (e.g., took some pain killers, asked someone to massage the painful area, took a hot bath). Finally, I would like you to note how effective your efforts to relieve the pain actually were. Rate how much you think your action helped, using the following scale: 0 = did not help at all; 1 = helped very little; 2 = helped somewhat; 3 = helped a lot; 4 = eliminated the pain completely.

2. I would like you to provide information about times when your pain is *least severe*: when this was, where you were, what you were doing, who was with you, and anything else you can recall about the situation.

Remember, this information is important if we are to understand your pain and to develop the most effective treatment for you. If you have any questions, do not hesitate to ask.

A Behavioral Trial

Another assessment technique that may be useful is a behavioral trial in which pain patients are exposed to laboratory-induced pain. A medical status report (e.g., from the referring physician) should be completed before the use of a behavioral trial. This medical report can provide information about realistic treatment goals as well as guidelines for the behavioral assessment.

Among the available means of safely inducing experimental pain, perhaps the most useful, because of their close similarity to a chronic pain, are muscle ischemia, with its slowly mounting deep pain (Smith *et al.*, 1966; Sternbach, Deems, Timmermans, & Huey, 1977), and cold water (the cold-pressor task), which produces a much more rapidly mounting pain (Kunckle, 1949; Lovallo, 1975). Sternbach and his colleagues (Sternbach, 1974b; Sternbach *et al.*, 1977) report that they routinely provide "a physical stimulus against which the patient may match his clinical pain" (Sternbach 1974b, p. 283). The behavior trial may be conducted in different ways.

Sternbach (1974b; Sternbach *et al.*, 1977) reported using a muscle-ischemic *tourniquet pain ratio,* calculated by dividing the matched tourni-

Severe pain

Name: _____   Date: _____

1. Time when pain was most severe: _____
2. Where were you? _____
3. What were you doing? _____
4. Who was with you? _____
5. What were you feeling and thinking just prior to and during the severe pain? ____
   _____
   _____
   _____

6. What did you do to try to reduce the pain? _____

7. How effective was this? (Circle the appropriate number.)
   0 = did not help at all
   1 = helped very little
   2 = helped somewhat
   3 = helped a lot
   4 = stopped the pain
8. Additional comments:

Lowest-level pain

Name: _____   Date: _____

1. Time when pain was at the lowest level for the day: _____
2. Where were you? _____
3. What were you doing? _____
4. Who was with you? _____
5. Additional comments:

FIGURE 9-2. *Patient diary.*

quet time (the elapsed time when the tourniquet pain matches the clinical pain) by the subject's total tolerance for the tourniquet. This is then used to indicate what ratio the clinical pain is to the maximum tolerable pain. A very low ratio is taken to suggest that the patient is overreacting to pain that is not very severe. For example, if a subject tolerated the tourniquet 10 minutes and indicated that at 5 minutes the pain was equal to his or her clinical pain, say back pain, then the pain ratio would be 50%.

There are some problems associated with this technique. The Sternbach *ratio* measure suggests that pain is a linear function of time, that the pain produced by the tourniquet after 20 minutes, for example, is one-half of that produced after 40 minutes, or 5 minutes is one-half of 10 minutes. There is evidence that this is *not* the case, but that the pain of muscle ischemia more closely approximates a power function (Fox, Steger, & Jennison, 1979; E. Hilgard *et al.,* 1967; Moore, Duncan, Scott, Gregg, & Ghia, 1979; Turk, 1977). As a result, the tourniquet pain ratio provides a misleading estimate of mild pain (the parts of the power function curve that vary the most from linear). Furthermore, as Sternbach has noted (Sternbach *et al.,* 1977), there is extreme variability in the tolerance for muscle ischemia, rendering comparisons among patients or subjects difficult.

Moore *et al.* (1979) have also noted that minor variations in procedure can have a considerable impact on the pain reported during the ischemia task. For example, prior to the administration of the muscle ischemia, the subject is asked to squeeze a hand dynamometer in order to deplete oxygen in the arm. This results in a more accelerated onset of the muscle-ischemic pain. Recent research by Moore *et al.* (1979) has indicated that squeezing the hand exercise for .6 seconds versus 2 seconds each time, or that using 30% of maximum effort to squeeze the dynamometer versus 50%, differentially affects the subject's pain tolerance. Such results do not preclude the use of the behavioral matching technique, but they do suggest caution in interpreting the results and invite further methodological investigations.

Although we do not see the behavioral assessment as crucial to the intervention, we have found its inclusion often quite helpful. Obviously, practical considerations such as the availability of laboratory equipment, space, personnel, and time will dictate whether such an assessment is included. We have treated patients both who have and who have not been assessed by means of the behavioral trial, but unfortunately, we do not have sufficient data to analyze what role this assessment procedure plays in the treatment regimen. Appendix A describes the specific equipment to be used and the steps and precautions to be followed in the cold-pressor and muscle-ischemic pain-induction procedures.

The behavioral test is introduced to the pain patient with elaboration depending on the patient's response:

> You are currently experiencing pain, and I have asked you to describe that pain in various ways, and that has been quite helpful for me in terms of understanding your pain. Something else that we have found helpful is asking a person to undertake a standardized painful task and to report what the experience is like. What I would like you to do, then, is to try immersing your hand and arm in circulating ice water, which causes some pain, but no actual harm to you, and to tell me in detail what that is like for you. You would simply place your hand and arm in the cold water and keep it there for

as long as you can, periodically reporting on the pain. Then afterwards, we will discuss what the sensations were like for you. In the past this has been helpful in understanding each individual's personal reactions to pain. [A similar format is used with the muscle-ischemic task.]

A behavioral trial on the muscle-ischemic or cold-pressor tasks provides the opportunity of making both the therapist and the patient aware of how the patient's thinking styles contribute to distress and pain. Following exposure to the laboratory-induced pain, the patient can be encouraged to discuss his or her pain in the context of the specific behavioral trial, in a similar way that the imagery procedure explored the situation, cognitions, and affect surrounding an imagined pain episode.

Meichenbaum (1977) has described this cognitive assessment procedure and its use in therapy, especially in a group session, as follows:

> The patient can explore in some detail his thoughts and feelings during the behavioral trial assessment situation. The clinician may try to have him ascertain what were the particular aspects of the environmental events that triggered specific thoughts and feelings, specific self-statements and images. At what point did the patient begin to feel pain? When was the pain most intense? What were the self-statements and images that the patient emitted at different points in the assessment? A group can explore common behaviors, thoughts, and feelings. A shared exploration of the common set of self-statements, and images, and feelings is quite valuable in having the patients come to appreciate the role thoughts and feelings play in the behavioral repertoire. The recognition that other individuals have similar thoughts and feelings, similar internal dialogues, provides an additional impetus for self-examination and self-disclosure. (p. 252)

In effect, what is being accomplished is a cognitive and affective analysis of pain behavior. A number of different assessment procedures may be used to help pain patients relate any thoughts and feelings they had in the behavioral test. One procedure is to videotape patients while they experience the experimentally induced stressor and afterwards to replay the videotape, asking patients to share any thoughts and feelings that they may have had before, during, and after experiencing the painful stimulus. In this reconstruction, the patient's pain intensity ratings and nonverbal behavior provide additional retrieval cues. If such videotape equipment is not available, then an imagery reconstruction may be used.

The following interview describes the procedures used to assess the flow of cognitions for the cold-pressor task. A similar procedure could be used for the muscle-ischemic task.

> One of the things we are interested in is what you were feeling and thinking while your hand was in the water. I am going to ask you a few questions

about thoughts, feelings, or anything that occurred to you while your hand and arm were in the water, and I would like you to answer in as much detail as you can. OK?

First of all, if you can, just imagine yourself back during the few moments just before you placed your hand in the water. What were you thinking and feeling at that time? Please tell me everything you can remember, even if your thoughts were brief or random, and even if they seem trivial. . . . Is there anything else?

If the patient reports being unable to recall anything when a question is posed, or if the patient responds to a question very briefly or with apparent difficulty in either formulating a response or remembering, then the therapist prompts with a question such as one of the following: "What were you thinking about?" "How were you feeling?" "Was there anything else going on?" "Can you tell me more about that?"

Also, if it is unclear whether a statement made during the interview is meant to be a report of a cognition that occurred during the cold-pressor task or is simply something that the patient is thinking of during the interview, the ambiguity should be resolved by a question such as "Were you thinking about that during the cold-pressor test?"

The interview continues with questions about the other phases of the behavioral trial. "Once you placed your arm in the water, what kind of thoughts did you have? Is there anything else that you can remember thinking about or feeling just before you took your hand out of the water?" Until the patient reports no new cognitions or feelings, the therapist would inquire, "Is there anything else?"

If one is conducting group therapy, then the patient's individual experiences during the behavioral trial may be shared later with the group. Both similar experiences and dissimilar responses are likely to be evident. The group can use these similarities and differences in reflecting on the range of behavioral and cognitive possibilities that is open to each of them: the shared problems and feelings, the various individual difficulties, and the alternative means of handling the situation. In this process, the group is continuing the translation of pain into controllable terms, relating it to cognitive and affective events that they can change themselves.

Comparing Clinical and Experimentally Induced Pain

Both the patient and the therapist can attend to how the experimental pain situation was similar to, and how it was different from, the patient's clinical pain. The therapist can, as a homework assignment, encourage the patient to carry out a similar cognitive and affective analysis of a particular episode of severe pain that occurred *in vivo*. The patient can then note how different cognitions and feelings may be elicited by different situations and how these may differentially affect the pain. The discussion of any such material can contribute to the emerging reconceptualization of pain in contrast to the previous physiological, stimulus–response view.

Sternbach noted that a group setting contributes to this enterprise: "Patients quickly realize that they are not alone, that others have been struggling and suffering and manipulating as they have, and that there is understanding of what they have been through" (1974b, p. 103). Perhaps most important, patients are likely to be encouraged, in the presence of similar patients, to be honest in reporting their thoughts and feelings and their recognition of the relationship of pain to cognitive, affective, and behavioral factors (e.g., Gottlieb *et al.*, 1977; Sternbach, 1974b). The comparative analysis of experimental and clinical pain may also provide an index of the dimension that has been termed "self-efficacy" (Bandura, 1977).

Self-Efficacy Ratings

A dimension of psychological functioning that has received attention is an individual's sense of his or her personal efficacy in dealing with problems. According to Bandura (1977), "self-efficacy" is the conviction that one can successfully execute the behavior required to produce a suitable outcome. This differs from "outcome expectancy," which is a person's estimate that a given behavior will lead to a certain outcome. One can have a high outcome expectancy for a specific cognitive or behavioral action plan, but if the individual does not believe he or she can execute that action at a particular time or in a particular situation, he or she may decide not even to try.

Imagine an individual who smokes two packs of cigarettes a day and who wishes to stop smoking. The individual may have sufficient information that smoking is hazardous to his or her health and may have information suggesting that a specific treatment procedure such as aversive conditioning is effective in terminating smoking behavior. (We are not endorsing this procedure.) This individual may, in fact, strongly believe that a particular treatment procedure is useful (high outcome expectancy), but still may not undergo this treatment because he or she does not feel able to complete the procedure successfully (low efficacy expectancy).

Perceived self-efficacy can have diverse effects on behavior, thought patterns, and affective arousal. The strength of people's convictions of their own effectiveness is likely to determine whether they will try to cope with a given situation. People tend to fear and avoid situations they believe exceed their coping abilities. They may imagine potential difficulties as more formidable than they really are. Such negative self-referent preoccupations may produce disruptive emotional arousal and impair performance by diverting attention from the task itself to self-evaluative concerns (A. Beck, 1976; Meichenbaum, 1977; Sarason, 1975).

Perceptions of self-efficacy influence one's choice of activities and settings as well as how much effort will be exerted and how long one will persist in the face of obstacles or aversive experiences. In the face of difficulties, people who entertain serious concerns and doubts about their capabilities tend to slacken their efforts or give up altogether, whereas those who have a strong sense of self-efficacy are likely to exert greater effort to master challenges. Because knowledge and competence are achieved through sustained effort, giving up easily precludes the occurrence of corrective experiences, which could, in turn, lead to enhanced perceptions of self-efficacy. In other words, low self-efficacy begets low self-efficacy.

We have recently begun to experiment with self-efficacy ratings with pain patients and experimental subjects. Our goal has been to develop an instrument that is sensitive to patients' changes in their assessments of their ability to tolerate, reduce, and avoid pain.

We ascertain self-efficacy ratings for a variety of events, especially those surrounding the achievement of specifiable goals. For example, with each patient we establish five goals in different domains of his or her life that have been affected by pain (e.g., social, marital, vocational, physical, medication intake). Sometimes there may be more than one goal within each category. We then have patients rank order the goals from the ones they feel will be the easiest to achieve to the ones they feel will be the most difficult to achieve. At this point we ask patients to rate on a 100% scale how confident or certain they are that they will meet each goal. This procedure is useful both in predicting treatment outcome and, more particularly, in examining patients' motivations for treatment. By comparing the ratings for each goal, the therapist and patient can consider what factors contribute to low self-efficacy ratings for a particular objective and then discuss what can be done to remove such obstacles. Figure 9-3 illustrates one scale we have used to assess self-efficacy ratings.

In addition, the following types of queries about self-efficacy have been useful:

1. Self-efficacy concerning the patient's ability to *prevent* pain. Can you ever prevent the pain from occurring (or from getting worse)? [It is important not to take a patient's reply to such a general question literally, but to follow it up either with an inquiry con-

The therapist should establish, in cooperation with the patient and his or her spouse, *specific* goals for each of the following areas: physical exercise program, vocational, recreational, social, marital/familial, and medication usage. The goals should be realistic, given the patient's medical condition, age, and environmental circumstances. Where appropriate, consultation with physical therapist and physician is advisable.

Once the goals are established, the patient should rank order them from the easiest to the most difficult. Following the rank ordering of goals by the patient, the therapist should record these goals in order from easiest to most difficult on the Self-Efficacy Rating Form. Once the specific goal has been recorded on the Self-Efficacy Rating Form, the patient will be asked to do two things. First, the patient will simply indicate (yes or no) whether he or she believes that he or she will be able to achieve each goal. Second, the patient rates how likely or how sure he or she is that he or she will be able to achieve each of the goals. Ratings extend from 0 (no likelihood of achieving goal) to 100 (complete certainty of success).

Example

Directions: Write "yes" or "no" in the space next to each goal, indicating whether you believe you will be able to achieve the specific goal during (or following) treatment.

Next, indicate on the scale provided how sure you are that you will achieve the specific goals.

Recreational area goals
1. Walk in the park for 15 minutes a day. _YES_ (yes or no?)
How likely is it that you will achieve this goal? Put an × on the scale.

/   /   /   /   /   /   /   /   /   /   / × /

0   10   20   30   40   50   60   70   80   90   100
No likelihood   Completely sure

2. Sit and play cards for one-half hour each day. _YES_ (yes or no?)

/   /   /   /   /   /   /   / × /   /   /   /

0   10   20   30   40   50   60   70   80   90   100
No likelihood   Completely sure

FIGURE 9-3. *Self-efficacy ratings: Instructions to therapist.*

cerning how the patient accomplishes this, if the answer is "yes," or with further questions such as the following, if the answer is "no."] Are there ever times when you are pain-free (or when the pain is quite low)? [If the answer is "no" here, then the patient likely has an inaccurate perception of his or her pain or is trying to present a certain image, since with almost all patients the pain does have peaks and troughs.] When does this happen? Can you predict these times? [This can be followed up to determine whether the patient has the impression of affecting the onset and intensity of pain.] For example: Do you ever think to yourself, "Now, if I do *that*, it will start again"? From inquiries such as these, the patient can be led to consider connections that he or she may not have made before between personal actions and the pain-related outcome.

2. Self-efficacy concerning the patient's ability to *reduce* pain. How much can you affect the degree of pain you are experiencing? [Again, follow-up inquiry is necessary, whatever response is given to the initial question.] Can you ever alter the intensity of pain or the kind of pain you are feeling? Do you ever have a sense that the pain is likely to get a bit better soon? Do you ever think to yourself, "If I just do this for a while (lie down, rub it, go for a walk, talk to someone, etc.), it might get a bit better"? Are you ever right in making such predictions? When was the last time you were able to predict that the pain (or knew that the pain) was going to go down? What kinds of things do you avoid (or do) in order to make the pain diminish somewhat?

3. Self-efficacy concerning the patient's ability to *cope* with pain. How well can you deal with the pain when it is severe? What kinds of things do you do just to get through a particularly bad time? What kinds of things go through your head when you are just trying to last through a bad episode? [Frequently, patients will actively engage in coping attempts, but not label them as such. Asking "What do you do?" is therefore often more productive than asking "How do you cope?" Nevertheless, the latter type of question is important in order to determine whether patients can identify their own activities as coping attempts and therefore their own resources as useful to them.]

4. Self-efficacy concerning the patient's ability to *change*. The therapist can assess the patient's ability to achieve the various specified objectives by asking about the areas in which the patient has received or is likely to receive some therapy or assistance. Instead of asking the patient to make a specific judgment on each component of the treatment at the outset, such efficacy ratings are obtained throughout the course of treatment as each component is considered. Initially, more general estimates of self-efficacy are sought. How helpful do you think this [particular] treatment will be for you? Do you think you will be able to use any help in this area? In what way will it be helpful? How do you think treatment could be changed in order to be of more help to yourself? Do you think you can learn anything that will make it any easier? Do you think that this procedure of relaxation, for example, will be of any use to you? Why? (or why not?) What will you learn from it? What

will it do for you? [Does the patient feel that he or she can be an agent in change or that change is solely the responsibility of an external agent or therapy?]

The inquiry suggested here is by no means exhaustive. We suggest that the clinician assess the constructs in whatever way seems most useful. It is the organization of such inquiry and the information it leads to under the constructs of self-efficacy that may constitute a fruitful new direction. There is much to be learned yet about how concepts of self-efficacy develop, how they are related across different content areas, and, most important, how they relate to treatment outcome.

Additional Assessment Procedures

The methods of performing a cognitive and behavioral assessment of the patient's pain, and of using that assessment to contribute to the reconceptualization, are by no means limited to those we have described. For further examples, the reader is referred to other sources: interview— Kanfer and Saslow (1969), Linehan (1977), Morganstern (1976); self-report inventories and checklists—Bellack and Hersen (1977), Cautela and Upper (1976), Rosenbaum, (1980a), Walls, Werner, Bacon, and Zane (1977); self-monitoring procedures—Mahoney (1977d), Nelson (1977); and other cognitive–behavioral methods—Meichenbaum (1976a), Merluzzi *et al.* (1981).

Additional procedures that have been used in the assessment of patients with pain and other medical problems include the Illness Behavior Questionnaire (Pilowsky & Spence, 1975, 1976a, 1976b, 1976c), Eysenck Personality Inventory (Barnes, 1975; Bond, 1971; Woodforde & Merskey, 1972a, 1972b), Pain Apperception Test (Petrovich, 1978; Ziesat & Gentry, 1978), Cornell Medical Index (Bond, 1971; Woodforde & Fielding, 1970), and Pain Survey Schedule (Cautela, 1977). The interested reader is referred to Bond (1971), Bradley *et al.* (1981), and Weisenberg (1977) for reviews of these measures.

Melzack–McGill Pain Questionnaire

In addition to the pain-report scales and methods we have described, other instruments and techniques for monitoring and reporting clinical pain are available. One of the most useful is the Melzack–McGill Pain Questionnaire (Melzack, 1975a; Melzack & Torgerson, 1971). This instrument provides a quantitative measure of the patient's description of pain intensity, as well as separate indexes of sensory, affective, and evaluative aspects of pain (Melzack, 1975a). The qualitative evaluation of pain using the Melzack–McGill questionnaire has been reported on by Agnew and Merskey (1976); Bailey and Davidson (1976); Bakal and Kaganov (1976); C. Graham, Bond, Gerkovich, and Cook (1980); Prieto, Hopson, Bradley, Byrne, Geisinger, Midax, and Marchisello (1980); and Reading (1979a). We have incorporated part of the Melzack–McGill Pain Questionnaire in the questionnaire included in Appendix C.

In recent years the Melzack–McGill Pain Questionnaire has served a variety of clinical and experimental purposes. These include (1) characterization of patients in chronic pain (Catchlove & Ramsay, 1978), (2) assessment of pain relief resulting from a variety of pain-reduction interventions (e.g., Melzack & Perry, 1975; Rybstein-Blinchik, 1979), (3) use with cross-modality matching in laboratory studies (Gracely, 1978), and (4) use as a potential diagnostic tool to identify specific disease categories (Dubisson & Melzack, 1976). Although the factor structure of this instrument remains unclear, it does appear to be a promising tool that should benefit from further refinements (Bradley et al., 1981) and that may be employed in conjunction with other, previously described procedures.

Minnesota Multiphasic Personality Inventory

The Minnesota Multiphasic Personality Inventory (MMPI) has been used in the evaluation of psychological contributors to pain (e.g., Bradley, Prieto, Hopson, & Prokop, 1978; Carr, Brownsberger, & Rutherford, 1966; Cox, Chapman, & Black, 1978; Maruta, Swanson, & Swenson, 1979; Sternbach, 1974b). Following an initial report by Hanvik (1951) that so-called functional pain patients and organic pain patients differed in their MMPI profiles (i.e., functional patients were reported to have elevated *Hs*, Hypochondriasis scale, and *Hy*, Hysteria scale, and low *D*, Depression scale—the "conversion V"), several studies continued to investigate this dimension (e.g., Calsyn, Louks, & Freeman, 1976; Carr et al., 1966; Dahlstrom, 1954; Louks, Freeman, & Calsyn, 1978; McCreary, Turner, & Dawson, 1977).

Findings have been inconsistent, and several of these studies have been criticized on methodological grounds (Bradley, Prieto, Hopson, & Prokop, 1978). It makes sense to investigate the psychological contributions to pain of any sort, and several studies have utilized the MMPI to this end (e.g., Bradley, Prokop, Margolis, & Gentry, 1978; Carr et al., 1966; Sternbach, 1974b; Sternbach et al., 1973). In a recent review of the area, Bradley et al. (1981) suggested the following:

Psychologists who use the MMPI to assess pain patients abandon the task of classifying patients as organic, functional or mixed and instead redirect their efforts toward the delineation of (a) replicable MMPI profile subgroups within their respective pain patient populations and (b) the pain-related correlates uniquely associated with each profile subgroup. (p. 16)

Sternbach (1974b), for example, has described four MMPI profiles common among patients suffering from chronic disorders, including pain. He characterized these as reflecting symptoms of hypochondriasis, reactive depression, somatization reactions, and manipulative reaction, and he outlined the problems specific to each type of patient.

SUMMARY

In this chapter we have described a number of assessment procedures that may be employed to obtain a detailed pain history and to assess patient's perception of their pain and the impact of pain on their lives. In the next chapter we will consider how significant others can be included in the assessment process.

CHAPTER 10

INITIAL PHASE OF
COGNITIVE–BEHAVIORAL TREATMENT:
PART II

The initial focus of this chapter is on the role of significant others in the assessment of patients' pain and on the impact of patients' pain on their relationships with significant others. The remainder of the chapter discusses the reconceptualization process of pain, using the assessment material obtained from both patients and significant others.

THE ROLE OF SIGNIFICANT OTHERS IN ASSESSMENT

The inclusion of the patient's significant others is an important element in both the assessment and the treatment phases of cognitive–behavioral therapy. There is a variety of approaches available for assessing the nature of the relationship between the patient and significant others. We will describe several procedures that we have employed to involve significant others in assessment and treatment.

As noted previously, chronic pain is the family's problem, often becoming the focus of all aspects of family life. The family's schedule may be altered by the demands of the patient, frequent visits to the physician, hospitalizations, and time-consuming therapeutic regimens. The budget is usually strained, since it is not unusual for a pain patient to spend $25,000 a year for medical and pharmacological treatments (Chapman, 1973). Recreation patterns are drastically altered, and vacation plans may be disrupted by instability in physical or psychological condition and the need to be close to established medical supports. The sexual relationship of a married couple may be altered, if not completely curtailed. And family role responsibilities are often dramatically changed, with other members having to assume tasks that were formerly carried out by the patient. Children may prefer to visit other homes rather than subject friends to an unpredictable and often irritable parent.

Initial sympathy for a patient often gives way to frustration, as the family finds itself unable to alleviate the patient's pain. Anger and resentment at altered life-styles are generally accompanied by guilt for experiencing such feelings toward a helpless and suffering person. The following excerpt from a letter sent by the wife of one patient after an initial family interview illustrates the processes we are describing.

> Since his back operation five years ago he has become increasingly impatient and progressively slower with no ambition at all to even try to help himself. He has made himself and invalid and it has become very difficult for me and my family to tolerate his constant complaining. He blames me, blames our two sons who he says don't help him around the house when in fact he does little or nothing to help himself. He does exactly the same things day after day with projects he starts and never completes and always because of health. . . . My husband cannot seem to forget his problems and put some effort into accomplishments instead of complaints. . . . We hope that perhaps you can convince him to get some work outside the home which I'm sure will help him understand the pressure the family has been under for five years now. . . . If you can convince him to get out of the lounge chair that he sits in half a day and sleeps the other half, we would be extremely grateful.

This letter needs little comment. The wife's sense of frustration and anger and her resentment and distress underscore our point about pain being a family problem. This letter is also consistent with the report by Turk and Kerns (1980) that the spouses of pain patients revealed as much distress as did the patients themselves.

An interdependent relationship characterizes the family interactions of pain patients, a relationship that often seems to reinforce the patient's pain behavior. Some family members we have worked with act as if they enjoy having someone dependent upon them, someone to cater to, to bring pills to, to feed. One woman had recently moved with her retired husband. They had few friends, and the husband had assumed all of the household chores. He viewed it as his "mission" in life to care for his wife. After all, he had little else on which to spend his time.

In other instances the patient–spouse interaction may take on a "conspiracy of silence." For example, it is not unusual for patients to report that they do not specifically tell others when they experience intense pain and for them to assume, therefore, that those around them are not aware of the severe pain they experience. Yet pain behaviors such as grimacing, walking in a shuffling manner, lying down, and so on, can communicate this message clearly, without the patient's verbalizing the suffering.

One patient at an assessment interview shuffled to a straight-back chair, turned slowly around, gripped both arms of the chair, and gingerly lowered himself into his seat, grimacing as he settled in and continually shifting his position in the seat throughout the interview. This same patient indicated that people did not really know when he experienced pain, and he made a point of stating that he did not like "bothering others with his problems." His distress was blatantly evident to all who observed him. The patient's wife confirmed that the behavior we observed during the interview was typical and that she was well aware when her husband was experiencing pain. Interestingly, the wife did not mention this to the patient because she did not want to "distress him." The patient, however, acknowledged that, at times of intense pain episodes, his wife responded to him differently. Both the patient and the spouse were deceiving each other with a conspiracy of silence. In such situations it may be useful to videotape patients and to show the tapes to them as vivid illustrations of the communnciation of pain by nonverbal means.

Family members may contribute to pain behaviors in other ways. "Shh! Daddy is having one of his headaches" (implying that if he is disturbed or asked to do something, it would exacerbate the pain). The family can assume and reinforce the patient's pain-related concerns.

Because pain has such a major impact on the life of families of patients, we view it as essential to involve family members in the assessment and therapeutic process. There are a number of different ways to involve significant others. Without having data concerning which way is best, or, indeed, whether the inclusion of significant others does or does not enhance treatment, we will indicate our clinical preference and call for research on these issues.

During the first meeting with a pain patient, we encourage the spouse, and on some occasions other family members or significant others (e.g., fiancé, coworkers, friends), to participate in the next session. There are two objectives regarding involvement of the significant other at this initial stage.

First, the significant other helps to clarify any ambiguities, to validate the patient's description of certain types of experiences (pain and otherwise), and to assess the potential role of the family and friends in the treatment program. Such information may be collected by interviewing the significant other separately, with the focus being essentially the same as in the interview with the patient. The therapist should first discuss this interview with the patient and explain why it is helpful to obtain a thorough, independent account from the spouse. The therapist should be careful to ensure that the patient does not become concerned or suspicious about the need for such a separate meeting with the significant other and that the patient agrees to the interview. The interview allows the opportunity to collect the details of the spouse's story and also to make a judgment about the possible cooperation that will be offered. It is essential to solicit and nurture the spouse's cooperation if the treatment regimen is to succeed.

A second objective of joint assessment is for the therapist to observe the interactional style of the patient and spouse (or significant others). Although one must be concerned about the generalizability of these behavioral clinical samples to outside settings, such observations may prove quite helpful. At such meetings issues concerning the appropriateness of the program for the patient, the duration of the program, probable outcome, and so on, can also be discussed.

The significant other may be seen not only at the assessment phase, but at regularly scheduled intervals during the course of the program. These sessions may occur on a weekly basis or less frequently. When treatment is conducted on a group basis, groups of couples (significant other and the patient) may be seen.

At this point we are not prepared to specify the best combination of patient–significant other meetings, whether they are to be conducted together or alone or in what sequence. Both clinical acumen and practical scheduling considerations have guided us in the past. The key point is that the involvement of the significant other has emerged in our clinical practice as an important ingredient of the treatment regimen. This does not mean that individuals without significant others or with uncooperative significant others cannot be candidates for intervention (although Fordyce & Steger, 1979, suggest that nonparticipation of the significant other is a contraindication for operant treatment of pain). But when a significant other is available, it is important to nurture this persons as an ally and collaborator in the treatment regimen.

Joint Definition of Goals

A key feature of the assessment is the design of specific treatment goals that the patient wishes to achieve. Usually the attempt to formulate treatment goals follows the reconceptualization process. We include it at this point because it fits nicely into a consideration of involvement of significant others. In establishing such goals, it is critical that they be realistic and that they consider a particular patient's limitations. The joint consideration of possible goals by both the patient and significant others is particularly valuable. A useful way to raise this topic is to ask a question that was asked of the patient when seen alone in the first session, namely, "How would your life be different if your pain could be relieved?" "What would you be doing if your pain was removed that you are not doing now?" In asking such questions, the therapist looks at both the patient and the significant other, raising the question generally for both of them.

It is interesting and clinically useful to compare the answer offered in session one, when only the patient was present, with the answer that emerges when the significant other is present in session two. The patient is likely to give more "socially desirable" responses during session one, whereas the presence of the significant other may provide an important counterweight. For example, one patient reported initially that the alleviation of pain would mean going back to work and working around the house. The therapist was a bit skeptical and minimally challenged the patient on whether these indeed represented desirable goals. The patient maintained a positive stance nonetheless. A somewhat different picture emerged once the wife was present, because she questioned her husband's goals, given his complaints about his job and household chores.

We are not suggesting that all pain patients deliberately use pain as a means of acquiring "secondary gains" or that they behave in a manipulative manner. Nevertheless, for most patients who have had an extended period of pain, a life-style emerges that helps to maintain pain behaviors.

The significant other's recollection and description of the patient's activities can help to clarify the specific stages of goal attainment as well as the details of the goals themselves. For example, one patient reported a treatment goal of spending more time with his grandchildren. His wife pointed out that he had a favorite granddaughter, with whom he now spent most of his visiting time, and that he often groused about seeing the other grandchildren, who were unruly and loud. Upon reflection, the patient agreed that the goal as he first stated it was undesirable, and he was able to modify his goals accordingly so as to accommodate his real desire, additional time with one grandchild and her parents.

The short-, medium-, and long-term treatment goals must be measurable. They may include such things as reduction of medication, less time lying down, specific tasks to accomplish at home and on the job, recreational activities and exercises, and reestablishment of social and sexual relationships. Figure 10-1, offered by Turner (1979), illustrates one procedure we have used to help patients specify specific treatment goals.

Physical Goals

Since the treatment goals should be attainable in light of the patient's physical condition, the patient may be informed that his or her primary physician or the referral physician will be asked to indicate that the patient has no medical problems that would interfere with the proposed

Name: _____

Please list below the five goals you would most like to achieve by participating in this program. These goals should be activities that you are now kept from doing as much or as well as you would like to because of your pain. Select goals you think you can reasonably attain. Define your goals in terms of specific behaviors. Pain relief, for example, is *not* an acceptable goal because it does not involve a behavior. Possible goals might be to be able to sit longer, return to a job, or participate more in social activities. For each goal, please describe as specifically as possible how much of the activity you do now, how much you consider to be a moderate improvement, and how much you consider to be the most improvement possible for you. (Behaviors [a] and [b] are given as examples.)

Behavior	Current status	Moderate improvement	Most improvement possible for me
a. Sitting in chair	Can sit 20 minutes at a time	Able to sit 45 minutes at a time	Able to sit 2 hours at a time
b. Participation with family in activities	Participate in activity (play games, go to movies, etc.) with family once every 2 weeks	Participate in activity with family once a week	Participate in activity with family 3 times a week
1.			
2.			
3.			
4.			
5.			

FIGURE 10-1. *Procedure for specifying treatment goals. Adapted from Turner, J. Evaluation of two behavioral interventions for chronic low back pain. Unpublished doctoral dissertation, University of California, Los Angeles, 1979, p. 172. Reprinted by permission.*

treatment program. The therapist may contact physicians who are not familiar with the program, describe the program to them, and enlist their support. A medical examination within the last 6 months is also advisable before a patient is accepted into the treatment program. In this way, the therapist can help match the treatment goals and exercise activities with the patient's abilities and capacities. For example, a coronary bypass patient with chest-wall pain is ill-advised to engage in strenuous exercise involving the extension of arm and chest muscles. Long walks, leg exercises, and other exercise involving muscle groups relatively unaffected by the surgery are more appropriate for such an individual.

Especially with chronic pain patients who have been quite inactive, it is recommended that an exercise regimen be introduced gradually, beginning with simple, easily manageable tasks and building up to more formidable tasks. A paced exercise and activity regimen that engenders a sense of mastery and self-efficacy can be followed. The likelihood of initial success is increased and enthusiasm is more easily maintained when demanding activities are introduced gradually. The use of an individually tailored activity-level chart for daily records of exercise also helps to engender a sense of accomplishment and self-efficacy (Fordyce, 1976). Consultation with the patient's physician and with a physiotherapist in setting up such exercise programs is essential. Such consultation is aimed at determining the optimal level of exercise and activity in light of the patient's physical status, age, and sex.

Monitoring by Significant Other

An important task when working with the significant other is training him or her in careful observation of the patient's pain behavior. There have been a number of suggestions concerning how the significant other should conduct such observation. Fordyce (1976) suggested that the significant other be asked to generate a list of pain behaviors, indicating the ways in which he or she is aware that the patient is "in pain." Fordyce suggested that the list contain between five and ten items. A list longer than this suggests that the significant other is attending to too much detail, and a list containing less than five items suggests that the significant other is not sufficiently attentive. After an adequate list has been generated, the significant other is asked to keep track of the amount of time that the patient exhibits pain behaviors. Following the development of such observational skills, the significant other is encouraged to monitor what he or she does in response to the patient's pain behavior. The use of videotape may assist significant others in identifying pain behaviors.

Although we have tried the Fordyce procedure, we have been experimenting with other monitoring procedures. For example, another means of involving significant others is to give them the assignment of rating the patient's pain behaviors, using the same index cards as those the patient has used. The significant other may rate each hour as the patient was asked to or may use whatever procedure is feasible. Significant others are asked to record their perceptions of the patient's pain, thus becoming sensitive to what cues are associated with pain. It may also be useful for significant others to record their own reactions (i.e., thoughts and feelings).

The therapist should impress upon the significant other the importance of diligently collecting information about the nature of the patient's pain experience and its impact on the family, friends, the boss, and so on. These data can also be used to note how the significant other's and other people's reactions affect the patient's behavior. In short, having the significant other monitor reactions to the patient's pain allows examination of the pattern of interpersonal reactions, their reciprocity, and their cycles, which influence the pain experience.

Instead of lecturing the patient and the significant other about the important role of the latter in unwittingly reinforcing the patient's pain behaviors, such as moaning, grimacing, lying down, and avoiding certain activities, the therapist will now be able to engage the couple in a discussion of the impact of such behaviors on the feelings of others and on the patient's pain experience, using data collected by both the patient and the significant other.

Significant-Other (Spouse) Diary

In many instances asking the significant other to keep a record of the patient's pain behavior by means of the pain intensity rating cards may prove too demanding or not feasible because of the unavailability of the significant other or some similar reason. Another means we have used, either in lieu of the pain rating cards or in addition to them, is a significant-other (spouse) diary that parallels the patient diary. Figure 10-2 provides an example of the significant-other diary that we have used.

To help us learn more about the nature of your spouse's pain, it is important that you keep careful records. The spouse diary is designed to provide detailed information about periods when your spouse's pain is severest, how you respond to your spouse when he is experiencing severe pain, and how effective your response is in reducing the pain. It is particularly important that we obtain this information so that we can design the most appropriate treatment program for your spouse.

Specifically, we would like you to keep a record of the times when you are

---

FIGURE 10-2. (Continued)

aware that your spouse's pain is particularly severe. Note the date, the time, and your location (e.g., home, in the car). Next, we would like you to record how you recognize your spouse's pain (e.g., he told you, he lay down, he asked you to bring him some pain medication, he looked very distressed and was moaning). Then note what you thought and how you felt at the time at which you noted your spouse's pain was severe (e.g., distressed, helpless, wondered why the doctors can't find some way to help him, frustrated). Then indicate what you tried to do to reduce the pain or discomfort (e.g., gave him pain medication, tried to talk to him, gave him a massage, left him alone trying not to bother him).

We would also like you to indicate how effective your attempt to reduce the pain was. That is, rate how much you think your action helped, using a scale ranging from 0 to 5 as follows:

0 = did not help at all
1 = helped very little
2 = helped somewhat
3 = helped a lot
4 = helped very much
5 = seemed to stop the pain completely

Using the numbers listed, try to rate how effective each of your attempts was in reducing your spouse's pain.

To illustrate what we would like you to do, we have included a sample. Use as much paper as you want to complete this diary between now and our next appointment. Thank you for your help.

Name: _____ Sample _____   Date: ____ August 10, 1981 ____

Time	Location	How you recognized spouse's pain	What you thought	How you felt	How you tried to help	Your effectiveness (0–5)
2:00 p.m.	At home in living room	He was lying down; face looked drawn; heard him breathing, moaning	It seems hopeless	Frustrated Angry at doctors	I asked him if I could get him some pain killers or make some tea	
					I rubbed his shoulder	0
					I made tea	4
11:00 p.m.	In bed at home	Husband got out of bed, paced the floor, and took some medicine		Frustrated Helpless	I didn't know what to do so I turned over and cried myself to sleep	

FIGURE 10-2. *Spouse diary. (A different form, changing pronouns, is used for husbands, wives, and significant others.)*

The patient's significant other is asked to keep such a diary for 1 week or 2 weeks prior to the pain management program. The diary may be employed at treatment termination and follow-up as well.

A Sample Exchange

The following excerpt illustrates the way in which the therapist can employ the patient's and significant other's monitoring and diary data and also shows that assessment and therapy are actually interwoven.

Therapist: Mr. Cox, let's examine your wife's recording of pain behaviors during the past week. Mrs. Cox, please read what you wrote down regarding a specific incident when you observed that your husband was experiencing severe pain.

Mrs. Cox: Well, last Tuesday evening around 9 P.M., John and I were sitting and watching television. Every time I asked him a question, he shifted his whole body in his seat to look at me rather than turning his head. I could tell that his neck must have been bothering him a lot.

Therapist: Mr. Cox, can you recall this incident? Were you experiencing a lot of pain Tuesday evening as your wife has indicated?

Mr. Cox: Well, I really can't remember.

Therapist: Let's look at your pain ratings. At the time your wife is referring to, about 9 P.M. last Tuesday, what rating did you give your pain?

Mr. Cox: Let me see, I rated it a 4, so it must have really have been bothering me. I can remember now, we were watching a documentary, but I couldn't concentrate.

Therapist: Well, it seems that your wife was aware you were in pain. Mrs. Cox, what did you do or how did you react to your husband when he moved his head stiffly?

Mrs. Cox: I didn't know what to do, so I just stopped asking questions; I really felt sorry for John, but didn't know what to do. I just tried to watch the show and not say anything to him. At those times I feel . . . so helpless.

Therapist: Mr. Cox, it sounds as if your wife tried to avoid talking about your pain. She sounds sort of helpless and frustrated because there was nothing she felt she could do. How did you feel about her response?

Mr. Cox: I think I got kind of mad at her because she seemed to be ignoring me, not really caring how I was feeling.

Therapist: Mr. Cox, what do you think she should have done at that time?

Mr. Cox: I don't really know.

Therapist: Mr. Cox, do you think there was anything she could have done to make you feel better?

Mr. Cox: Not really.

Therapist: So, Mr. Cox, there really is not much your wife could do to help. Perhaps at such times ignoring your pain may be the most she can do, since talking about it and focusing on how bad you feel may serve only to make it more unpleasant, preventing you from trying to ignore your pain yourself.

Mr. Cox: Perhaps.

Therapist: Perhaps?

Mr. Cox: Well, maybe she did know how I was feeling, but I felt upset that she didn't tell me.

Therapist: It looks as if pain can be communicated even without your saying that the pain is present. I think we can also see that at times there is little others can do to help someone who is in pain and that they really have to learn ways to cope by themselves. At the same time, one may misinterpret the ways others cope with the situation and view it as not caring when in fact they really do care. . . . Do you have other examples written down in your diary, Mrs. Cox?

Mrs. Cox: Let me see, yes, on Saturday we were going to visit some relatives, and John said he didn't want to go, but preferred to stay home.

Therapist: Mrs. Cox, how could you tell that your husband was in pain?

Mrs. Cox: Well, we had been talking about going all week, and Saturday morning he was lying down with a pained look on his face. I can't describe it, but I always know when I see that look that his neck is bothering him. So when he said he didn't want to go, I knew it must be because his pain was bothering him.

Therapist: Mr. Cox, was your wife correct in her view of your pain and the reason you didn't want to go to visit your relatives?

Mr. Cox: Yes, my neck was hurting, and I really don't like seeing her cousins all that much.

Therapist: Your neck pain, your not wanting to see your cousins—how do these two things go together? The pain, it kept you from having to visit with relatives that you really didn't care to be with?

Mr. Cox: Well, my neck really did hurt.

Therapist: I am *not* suggesting that your neck didn't hurt, but I am wondering whether sometimes pain allows us to avoid doing some things we don't want to do. Similarly, I am *not* suggesting that you were faking the pain, but only that sometimes the consequences of having pain can be somewhat rewarding. Mrs. Cox, what did you say when your husband indicated that he didn't want to go visit your cousins?

Mrs. Cox: Nothing, just that I guessed I would call them and let them know we weren't coming.

Therapist: Did you say anything else to your husband?

Mrs. Cox: No.

Therapist: How did you feel about not going?

Mrs. Cox: Disappointed.

Therapist: I get the sense that you were not only disappointed, but perhaps a little angry.

Mrs. Cox: John's pain often interferes with our plans. It's hard to make any arrangements because we have to cancel so often.

Therapist: Mrs. Cox, have you ever told John how you feel when you have to cancel your arrangements at the last moment?

Mrs. Cox: No, he feels bad enough with the pain and all.

Therapist: The feelings you have been experiencing, Mrs. Cox, are not unusual. Many families with pain problems are hesitant about sharing their feelings because they are afraid to add additional problems. Such lack in communicating often leads to stress in the family, and the stress may be picked up by the patient, and at times this may make the pain worse. It is important to address such problems and not cover them up . . . like a lid on a pot because eventually they may boil over.

Discussions such as these provide a basis for considering any hidden agendas that the patient or significant other might have concerning the change in behavior. By asking the spouse to describe the feelings and thoughts that precede, accompany, and follow the patient's pain experiences, one can look for cues and themes that indicate current concern. How would the alleviation or reduction of the pain change the life-style of the significant other? Are such changes seen as desirable by the significant other? Certainly, not all instances of pain are maintained by significant others, nor do all pain patients require marital counseling or psychotherapy. But in the course of assessment, it is both prudent and helpful to consider such interpersonal factors in the maintenance of pain, especially in the case of chronic pain.

In short, there is a need for a thorough analysis of the pain patient and his or her social situation. Although we have highlighted the need to identify psychological factors as causes of pain behavior, it is important to remind ourselves that pain behavior may be caused by a host of factors. For example, in the case of headaches, a wide variety of physical as well as psychological events can act as triggers. These include such factors as barometric pressure, consumption of foods that contain tyramine, flashing lights, and temporomandibular joint misalignment. In the psychological domain, Reeves (1976) reported a case in which the headache patient had cognitions involving the anticipation of punishment, feelings of inadequacy, and "catastrophizing" thoughts about forthcoming events as well as possible loss of status and esteem.

Given the low relationship between the various pain measures that we have discussed, it would seem advisable to employ objective and multiple subjective measures. Pain is not a unitary phenomenon, and the recognition of this should guide the assessment approach.

RECONCEPTUALIZATION

The initial phase of treatment ends with the presentation of the specific treatment rationale that consolidates the reconceptualization process. As noted, the entire assessment and therapy process is designed to engender a reconceptualization of the patient's pain. The aim is not to *convert* patients to a "true" conception of their problem, but simply to encourage them to adopt a way of looking at it that inherently allows for change.

A central feature of this reconceptualization process is the establishment of a collaborative, participatory relationship between the health care provider and the patient and his or her significant others, with the patient assuming more responsibility. The goal of the reconceptualization process is to recast the pain experience in terms that imply hope and resourcefulness. Instead of the patient's viewing pain in global terms, the therapist works with the patient to develop a more differentiated view— one that implies voluntary control by the patient over components of the pain. These components include (1) unpleasant physical sensations over which the patient may exert control, (2) pain-related thoughts and images, (3) pain-related feelings, and (4) pain-related behaviors.

To illustrate each component, the therapist should use the patient's own experience or own data as collected in the interviews, questionnaires, and diaries. Each time the therapist provides a component of the pain model, he or she should immediately offer an example from the patient's own experience to illustrate that component. When the treatment is conducted on a group basis, the therapist can offer examples from several patients or, preferably, encourage patients to offer their own examples. For example, in the case of pain behaviors, the group can refer to the use of medication, their inactive life-styles, and their preoccupation with pain as evident in grimacing, moaning, and complaining.

This reconceptualization process underscores the point that patients need not be passive and dependent upon others for relief, but can take on much of the responsibility to alter the elements of the pain experience. In short, reconceptualization chunks the pain into manageable units, units that can be subjected to change. This encourages patients to become active problem solvers with regard to both pain and other problems (e.g., interpersonal conflicts). To facilitate this process, each aspect of the treatment regimen is made explicit and is explained to the patients.

Groundwork

From the outset, we wish to convey to potential patients that *this* therapeutic opportunity is most likely different from others they have experienced with health care providers: That is, they can be helped, but only if they are prepared to participate by taking an active role in the intervention and in reshaping their lives. As an example, at an early point, the therapist may say something like the following:

> You have been to several doctors and clinics before you came here, so when you arrived this morning, you probably had some idea of what to expect. At the same time, you might have been wondering whether we would do anything differently here, perhaps hoping that finally something could be done to help. Well, I don't know yet how much assistance we can offer you; finding that out will be our first task. But I do know that we do things differently here.
>
> Here we don't do things to you or give you *things* to change your pain. We we will be doing is helping you to use the resources *you* have to affect your pain. Now, you may think you have already tried everything, done everything you can to help yourself. And I know that you do indeed want to reduce your pain and do what you can for yourself. What we are going to look for is resources that you may not be aware of and ways of using your abilities in a different manner. We can offer some help for most people, but that help is useful only through your own efforts to put it to use. We will want you to participate in everything, from learning more about your problem to the stages of doing something about it.

We have found this emphasis to have a sobering effect on the patient, placing the treatment program's responsibility in the hands of both the patient and the therapist.

To prepare the patient and the significant other for the need for a collaborative venture, the therapist may consider some of the myths that patients may hold about pain. The most succinct presentation of these myths has been offered by Malec, Glasgow, Ely, and Kling (1977), in a cognitive–behavioral bibliotherapy manual for pain patients. This material either may be discussed in the therapy sessions with both patient and significant other or can be presented in written form as Malec *et al.* have done. In either case, a consideration of these points helps to establish a common conceptualization between the patient and therapist. For example, the therapist states:

There are various false ideas or myths about pain that patients and their significant others often have. I am not sure if you believe these, but they are worth our going over and considering where they fit and do not fit with your own notions.

Malec *et al.* offer the following myths about pain:

1. Pain always means that you are hurt and need to rest and take care of yourself until you get better. *FALSE.*

   Many people feel that pain is a signal that something is going wrong with their bodies. Scientists also used to think pain was a simple matter of something hurting your body and you feeling it. It is *not that simple.* This is the way pain should work and usually it does. But sometimes this system goes haywire. The pain can still be there even after the damage to your body has stopped.

   Pain often starts as a danger signal. But some pain lasts even after your injury has healed. This pain is like a scar because it is still there even after the injury that started it has healed. Using the methods we will discuss you can learn to reduce this pain. But you can't count on the pain going away by itself because your body has probably healed as much as it's going to.

Or, as we have conveyed to patients, the following:

We have now seen that pain usually acts as a warning sign, and that rest is beneficial when pain is acute and short-lived; but in the case of chronic pain such as your own, the presence of pain is not a sign that something bad will happen.

Malec *et al.* continue:

2. If physicians can't cure your pain or find out exactly what is causing it, then your pain must be in your imagination. *FALSE.*

   Besides, looking at it another way, *all* pain is "in your head." After all, your brain is in your head. The brain is what tells you if you hurt, how much you hurt, where you hurt, and what to do about it. Even when you hurt because you hit your thumb with a hammer, that pain is "in your head." The reason psychological methods of pain control work is because you can learn to keep pain from bothering you.

3. Someday, someone, somewhere will find a cure that will quickly make your pain go away once and for all. *TRUE???*

   Maybe someday someone will. We sure hope so. But do you really want to wait around? Wouldn't you rather work *now* to reduce your pain by using the methods we know about *today*? Even if you are working to control your pain, you can always take advantage of a miracle cure if one comes along.

4. If you can make your pain less by psychological self-control, then the pain was "all in your head" to begin with. *FALSE.*

Many people who have good control of their imagination use psychological self-control to improve their lives. The best athletes "psych" themselves up to their best game. The best businessmen use special methods to stay cool under pressure. If you learn to control your pain, it doesn't mean you were crazy to begin with. It means you have learned skills to overcome your pain and lead a happier life. That's smart, *not* crazy.

In short, in our approach we are reluctant to tell patients that there is nothing physically wrong with them and that their pain is not physiological. Such a message to pain patients often has a negative effect.

5. I've had pain so long and suffered so much that I'm beyond help. I've tried everything and nothing works. I've tried "tricks" like the ones you will describe and they didn't work. I must be hopeless. *FALSE.*

You probably have tried a lot of different ways to make your pain go away. Different things work for different people. The treatment is especially made to help you find those methods that work best for you. It is worth a shot—if you'll work at it. You must keep working to learn. You need to learn a number of skills and use them together. It's a gradual process but with work you can learn to hurt less. (pp. 11–13)

We offer the excerpts from Malec *et al.* (1977) to convey the flavor of the messages to be offered to pain patients. There are a number of ways to cover these same points or to facilitate the reconceptualization process with the patient and his or her significant other, some less didactic than this. For example, the following message may be offered to patients and their significant others:

If you think of trying to convey to someone the sensations that you felt during some particular painful experience that you have had, you will realize that pain is a very individual experience. It can be next to impossible to explain *exactly* how you felt—something like trying to describe the color "green" to a man who has been blind from birth. One of the most common things for a person experiencing pain to say is, "You don't *know* how painful it is. I just can't tell you how much it hurts." Not only is it hard to say how *much* it hurts, it is practically impossible to describe exactly *how* it hurts. We have words such as "burning," "pricking," "searing," "tearing" that attempt to define the sensations of pain, but sometimes they don't seem adequate. Although some of the outward signs of pain may be visible, pain is a private, individual experience.

And because it is so private, so individual, no two people undergo exactly the same feelings of pain from the same source. Many things besides the *intensity of the stimulation* contribute to the experience of pain. On two different occasions, you may experience quite different "pain" from exactly the same external stimulation.

Think of someone receiving a minor wound to his face during an active game, such as football or hockey. He would probably not even notice the cut and would go on playing, feeling little, if any, pain. However, if he had received exactly the same degree of injury while working around the home, or shaving, or engaging in some such activity, he would probably notice the cut immediately, take steps to stop the bleeding, and find it uncomfortably painful. (It is only *after* the football or hockey game that the player is likely to find that the wound causes some discomfort.) Or, consider cutting your finger on the edge of a newspaper that you are reading. During some active game, you probably would not notice much pain from a minor cut like this.

Still another example: In several tribes, women in labor apparently experience no pain. They simply stop their work to have the baby and return to work immediately afterwards. In North America the average hospital stay after birth is from 5 days to 7 days. But in these primitive cultures, the husband stays in bed with "labor pains" while his wife is having the baby. Perhaps these men are not really experiencing the pain of labor. They say that they are! In any case, the women are not experiencing the intense, debilitating pain that is usual in our culture. Obviously, pain is influenced by many things.

Similarly, Turner (1979) conveys the message like this:

> Pain is not a thing. Having pain in my hand is *not* like having a splinter in my hand. If pain was a thing, you'd feel it every time you had an injury. But football players or soldiers who are injured or wounded often don't feel pain while they're in the midst of action, only when they've gone off the field or out of battle.
>
> Further, there is not necessarily a direct relationship between the amount of the injury and the amount of pain experienced. [Examples are offered of a tiny cavity causing excruciating pain and extreme cancer with extensive physical damage sometimes causing little or no pain.] (p. 105)

Patient Collaboration in a Conceptualization

It is worthwhile to have the patient and the significant other help generate, in a collaborative fashion, evidence from the patient's own experience that supports the contention that pain is more than a consequence of the specific so-called physical cause. Data from the patient's questionnaire, interview, imagery reconstruction, pain ratings, diary, and behavioral test, and the significant other's data, can be used to illustrate the variety of factors influencing the patient's pain. The patient can use these data as evidence to confirm the therapy rationale that is being offered by the therapist.

> As I listen to you describe your pain experience, there seem to be a number of different things going on. Correct me if I am wrong or if I am missing something, but it seems that the pain you are experiencing is made of several components.

A Conceptual Model

At this point the therapist conveys a conceptual model of pain using the patient's own symptoms and complaints to illustrate and document each of the proposed components. In our work we have employed various conceptual models, each offered in quite simple lay terms in order to help the patient understand the nature of pain. Patients have been introduced in a simple fashion to Melzack and Wall's (1965, 1970) gate-control model of pain, with its three interactive components of sensory–discriminative, motivational–affective, and cognitive–evaluative components, or to Beecher's (1959) model of pain, which assumes two elements, the sensory input and one's reactions to the sensory input.

An example of how a conceptualization of pain can be used to develop a treatment regimen is offered by Karol, Doerfler, Parker, and Armentrout (1981), who adopt Melzack and Wall's gate-control theory of pain. They point out that pain may begin with bodily damage or injury or with disease. A pain message from the site of injury is sent through a mechanism that works like a "gate to the brain." The brain then interprets this message. Karol *et al.* indicate that this gate can be partially or fully opened or closed, determining the amount of pain. In terms of implications for treatment, Karol *et al.* discuss various physical, emotional, and mental factors that may open or close the gate. The following list, taken from Karol *et al.*, indicates the variety of factors that are discussed with the patient:

Factors That Open the Gate
1. Physical factors
   a. Extent of the injury.
   b. Readiness of the nervous system to send pain signals.
   c. Inappropriate activity level.
2. Emotional stress
   a. Depression.
   b. Anxiety.
   c. Worry.

    d. Tension.

    e. Anger.

3. Mental factors

    a. Focusing on the pain.

    b. Boredom due to minimal involvement in life activities.

    c. Nonadaptive attitudes.

Factors That Close the Gate

1. Physical factors

    a. Medication.

    b. Counterstimulation (heat, massage, transcutaneous neural stimulation, acupuncture).

    c. Appropriate activity level.

2. Relative emotional stability

    a. Relaxation.

    b. Positive emotions (e.g., happiness, optimism).

    c. Rest.

3. Mental factors

    a. Life involvement and increased interest in life activities.

    b. Intense concentration (distraction).

    c. Adaptive attitudes.

In considering such factors that influence pain, the therapist should encourage the patient and the significant other to provide specific personal examples that illustrate each factor. We believe it is important that this discussion of factors that open and close the gate does not come across as a lecture to an introductory psychology class, giving the patient and the significant other the feeling that they will have to pass an examination. Rather, personalizing and illustrating the factors will assist the patient in entertaining the notion that his or her own pain may be viewed within the conceptualization of a gate-control model. A pictorial representation of this model may also help, showing sensory input, the brain, and a gate that can be opened or closed between the sensory input and the brain.

What is important to keep in mind about these models is that, from the viewpoint of therapy, the key feature is not the scientific validity of a given conceptualization, but the aura of its plausibility to the patient and its heuristic value in providing a basis for specific interventions that follow from that specific model. The aim of this reconceptualization phase of treatment is not to impart precise, scientific information, but rather to provide a conceptualization that will facilitate therapy and make its rationale comprehensible.

More specifically, the goal of the conceptualization phase is to have patients and significant others talk to themselves differently about the presenting problems, in this case, pain. An attempt is made to have patients and significant others change their perceptions, attributions, appraisals, expectations, sense of control, and sense of helplessness, hopelessness, and victimization. In short, the rationale that is offered to the patient and the significant other contributes to the translation process. Once again, we must stress that this translation process is *not* a didactic presentation or a lecture, but rather a Socratic-type dialogue, always using the patient's own behavior, feelings, and thoughts, and others' reactions, to provide consensual validation for the model being presented. The following excerpts illustrate the use of a patient's own material in fostering a reconceptualization:

> As I listen to you describe your situation, it seems as if there are two main aspects to your pain experience. The first is the sensory input, and the second, your reactions to these sensations, especially the way in which you focus your attention. By the sensory input I am referring to the actual intensity of the stimulation, the physical symptoms that you experience.

Here the therapist refers to the specific bodily symptoms that have been previously discussed, using the descriptive words offered by the patient on the pain questionnaire and in the interview. These may include descriptions of the degree of physical pressure, throbbing, cold, or whatever sensations the patient has experienced. The therapist continues:

> In addition to the actual physical sensations, another aspect of the pain you experience seems to be the reactions you have when you notice these sensations. The kinds of thoughts, images, and feelings you have also help to determine the pain experience, as well as the reactions of others.

Once again, the therapist uses the patient's previous descriptions to illustrate the role of such interpretations of sensations as contributors to the pain reactions.

One of our patients, who experienced severe back pain that was related to muscle spasms, indicated on the pain questionnaire that, when he suffered an attack, he would lie down and become very tense and nervous, wondering what was going to happen to him and whether he was going to die. He often thought that people did not care about him, and this made him very irritable, often resulting in his shouting at family members and subsequently feeling guilty. During our interview with the patient, we asked him what sensations he noted when he lay down. He noted that the pain was aching and radiating from his lower back down his left leg. He was then asked what thoughts he had while lying down. The patient noted that he felt anxious and became aware of his pulse racing.

When he was questioned further, he acknowledged that the feelings of helplessness and guilt about yelling at his family made him very tense.

We used this situation to illustrate the difference between the initial sensory sensations and how his reactions to the sensations—his feelings of helplessness and of no one caring, his thoughts that he was going to die, and his irritability and the resulting guilt—actually contributed to the pain by making his muscles even more tense and the resulting spasm even more distressing. In this way, we were able to demonstrate to the patient that his pain and response formed a vicious circle, with painful sensations influencing how he felt and with what he thought about these thoughts and feelings in turn exacerbating the pain. We also discussed how lying down and doing nothing reduces sensory stimuli and leads to an increased focus on pain sensation and self-preoccupation.

A common theme that emerges in a number of treatment manuals (e.g., Karol *et al.*, 1981; Malec *et al.*, 1977) is the need to help the patient distinguish between acute and chronic pain. Whereas several types of interventions may be helpful (e.g., medication, decreased activity) with acute pain, which is usually time-limited, these same interventions may have the opposite effect in the case of chronic pain. For example, inactivity may exacerbate chronic pain.

The interaction of behavior, cognitions, motivations, and sensory aspects of a situation can be presented in a clear, understandable fashion, with the therapist and the patient noting fluctuations of pain in stressful situations and changes in the course of pain over time. For example, one coronary patient, who had been seemingly unaware of a connection between periods of tension and the intensity of his pain, attributed the pain instead to changes in the state of his heart. This attribution further enhanced anxiety, leading to a cycle of more pain, further misattributions, more anxiety, pain, and so on. As we examined the details of his situation, it became clear that the source of pain had been incorrectly identified. Muscle tension in the chest and shoulders increased when he was under stress, but the heart rate and apparent pulse volume remained essentially unchanged. His misattribution prevented appropriate action from being taken to reduce the muscle contractions that aggravated the chest-wall pain. The reappraisal of the pain stimulus improved both his ability to control his pain through timely and target-appropriate interventions and his accompanying sense of self-efficacy.

Manageable Phases of Pain

Fluctuations in the pain ratings also provide a basis for fostering a reconceptualization. The therapist can introduce the notion that the patient's experience of pain can be broken down into several manageable phases rather than being considered as one overwhelming assault. For example, the therapist might say the following:

As I listen to you describe your pain, it seems that it goes through different phases or steps. I have the sense that there are times when you can almost *prepare* yourself for the pain. You may have occasions when the pain is not yet intense and when you rate it as 0 or 1 (no pain or a fairly low level of intensity). The second phase is when you feel that you are about to confront or handle the pain, when you may be offering ratings of 2, 3, and 4, and a third phase represents critical moments when you are feeling intense and excruciating pain comparable to your rating of 5. . . . Finally, there is the phase when you reflect about how you coped or failed to cope with the pain. At these points you consider how things went, how well you handled it.

Although some of our patients, for example, those suffering from trigeminal neuralgia and rheumatoid arthritis, describe their pain as having a relatively sudden onset, a substantial proportion have indicated that they could feel the unpleasant sensations and discomfort building up over several hours and eventually reaching a peak, or acute, stage. For this latter group of patients, we have found it most useful to illustrate this exacerbation of pain by examining with them the pain intensity rating cards.

When one migraine-headache patient described the intensifying of her pain over a period of several days, this was confirmed in the pain intensity ratings. The therapist conveyed the notion of there being several steps in her pain evolution and examined her thoughts at each stage. The patient noted that at the earliest points her usual reaction was, "Oh no, here it goes again; I don't think I can stand it." This response usually resulted in increased anxiety, which seemed to increase as the sensations mounted, until she became incapacitated. The therapist suggested that when she first experienced the beginning of the attack was the time that she could begin to take control and prepare how she was going to respond should the sensations continue to intensify. The Socratic-type probes helped her appreciate how her anticipation of increasing pain and the building of tension contributed to the pain's increasing.

The therapist noted that at these early stages it might be possible for her to learn some techniques that would help her short-circuit the pain. Even if the pain began to intensify during the second and third days, she could still maintain some control over the sensations by engaging in a number of coping techniques that she would learn in later training sessions. The therapist acknowledged that at times the pain might reach points of extreme intensity, "critical moments," when it seemed out of control; feelings of despair, however, would only make things worse. Some of the coping strategies might still help to keep emotional distress from making the pain even worse. The therapist indicated that, during the early stages, the patient could begin developing her "plan" to deal with subsequent sensations and noted the importance of her preparing prior to the development of the most intense sensations. At the most intense point in the cycle, she would likely find it most difficult to try to think of coping strategies. She would find it much easier if she could implement her already well-rehearsed coping techniques. Indeed, at this point it would be unlikely that she could think of and implement *new* ways of coping.

Thus the patient begins to view his or her pain differently. Prior to treatment, patients often view pain as an "all-or-none" phenomenon that just happens, based totally on some physiological process. The consequence of this view is feelings of victimization, helplessness, hopelessness, demoralization, and, quite often, depression to the point of considering suicide. The purpose of the reconceptualization process is to change the patient's view of his or her pain.

Using the data collected from the patient, the therapist suggests that the pain is made up of at least two components that go through four phases and that it also varies over time and settings. It is not as if the patient is asked to endorse in writing that this altered view has been accepted; rather, the tenor of the therapist's questions, rationale, and reflections contributes to this emerging reconceptualization. Moreover, the reconceptualization, with its various components and phases, will provide the basis for the specific interventions. The next phase of therapy is designed to help the patient, by bolstering various skills, to undertake personal experiments and to consider the data and implications from these experiments.

SUMMARY

The major objective of the reconceptualization or translation process is that the level of pain that one experiences at any given moment should be viewed as being influenced by many factors, which may include a physiological disorder, intentional or unintentional cognitions, reactions of others, and so on. Not only is there evidence to support this contention, as has been noted, but also viewing pain solely as a physiological event is not conducive to therapy. If the pain is regarded by patients as completely beyond the control of any intervention, save intrusive medical ones, they will not be amenable to other kinds of assistance. The cognitive–behavioral model, therefore, encourages the therapist to focus on the patient's cognitions concerning pain and on his or her expectancies concerning the therapy process as they are revealed during the assessment tasks. The cognitions can then be incorporated into the intervention; that is, the therapist can plan to modify whichever cognitions need to be modified and to capitalize on useful ones. Therapy can thereby attempt to subsume patient's resistances and maladaptive behaviors so that the patient comes to entertain the possibility that cognitive events, social stimuli, and learned patterns of responding are all important influences on the experience of pain, *in addition to* somatic factors.

We have focused on the initial assessment and conceptualization phases in the last two chapters because we have found that in most presentations of therapy procedures the description of these aspects of treatment is usually overlooked. There is usually much attention directed at specific treatment procedures (e.g., biofeedback, hypnotic induction, operant conditioning) as we are also about to describe, but exactly what preceded these procedures—how the patient was prepared for such interventions—is given short shrift.

From our perspective, the initial assessment and conceptualization phases constitute an important part of the therapy process. There are *no nonspecific* factors in therapy; insofar as they remain, we have simply failed to explicate how these so-called nonspecific factors operate. Our discussion of the role of the initial phase of therapy reflects our attempt to begin to explicate these. Moreover, we believe that the processes we have described in this initial phase are common to all therapeutic interventions, be they psychological or medical in nature.

Whether this initial phase is sufficient, in and of itself, to alter behavior is doubtful, as illustrated in several studies (Girodo & Wood, 1979; Holroyd & Andrasik, 1978) in which the initial phase, in the absence of the specific treatment techniques, was found to be less efficient than the total treatment package. It is not that conducting assessment and providing a treatment rationale are not effective in changing behavior; rather, the assessment and conceptualization in combination with the remainder of the treatment package was found to be that much more effective. But more such dismantling-type studies with pain patients are needed in order to measure the therapeutic value of the initial phase of treatment per se. Indeed, we described several cases in which significant changes followed from aspects of assessment such as self-monitoring and inclusion of the significant other.

Let us now turn our attention to some of the specific techniques that are used, and treatment issues that are raised, in the second phase of the cognitive–behavioral treatment of pain patients. Many of the points discussed in relation to assessment will be reiterated as we describe specific components of treatment.

CHAPTER 11

SKILLS-ACQUISITION AND
CONSOLIDATION PHASE: PART I

In this and the next two chapters, we discuss the second phase of cognitive–behavioral treatment, which focuses on skills acquisition and consolidation. The task is to encourage appropriate and successful implementation of the patient's existing coping skills and to arrange acquisition of any essential skills that are absent. In a collaborative fashion, the therapist introduces rationales and examples encouraging the patient's initiation and development of each coping method. Following practice within the therapy session, the patient tries out the specific procedure in vivo, and the results are examined in treatment.

In this chapter we focus on the use of relaxation as a coping skill and on the clinical issues surrounding the training of such a skill. The use of homework assignments is also considered.

"A little island of pain floating in a sea of indifference" was how one man described the cancer in his jaw. He underwent 30 operations in 16 years, and the prosthesis he wore to replace portions of his mouth that had been removed was constantly painful and awkwardly distorting his face and speech. Yet he refused medication, only finally consenting to take aspirin. The patient was Sigmund Freud.

"A sea of indifference" may seem a very unusual reaction to pain of such severity. But there are many examples of individuals who have adopted a certain attitude, employing a particular set of attentional, behavioral, and interpersonal coping skills, and who have functioned in spite of their pain—in some cases having reduced or avoided the pain. These individuals have not been studied adequately and represent a population in need of investigation.

Because the field has focused so much on those who continue to have difficulty coping (chronic pain patients), and because those research studies that have evaluated cognitive–behavioral approaches are mainly limited to demonstration studies, our data base for offering positive treatment advice is limited. We have a good deal of information about how people *maladaptively* deal with their pain, but much less information about how people *adaptively cope* with pain. Recently there has been some shift in attention to the study of those who have successfully coped with stress (Weisman & Sobel, 1979; Turk, Sobel, Follick, & Youkilis, 1980), but our efforts in this area have only just begun. We therefore offer our treatment advice, as we have offered assessment recommendations, cautiously. We shall describe in some detail a set of treatment procedures, but we are aware of the limited empirical data upon which these procedures rest (as do, of course, many other modes of intervention). We do think, however, that the treatment procedures discussed herein, based on the material we examined earlier, reflect our current best knowledge about the role that psychological variables play in stress and pain, and we hope that they will stimulate additional research.

This chapter combines the specific details of cognitive–behavioral treatment procedures with accompanying rationales used to introduce these procedures. The emphasis placed on the rationales underscores a point made earlier: Treatment procedures, whether medical or psychological, are not merely *administered* to patients who are assumed to be passive recipients. Rather, procedures are implemented in the context of a collaborative relationship in which the rationale for treatment plays an important role.

INTRODUCING SKILLS ACQUISITION AND CONSOLIDATION

The detailed discussion of rationales and treatment procedures may mislead the reader into the impression that the cognitive–behavioral approach is didactic, that the therapy is in some way similar to a lecture presentation. Nothing could be further from our intention. Although we recognize the importance of education in the change process, we view the *patient as an active collaborator* in the generation, selection, implementation, and evaluation of treatment procedures. Ideally, the patient should generate the program that the therapist would like implemented.

To achieve this goal, the second phase of treatment (skills acquisition and consolidation) begins with a question that was raised previously: What suggestions does the patient have about ways to reduce and avoid pain? At this point the therapist is soliciting the specifics of what the patient has done that has worked or failed in the past. Are there any instances in which the patient had to cope with pain other than the referral pain? For example, has a patient with headaches or back pain had to deal with pain in a dentist's office or with childbirth pain? Or, since the chronic patient is in some ways an "expert" on pain, what advice, if any, would the patient have to offer someone else who has similar pain in order to reduce, avoid, or get through the worst moments? What kind of things (thoughts, feelings, etc.) might get in the way of this other person's effectively using such suggestions to reduce pain?

Addressing such questions increases the patient's awareness of the availability of a *variety* of potential coping skills in his or her own repertoire. The therapist can then encourage the patient to consider whether such techniques could in any way be applicable to dealing with his or her current pain problem(s). In this way, the therapist tries to potentiate and consolidate those coping skills that the patient already possesses.

Another purpose for this inquiry is that the therapist wishes to tap the patient's attitudes, self-statements, and expectancies about specific treatment procedures. For example, the patient may indicate that he or she has already tried relaxation, but that the procedure did not work. It is important for the therapist to understand exactly what the patient means by the judgment "tried relaxation" and also by "it did not work." The therapist is listening for such parameters as the type of relaxation, timing, criteria for success, duration of efforts, how and when the patient was trained, and the nature of the patient's self-statements about the utility of relaxation and his or her reactions following failure.

It is important to have information about the patient's existing attitudes toward, prior experiences with, and knowledge of particular treatment techniques before any procedure is introduced to the patient. Given a prior negative attitude, for example, some patients will "turn off" when the therapist suggests that the patient employ relaxation or some other technique. A dubious attitude about one element of the treatment program may lessen the credibility of the entire program and increase the likelihood of resistance and nonadherence. Once the therapist appreciates the patient's "set," he or she can anticipate and subsume the patient's concerns in the therapy rationale. The therapist can, for example, highlight the distinction between what the patient has tried in the past and what is being described and suggested at this time.

This example illustrates that assessment should not be equated with formal testing or a particular phase of intervention. It is necessary to continually conduct *metacognitive assessments* (see Meichenbaum *et al.*, 1980). By "metacognition" we mean thinking about thinking, or higher

cognitive processes. Metacognition comes into play when routine automatic modes of processing and stereotyped action plans are ineffective or
inadequate. Metacognition is also evident when standard modes of
processing are unavailable for use in handling novel information. In
short, metacognition plays an important role when reflexive responding is
inadequate. As applied to pain patients, metacognition refers to the
patients' thoughts and feelings about the cognitive and behavioral strategies they use, as well as to patients' implicit personal theories and knowledge about health care providers, pain, and how to cope with pain. The
important point is that both the particular treatment techniques and the
patient's views of them are central to the therapeutic process.

Given the importance of the role of metacognitions in the treatment,
let us illustrate this point by way of analogy. Imagine yourself at a party,
and in the course of conversation you block on someone's name. "What's
her name? You know the one I'm talking about." Let us say at this point
you were then asked what you would do to retrieve the missing name. It's
on the tip of your tongue. You might say: I would (1) try to imagine the
person, where I last saw her, and so on (this is recall by means of
association); (2) go through the alphabet systematically, using each letter
as a retrieval cue; (3) decide to find the right person to ask, giving cues
such as "You know, the one I really don't like"; and many other recall
strategies. Your answer to the query about what you will do to retrieve the
missing name is what we are referring to as metacognition (i.e., reflective
knowledge and ability to control your cognitive strategies).

Now imagine someone teaching you a particular strategy to improve
your memory recall. Obviously, your attitude about that strategy, your
own ability and motivation to improve your memory, and so on, will
influence whether you adopt the proposed strategy or not. No matter how
good the skill that is being taught, your thoughts and feelings concerning
that skill will influence its successful implementation.

A similar process occurs in the teaching of coping strategies to pain
patients, and for that matter, to any patient. The therapist should adopt a
style that encourages the patient to disclose his or her concerns and
doubts about the treatment techniques and should avoid turning the
interview into a cross-examination. Instead, the therapist uses subtle
means—intonation, nonverbal cues, few words—to convey a questioning
attitude, a searching for the patient's data without being oppressive or
accusatory. We believe that these stylistic qualities contribute to treatment adherence and are often overlooked by health care professionals
interacting with patients, regardless of patients' problems (e.g., obesity,
hypertension, arthritis). With these general concerns stated, let us now
consider some specific treatment procedures.

HOMEWORK ASSIGNMENTS

An essential component of our approach to pain management is the active involvement of the patient and significant others *outside of the therapy sessions.* Tasks to be carried out between sessions begin during the assessment phase of treatment and continue throughout the therapy process. Homework assignments fulfill a number of purposes:

1. To assess various areas of the patient's and significant others' lives and how these influence and are affected by the pain problem.
2. To examine the typical responses of significant others and the patient to pain and pain behavior.
3. To make the patient and significant others more aware of factors that exacerbate and alleviate suffering.
4. To help the patient and significant others identify maladaptive responses to pain and pain behavior.
5. To consolidate the use of coping procedures discussed during therapy sessions.
6. To increase physical activity.
7. To illustrate to the patient and significant others that progress can be made in living with pain.
8. To serve as reinforcers and as enhancers of self-efficacy as the patient achieves goals.
9. To assist the therapist and patient in assessing progress and in modifying goals and treatment strategies.

Each homework assignment is geared toward observable and manageable goals, starting with those that are most readily achievable and progressing to more difficult ones. The purpose of such graded tasks is to enhance the patient's sense of competence and to reinforce his or her continued efforts. The therapist uses the assessment procedures, especially self-efficacy ratings and diaries, to establish short-, medium-, and long-term goals and the accompanying tasks designed to achieve these goals. Goals and assignments are individually tailored to meet the needs of each patient.

One of our patients who suffered from low back pain indicated that he could not sit in a chair for more than 1 hour because of his pain. Because of this problem, the patient spent great amounts of time lying down and was essentially homebound. One of the pleasures for this man and his family before his injury was going out to dinner or the movies. Since the time of his injury, 7 years before he entered our pain treatment program, the patient and his family had not been out to dinner or a movie. For this patient we negotiated a set of goals that were specific to his problems and interests, combining physical and recreational activities. The development of goals in this area was conducted in the following manner:

Therapist: As we have talked, Mr. Murphy, I could tell that spending so much time at home and in bed had taken a lot of joy out of your life.

Mr. Murphy: Yes, each day is much the same, and I don't have anything to look forward to. I wish I could just go out with my family like I used to.

Therapist: This seems to be one area that we can work on, and together we can try to set up some goals. Let's be specific; what would you like to be able to do in this area by the end of therapy?

Mr. Murphy: I would love to go out to dinner or a movie at least once a week.

Therapist: That sounds like a reasonable goal to work toward. To achieve it, we need to set some daily and weekly goals. One area we can work on is increasing the amount of time you can sit in a chair. I believe you indicated that you could sit for about 1 hour before your pain became too severe. Am I correct? [Obviously, goals must be based on the patient's physical condition, in consultation with the patient's physician and physiotherapist.]

Mr. Murphy: Yes, I could just about make if for an hour without having to lie down.

Therapist: OK. Let us consider how we can work together to increase your ability to sit. One way that patients like yourself have done this is to gradually increase the length of time they practice sitting in a chair. One could begin with a comfortable amount of time and then slowly and gradually increase the time each day. We can also consider some physical exercises that might help strengthen your muscles and increase your sitting time. What would be a reasonable beginning sitting time in your case?

Mr. Murphy: I'm not sure. The pain just comes. I guess I could sit for 30 minutes or so.

Therapist: Thirty minutes. That sounds like a reasonable place to begin. Let's set a goal of sitting for 30 minutes tomorrow, and then let's increase that by 5-minute intervals. You could try to increase by 5 minutes every other day. In this way, you will be able to increase your sitting tolerance gradually. How does that sound?

Mr. Murphy: OK.

Therapist: Good. Let's set up a chart so that you can keep track of your progress. On this piece of paper, I will list the days of the week along

the bottom line. On the vertical line I will indicate times, beginning with
30 minutes and moving up by 5-minute intervals. Each day you should
mark on the sheet the amount of time you sat in a chair. Don't try to
increase more than 5 minutes every other day. What we want to do is to
gradually build up your tolerance for sitting. [At this point the therapist
shows Mr. Murphy the chart, making sure he understands how it is set up
and what he is to do.] How does this sound?

Mr. Murphy: I think I can do that.

Therapist: Good. Are there any difficulties you can see in working
on this goal?

Mr. Murphy: No.

Therapist: OK. Let's make sure this is clear; how are you going to go
about working on your sitting this week?

After the patient reviewed the task for the week, the therapist
continued.

Therapist: OK. Increasing your sitting time will help in getting you
to be able to sit in a movie or a restaurant. Let's think about sitting at a
restaurant for a moment. How long do you think you sit in a restaurant?

Mr. Murphy: Oh, about 2 hours.

Therapist: Is that true for all restaurants? What about some fast-
food places like McDonald's?

Mr. Murphy: Not those kind of restaurants; in those you're in and
out quickly.

Therapist: That's right; probably in fast-food restaurants you are
out in a half hour or less. Have you thought about taking your family to
one of these types of restaurants?

Mr. Murphy: No, not really.

Therapist: This would be one way you could spend time with your
family right now. How about setting a goal that you go out with your
family to a fast-food restaurant during the next week?

Mr. Murphy: Yes, I could do that, but . . .

Therapist: You sound a little hesitant. What problems are you
thinking of?

Mr. Murphy: Well, what happens if I go and my back starts to hurt?

Therapist: Well, what could you do if in fact that did occur?

Mr. Murphy: I guess I could get up and leave. Since I can already sit
for 30 minutes now, this should be something I can try. What have I got
to lose?

Therapist: You're right; you can give it a shot.

The therapist would continue to work with Mr. Murphy in establishing several goals for him to work on during the week between sessions. The use of charts, asking the patient to report what it is that he or she has to do, and setting reasonable, achievable goals is illustrated in the preceding example. A similar process is carried out during each therapy session. As the sessions progress, the patient is given more of an opportunity and responsibility in formulating problem-solving strategies about how to handle possible problems surrounding homework assignments.

One point to note about the use of charts is that only one goal should be included on each chart so that the patient does not become confused. If several charts are being used, the therapist should label the specific goal and tasks on each one. Patients are asked to bring charts with them each week so that progress can be reviewed and problem areas identified. In addition, the therapist should discuss with the patient what to do if a daily goal is not met. Emphasis is placed on not giving up, on considering what may have contributed to the lack of success, and on the importance of continued effort, with reinforcement for the effort, not just for success.

Finally, an important point to make before we describe different behavioral and cognitive coping techniques (relaxation, mental distraction, imagery) is that patients who have experienced chronic pain for long periods are likely to have little initial confidence in such techniques. They usually believe that such techniques are unlikely to reduce severe and long-standing pain (McCaffrey, 1979). Moreover, they may believe that suggesting such techniques to alleviate pain implies that their pain is only in their "heads." We noted the importance of these patient beliefs in the last chapter, but it needs to be reiterated here.

The therapist must be cognizant of such beliefs and must address them, even if the patient does not raise them. The therapist–patient relationship is critical if patients are to be expected to try techniques despite their skepticism. We use concrete examples, metaphors, and demonstrations to illustrate the potential utility of the various coping techniques. We will describe some of these as we introduce the different techniques.

CUE-CONTROLLED RELAXATION AND CONTROLLED BREATHING

We usually begin skills training with relaxation and controlled, diaphragmatic breathing exercises. Relaxation is especially useful early in the skills acquisition phase because it can be learned readily by almost all patients and has a good deal of face validity. Russo, Bird, and Masek (1980) characterized relaxation as the "aspirin of behavioral medicine," since it is used so widely across disorders. Our use of relaxation procedures has been influenced by the suggestion that their major contribution to such treatments as systematic desensitization is inducing *mental*, rather than just *physical*, relaxation (Rachman, 1967) and that one can be muscularly relaxed, yet autonomically aroused (Lader & Mathews, 1968; Van Egeren, 1971).

We have altered the "traditional" Jacobsonian (Jacobson, 1962) mode of relaxation as employed by Paul (1966) by adding a cognitive, cue-controlling procedure (R. Russell & Sipich, 1973). In addition, we emphasize controlled breathing exercises, which aid in the reduction of anxiety and tension. The training is designed not only to teach a response incompatible with tension and anxiety, but also to provide the patient with a behavioral coping skill to employ in any situation in which adaptive coping is required. Practice strengthens the patient's sense of having some control over periods of stress and pain and reduces the feelings of helplessness.

Before describing these relaxation procedures, a warning should be offered: There are pain populations for whom *relaxation exercises of tensing and releasing certain muscle groups may be contraindicated.* Some of our patients with migraine and tension headaches have reported that tensing and relaxing the face muscles exacerbates their pain, a finding also reported by Bakal *et al.* (1981). In these populations one can instead focus upon cue-controlled breathing and autogenic suggestions. Furthermore, some patients report an increase in anxiety during relaxation exercises, sometimes because their minds wander to anxiety-provoking thoughts or images, or sometimes for reasons that are not clear, perhaps related to an initial antipathy for the exercises or to a fear of losing control.

We have found it helpful to discuss these potential difficulties with patients, noting that they are not uncommon and that they could be combated by keeping one's eyes open instead of closed, refocusing thoughts to more acceptable ones, generating pleasant images, focusing on the pattern of breathing, and so on. If problems persist, we encourage patients to discuss this with us so that we can help. In some cases the therapist has even suggested that the ability to let one's mind wander is a sign that the individual is in fact becoming more relaxed.

Although there are a number of different treatment manuals and audiotapes on relaxation, we are including our own guidelines and instructions for the therapist since our procedures have been adapted to pain patients and we have altered the relaxation procedure from a cognitive–behavioral perspective. Also, although our presentation will involve the tensing and releasing of various muscle groups and controlled breathing, one could relax by means of meditation or by engaging in strenuous activities such as walking, swimming, and other sports. In short, relaxation is as much a state of mind as it is a physical state. And both the state of mind and the physical state can be induced by a variety of stimuli and activities.

Relaxation training need not be terminated because a patient reports that he or she finds it "impossible to sit still through that damn tape." Such a reaction provides the occasion for the therapist to elicit what activities, situations, and so on, the patient *does* find relaxing. A week or two of self-monitoring may be necessary to sensitize the patient to these. Whatever the outcome of this investigation, it can be incorporated into the therapeutic regimen.

A RELAXATION PROTOCOL[1]

Before any treatment technique is offered, the therapist first provides a rationale or explanation of why the specific procedure will be used. As Hockersmith (1975) noted with regard to chronic back-pain patients, even though the original insult may have been resolved, the complex pain-tension cycle is quite capable of perpetuating the pain itself. A response to organic insult results in the tensing of muscles surrounding the area. This further antagonizes the insult and increases pain. Very often with an increase in pain, the neighboring muscle groups will also be tensed. This, too, will increase pain, and before long a pain–tension cycle has been established. The therapist explains to the pain patient the relationship between pain and tension and anxiety, and the role of relaxation.

For example, Turner (1979) has illustrated the contribution of this pain–tension cycle to back-pain patients by asking them to tense and hold the muscles of the fist and biceps and then to notice the impact on other portions of the body, such as the back. "How did tensing affect your back? I think you can see how, when one muscle group is tense, for whatever reason, it can quickly affect your whole body." The therapist can use experiential examples to illustrate each point.

To introduce the relaxation exercise, the therapist may begin by conveying the following:

---

1. We do *not* suggest that the therapist memorize this protocol, but instead we offer it in order to convey the general approach and the flavor of the intervention.

One of the most effective means of affecting the *sensations* of pain is through *relaxation.* If you are experiencing pain, the accompanying feelings of being tense, depressed, angry, frustrated, or anxious often can make your pain worse. One way to reduce the impact of these feelings is by learning to relax various parts of your body.

How can you actually reduce the physical sensations and control your feelings? One suggestion comes from methods of childbirth. You may be familiar with some of the methods of natural childbirth, that is, childbirth with the aid of few, if any, drugs. A primary feature of these methods is *relaxation.* Physical tension—the tightening of muscles—makes you feel more anxious and upset, and it increases physical sensations such as pain. And pain tends to cause tension. This sets up a vicious circle: Pain leads to tension, leading to anxiety and more pain, leading to more tension, and so on.

How do you stop the pain–tension–anxiety–pain circle? By relaxing.

A woman attending her first childbirth class could have the same response to this suggestion that you may have now: "Sure! Relax! That's easy to say. Just try to relax when you are in severe pain. Relaxing is the *last* thing you feel like doing. All you can do is tense up and try not to scream." It isn't usually quite so simple just to "relax" under such difficult circumstances.

It isn't simple, but it is *possible.* Witness to this fact are the thousands of mothers-to-be who take childbirth preparation classes each year and who report much less pain from labor than those women who do not engage in the training. Further evidence is provided by the popularity of this approach, which is growing by leaps and bounds every year. Classes are being held in hospitals everywhere, and doctors are routinely suggesting that patients attend. So *it is possible* to relax, even under circumstances that are normally as uncomfortable (or downright painful) as childbirth. *And,* most important, it has been found that this relaxation *lessens the actual sensations of pain,* despite the fact that these sensations have a clear-cut physical origin.

How Relaxation Works

Relaxation does several things.

1. Muscle tension increases painful sensations. Anyone who has experienced a charley horse or muscle spasm needs no convincing of this. Relaxation is incompatible with tension—you cannot mentally and physically relax and at the same time tighten your muscles. Therefore *relaxation reduces the amount of pain that is directly caused by tense muscles.*

2. When you are experiencing pain, it takes a lot of concentration to stay relaxed. You can learn specific techniques to stay relaxed under these circumstances, but they do take some effort. As a result, while you are concentrating on relaxing, you are *unable* to *attend* much to the experience of pain.

Consider that your brain is capable of paying primary attention only to one thing at a time. You know, for instance, that you cannot concentrate on doing very many tasks at once without getting rather confused. If you are filling all of your brain's capacity for attention with one kind of information, you cannot accept much information from other sources. This is precisely what happens when you are concentrating very hard on relaxing. While you are taking up a great deal of your powers of attention with staying relaxed, you have little attention left over to experience the pain, except on the edge of your awareness.

You will probably still "feel" your pain to some extent—that is, you will be aware that it is there. Women well prepared for labor sometimes speak of knowing that the pain is there, but finding that it is not overwhelmingly important; they were concentrating on the relaxation–breathing techniques so much, that the pain was merely in the background—and not so "painful." Thus, *by occupying your attention with something else, relaxation reduces the amount of pain you experience.*

3. When you are relaxed, you are *not* as likely to become anxious and depressed as when you are tense. Such feelings tend to increase muscular tension, and this, of course, leads to an increase in the pain. *Relaxation reduces such feelings of anxiety, frustration, and tension and therefore reduces your pain.*

4. Another use of the relaxation exercises is to help you become aware of and control various muscles that become tense and contribute to your pain. Even though you are not aware of it, various muscles may become tense prior to the actual onset of the pain or may increase the intensity of pain already present. Many people think that they are relaxed when they really are not. Muscles can be tense even when they are not in movement. This tenseness contributes to your pain. You can learn to counteract this tenseness. You can learn to use this tenseness as a cue, a bell ringer, to begin your relaxation and other coping responses.

5. Relaxation helps with sleep disturbance that may affect one's capacity to tolerate pain. Many patients tell us that it is hard to cope with pain when they are tired.

To summarize, relaxation reduces pain in several ways: (1) It reduces muscular tension, thereby reducing some pain; (2) it occupies your attention, short-circuiting much of the discomfort; (3) it reduces anxiety, which further helps reduce tension; (4) it provides you with something you can do before, during, or after you experience pain, especially when the pain is at low intensity (pain intensity ratings of 1, 2, and 3 on the 5-point scale you used earlier); and (5) it helps you get needed rest and sleep.

In addition to your being physically relaxed, relaxation helps to create a feeling of emotional calmness. Thus we can use these relaxation exercises as a way to help us close the pain gate, reduce the discomfort. In contrast, when you are tense, you tend to open the pain gate.

Whenever the opportunity occurs, the therapist relates the current training procedure to the conceptualization model, in this case the gate-control model of pain. Also, each time an experiential exercise is conducted, the therapist checks in with the patient to see how he or she felt about it and how the patient sees the exercise or activity relating to the conceptualization.

Learning to Relax

Now let us turn to the specific techniques that can be used to encourage relaxation. You may already have engaged in some relaxation exercises. They are commonly used in the practice of transcendental meditation, yoga, or biofeedback, for instance. Complete relaxation does not come easily for many people; it is a skill that needs to be practiced. It can be achieved without a great deal of difficulty, but it takes time to engage in some exercises, at least until the response of complete relaxation can come more automatically.

The technique that will be presented now involves intentionally tensing and then relaxing various muscle groups, controlled breathing, and using certain relaxing words and images. Let us consider each of these different ways of learning to relax. We will try each of these methods in order to see which ones help you to relax the best. After you have learned some relaxation techniques, you can choose which ones to try out. Some patients have told us that different techniques were more effective at different times. Other patients have told us they were surprised when some techniques they did not think would work actually helped.

At this point the therapist answers any queries and ensures that the patient understands what he or she is going to do and why. The therapist continues:

Muscle relaxation is a way to relax your whole body a little at a time. People usually find that it is easier to relax little by little than all at once. So, in muscle relaxation you will be relaxing all the muscles in your body one group at a time.

Muscle relaxation involves three steps:

1. Turning your attention to the muscles to be relaxed.
2. Tensing the muscles (not so that it hurts, but enough so that you can feel the tension).
3. Gradually letting the tension go and feeling the muscles unwind.

We usually begin with the muscles of the dominant hand and arm and then proceed to various muscle groups, as described by Paul (1966). Patients are often unaware of tense muscles, and thus we incorporate muscle-tension perception within the relaxation training (as described in the next two sections of this chapter). (See also Fowler & Kraft, 1974, for a discussion of such focusing exercises.) Particular attention is given to muscle groups that are related to the patient's pain problem. Since the basic relaxation procedure is quite well known, let us compare and contrast the usual script with one that has a cognitive–behavioral focus. First, here is an excerpt from a tension–relaxation induction that was adapted from the clinical work of A. Lazarus by Goldfried and Davison (1976):

> Once again now, clench the right fist, clench it tight. Study the tensions. Study them. And now relax the right fist. Let the fingers spread out comfortably. See if you can keep letting go a little bit more. Even though it seems as if you've let go as much as you possibly can, there always seems to be that extra bit of relaxation. Note the difference once again between the tension and relaxation. Note the looseness beginning to develop in the left and right arms and hands. Both your left and right arms and hands now are a little bit more relaxed. (p. 88)

Next is the comparable portion of a cognitive–behaviorally oriented relaxation exercise. Notice that the two scripts have much in common, but that the second one takes more account of the many possible physical and mental reactions that the patient may be experiencing during the exercise:

> Once again, make a fist with the right hand. Feel the pulling across the top and bottom of the hand. This is what we mean by tenseness. Hold it, and observe the sensations in your hand. Now, go ahead and relax the muscles of the hand. Slowly let your fingers come away from your palm, your fingers separating a little, gradually resting on the arm of the chair. Feel the changes; notice your hand, how the tenseness is beginning to disappear, slowly the tightness fading, as *you* bring forth a sense of calm and relaxation. Note that your hand is becoming more and more relaxed and that this feeling of calmness can being to spread. . . . Notice the changes you bring about.

A difference in these two excerpts is in the use of the present participle. In the second version, "is becoming" and "beginning to develop" are much less susceptible to disproof than telling the patient he or she is relaxed. Whereas a patient may not view his or her hand as relaxed, it is unlikely that he or she will fail to notice any changes at all that could be interpreted as becoming more relaxed. Moreover, we emphasized that relaxation is under the patient's own control. Such emphasis on control is important to enhancing generalization.

The therapist attempts to have the patient attend to the sensations he or she is experiencing and to interpret these as changes toward relaxation.

To do this, of course, maximum use should be made of the cues the patient provides during the exercise, and a strict protocol should *not* be adhered to. An attempt is made both to be suggestive and to avoid potential sources of resistance, incorporating any difficulties the patient experiences as perfectly normal steps on the road to mastery of the skill.

A BREATHING EXERCISE

The following illustrates instructions for a slow deep-breathing exercise:

> Now that we have relaxed the muscles of both hands and both arms, I want you to tense and hold the muscles of the chest and back. You can do this by filling your lungs slowly, with short, deep breaths. Let's begin by taking short, deep breaths, holding each one and then slowly exhaling.

At this point, while the patient is seated and in a relaxed state, the therapist demonstrates the breathing exercise. The pattern of inhalation modeled by the therapist involves filling the chest, then holding for a few seconds, and, finally, slowly exhaling. The therapist should ensure that the patient does not hold his or her breath to the point of breathlessness, but rather leaves sufficient time for slow, deep inhalation and exhalation. The therapist notes the distinction between a sudden, sharp inhalation-exhalation, which causes the heart rate to increase, and the slow inhalation-exhalation cycle, which causes a quieting of the bodily processes. The relaxation exercise continues:

> Fill the chest and hold the breath. Now, part your lips slightly and slowly exhale. Slowly. Good. Note, as you slowly exhale, the sense of relaxation and warmth you are able to bring forth. Good. [Pause, letting the patient return to a normal, even breathing pattern.] Now, once again, let's make the muscles of the chest and back tense by filling the lungs, using slow, deep breaths. Now hold the breath, feel the tenseness across the top of the chest and throughout the upper portion of your body. Now bring forth a sense of relaxation by slowly exhaling, parting the lips and letting the air out slowly, slowly. Good. Note the distinction between tenseness and relaxation that *you have been able to bring forth.*

To convey to the patient the idea of slowly inhaling and exhaling, the therapist can suggest to the patient:

> As you exhale slowly, imagine that you are gently blowing across the top of a spoon of hot soup so you do not spill it or that you are flickering a candle without blowing it out.

The therapist can suggest that the patient picture a feather slowly floating in the background; as the feather approaches the ground, the patient is becoming more and more relaxed.

The purpose of imagery-based techniques is to facilitate and embellish the relaxation exercises. It is important to ask the patient afterwards how things went, what difficulties (if any) were experienced, and so on. One patient reported that the relaxation went quite well, until the therapist suggested the image of hot soup. The patient disliked soup intensely and suggested that in future sessions he employ the image of a blob of gelatin dessert on a spoon. Such minor obstacles can have disproportionate influences. The patient collaborates in guiding the individual tailoring of the treatment program by describing personally relevant scenes that are relaxing and vivid. (See McCaffery, 1979, p. 150, for a description of additional slow, rhythmic breathing techniques.)

While the patient is sitting quietly, the therapist says:

> You can bring forth a feeling of relaxation and reduce your pain by using such breathing exercises. By using slow, deep breaths, and by inhaling and exhaling slowly, you can control feelings of pain and tenseness. The breathing technique is especially useful because of the effect breathing has on heart rate and upon the rest of the body. Breathing right slows the bodily processes, lowers arousal, and in turn reduces pain. Once again, let's try the breathing exercise. This time try it on your own, breathing in slowly, holding each breath, and then parting the lips and letting the air out slowly. Take your time and try it.

This cycle is repeated several times as the patient is given increased control over the relaxation. The therapist can also suggest to the patient the following:

> You can deepen the relaxation and remove feelings of tension by thinking silently to yourself the words "relax," "calm," or "peace" as you slowly let out your breath. Choose a word that you like and that helps you feel relaxed and pleasant. Say your word silently to yourself or even picture these words in your mind as you slowly let out the breath. This is especially helpful between sessions when you practice relaxing and slow, deep breathing, or when you begin to experience pain, or even when the pain becomes intense.
>
> Now, breathe naturally and listen to the normal wavelike flow of your breathing, breathing evenly and easily. Take a few moments to enjoy the pleasurable sensation of relaxation that you have been able to bring forth.
>
> If you notice that your mind has wandered and you are thinking about something besides relaxing, don't worry about that. This is natural. Everyone's mind wanders sometimes, and this may happen when you are relaxed. Just bring your attention back to your breathing and repeat your relaxing word each time you breathe out. . . . Good. Now take a few moments to

enjoy the pleasurable sensation of relaxation that *you have been able to bring forth.* When you are ready, just take a slow, deep breath, and as you exhale, open your eyes, sitting relaxed, but at the same time alert and awake.

The therapist should ensure that the patient does not view the lack of immediate success with the exercises as evidence of personal failure and treatment inappropriateness. It is important to short-circuit this possibility by preparing the patient for possible "failure" and offering alternative interpretations (such as the preceding suggestion that a wandering mind may constitute evidence of relaxation).

Some patients have reported that relaxing made them more aware of their pain. We have found it helpful to make relaxation more active in some cases. We have encouraged patients to incorporate engaging mental images (to be described later), to use slides or photographs of pleasant scenes, and to play pleasant, soothing music to increase distraction. There are many different types of relaxation and a number of variations available. The therapist should be familiar with a variety of them and should practice several different ones with patients (see Benson, 1976; Goleman, 1977; McCaffery, 1979; Shealy, 1976).

Teaching patients to use several relaxation techniques increases the sense of multiple resources being available for combating feelings of helplessness in the face of pain. Moreover, encouraging patients to select from a number of techniques also increases their sense of control. We have found it helpful to inform patients that different techniques may prove beneficial at different times. Thus patients are encouraged to try out techniques that may not have been helpful at other times, for they may prove effective in different circumstances.

RELAXATION AS A SKILL

The instructions to patients emphasize how they can bring forth the sense of relaxation or tenseness. This is consistent with the notion of viewing relaxation as a process in learning self-control (Goldfried, 1977). The following instructions further illustrate this point:

> Notice any differences in feelings you may have at the end of the relaxation exercise compared to those you were having when you began or when you first entered this room. Essentially, this difference is a result of *your own ability to control your body. You can slow your body down,* actually voluntarily relax, even though you may have been tense to begin with.
>
> Keep in mind, however, that relaxation is a skill, and like any other skill, it has to be learned. For some people it comes easily; for others it takes

longer and more work. As a result, the degree of relaxation that you achieved today may not be the most that you are capable of. I have prepared a summary sheet that may prove helpful in your trying out the relaxation exercise at home, at a speed that is appropriate for you. The relaxation skill is one that will be of benefit not only in dealing with pain, but in many everyday situations that you encounter.

A summary sheet (Figure 11-1) is given to patients in order to consolidate the training. Patients are encouraged to read over the relaxation summary sheet several times and to keep it available for review whenever necessary.

In some cases we have provided the patient with an audiotape of relaxation instructions in order to facilitate training and have even, on occasion, included the patient's significant other in the joint relaxation exercises, when mutual tenseness was evident. For one patient who reported particular difficulties with her mind wandering and an inability to

---

The point of relaxation exercise is that you can help yourself control your pain. Briefly, the three things to concentrate on in relaxing are:

1. Tensing and relaxing various muscles.
2. Slow, deep breathing: inhaling, holding the tension briefly, and then slowly letting out your breath between slightly parted lips. As you breathe out, just let the tension go as well.
3. Thinking of a pleasant, relaxing image or word while exhaling, such as a picture of a feather or cloud gently floating and any relaxing thoughts.

Since relaxation is a skill, practicing at least once a day for 10 or 15 minutes would be most helpful. Find a comfortable, quiet place and go through the exercises, especially the breathing exercises. This practice will enable you to become better at directing your own relaxation. If time permits, you can practice twice a day.
Recall that relaxation

- Reduces pain caused by muscle tension.
- Reduces pain by filling your attention.
- Reduces anxiety-related pain.
- Gives you something to do before, during, and after the experience of pain.
- Helps reduce disturbance of your sleep.

Practice first under calm conditions. When you develop the skill, you can try relaxing at more difficult times. Settle in a comfortable chair and take a relaxing position. Make a tight fist with your right hand. Hold it. Gradually let your hand relax, let the fingers open slowly and your hand once again rest comfortably. Notice the clear difference between muscle tension and relaxation. Relax the muscles as much as you can and enjoy the feelings you have been able to bring forth. Repeat this tension–relaxation exercise with the other muscles of your body: your right arm, left hand, left arm, shoulders, legs, and other muscles that feel tense.

FIGURE 11-1. (Continued)

Take in a slow, deep breath and hold it. Note how the muscles pull. Part your lips and gently exhale slowly, as though flickering a candle flame or blowing on a spoon of hot soup. Feel yourself becoming more and more relaxed and comfortable. Repeat this pattern several times, using a picture, such as a feather gently floating to earth, as you exhale. Notice the increasing state of relaxation that you have been able to bring forth.

If your mind wanders, just try to bring it back to the task of relaxing. If you do these relaxation exercises regularly, you will gradually find it takes less and less time and effort to relax on each occasion and that you can stay relaxed longer each time.

Relaxation may stop or slow down your pain that is just beginning, it may reduce the intensity and duration of your pain, and it may also prevent pain onset, if you can achieve greater degrees of relaxation in your daily activities. After you have practiced relaxation, keep the following points in mind:

1. PRACTICE
   Continue practicing relaxation using the exercises. Try to achieve deeper and deeper levels of relaxation.
2. SCAN
   Note signs of muscular and mental tension during the day. Notice such signs as stiffness in your back, tightness in your neck, sore muscles, clenched teeth, or any personal signs of tension. *Scan* your body at least two times each day for these signs. Pick specific times or places to use this scanning (e.g., as you sit down to a meal, while you are listening to someone in a conversation).
3. RELAX
   If you find any signs of tension present, take the time necessary to relax sufficiently so that they decrease. Take a slow, deep breath to control your tension and bring forth relaxation. If you do this regularly, you will gradually find that it takes less and less time to relax on each occasion and that you stay relaxed longer each time.
4. GENERALIZE
   When you are relaxed, pay attention to the pleasantness of your feelings. Try to keep this state of relaxation, even when you are active as well as when you are passive. Your whole body does not need to be tense when you are walking or sitting, for example.

FIGURE 11-1. *Relaxation summary sheet.*

imagine pleasant scenes, we suggested that she place posters of pleasant scenes on her walls so she could focus on these while she tried to relax.

In any case it is important for the therapist to ensure that the patient understands the rationale for the relaxation procedures and then discusses in detail how, when, and where the patient will implement the daily practice sessions. As noted before, the therapist should not assume that the patient will readily or willingly employ the treatment suggestions. Exactly what problems does the patient foresee in implementing the exercises? How can these problems be anticipated, avoided, or handled when they occur? We discuss these before the patient tries practicing relaxation at home in an attempt to prevent potential problems from arising. In future sessions, as the patient begins to develop some proficiency with relaxation, the therapist can begin to tap the patient's sense of efficacy about using relaxation as a means of reducing and tolerating pain.

In addition to providing detailed instructions and practice with the exercises, then, the therapist and the patient should be explicit concerning how the exercises will be used on a day-to-day basis. As noted in Figure 11-1 (the relaxation summary), there is a good deal of concern about how the patient will apply the relaxation procedures in his or her natural environment. Such generalization is *not* expected to occur without planning; rather, the therapist explicitly engineers such transfer into the treatment regimen.

Finally, the therapist should attempt to anticipate and subsume any doubts and concerns that the patient may have with regard to the relaxation exercises. For example, Turner (1979) compared the effects of someone learning to relax to someone going on a diet—one may not see results in a few days and may feel like quitting, but if one stays with it and practices the relaxation procedures, benefits will follow. In fact, learning such skills may result in less frequent, as well as less severe, episodes of pain over time. The therapist should also indicate that some patients at first even notice pain a little more because they have become aware of feelings in their bodies. But this awareness will eventually prove quite helpful, since the patient will be able to notice such tension and then relax.

Another problem with relaxation exercises, noted by McCaffery (1979), may be boredom. We deal with this by teaching patients a variety of relaxation techniques and suggesting that, if they find themselves becoming bored, they switch to a different technique and improvise by adding to the relaxation, by using music, mental images, and so on.

The therapist should discuss the times when relaxation will be practiced. The pain intensity rating cards may provide helpful information. The patient should not plan to begin practicing relaxation at times of the day when pain tends to be most intense. As the patient becomes more skilled at relaxing, practice may be encouraged prior to times of most intense pain in an attempt to short-circuit the pain. Relaxation practice should not be scheduled at times when the patient is likely to be interrupted (e.g., just before dinner). Patients should be asked to think of any problems that might interfere with the relaxation schedule. Finally, patients should be asked what they would do if their relaxation time were interrupted (e.g., by a telephone call). Since it is possible that some interruption is likely to occur, preparation for how this will be handled will reduce nonadherence.

SUMMARY

We have considered the relaxation procedure in some detail in order to convey the clinical sensitivity needed in conducting such interventions. Our discussion highlighted the important role of the treatment rationale; the patient's expectations, self-efficacy, and metacognitions; the role of homework assignments or practice; and the issues surrounding transfer or generalization. It should be apparent that treatment entails more than providing someone with a relaxation tape and a directive to practice. Sensitivity and concern are needed along with the other skills-training procedures discussed in the next chapter.

CHAPTER 12

SKILLS-ACQUISITION
AND CONSOLIDATION PHASE:
PART II

For a year I have been troubled by morbid inclination and very painful stimuli which from other's descriptions of such symptoms I believe to be gout, so that I had to call a doctor. One night, however, impatient at being kept awake by pain, I availed myself of the stoical means of concentration upon some different object of thought such for instance as the name of "Cicero" with its multifarious associations, in this way I found it possible to divert my attention, so that pain was soon dulled . . . Whenever the attacks recur and disturb my sleep, I find this remedy most useful.—*Immanuel Kant (cited by Fulop-Miller, 1938)*

This chapter focuses on the development and consolidation of a number of additional coping skills. Attention diversion by such means as imagery, mental activities, and control of appraisal processes is considered.

CONTROLLING ATTENTION

Although the image of Cicero may not serve the same function for us today, Kant's example highlights the potential of the cognitive strategy of attention diversion to reduce pain. Such attention-diverting coping strategies have been employed probably since humans first experienced pain. Consider another example. Arthur Koestler, in his book *Darkness at Noon*, describes Rubashov's reaction to the forthcoming interrogation by his prison officials:

> Rubashov had been beaten up repeatedly during his last imprisonment, but of this method he only knew by hearsay. He had learned that every known physical pain was bearable; if only one knew beforehand exactly what was going to happen to one, one stood it as a surgical operation—for instance the extraction of a tooth. Really bad was only the unknown, which gave no choice to foresee one's reactions and no scale to calculate one's capacity of

resistance. . . . He called to memory every particular he knew about the subject "steambath." He imagined the situation in detail and tried to analyze the physical sensations to be expected, in order to rid them of their uncanniness. The important thing was not to let oneself be caught unprepared. (1940, pp. 55-56)

In a more clinically relevant case study, Levendusky and Pankratz (1975) treated a 65-year-old male patient who was manifesting symptoms of chronic abdominal pain. The patient was taught to control his pain through relaxation, cognitive relabeling, and the use of the cognitive coping strategy of imaginative transformation of pain (which was specifically tailored to the patient). Levendusky and Pankratz described the cognitive strategy as follows:

Images were devised that were familiar and meaningful to him because of his engineering background. For example, he visualized his pain sensations as being caused by tightening steel bands, which he could loosen, and as electrical impulses traveling over circuits, which he could manipulate. After a short period of visualization training, Mr. X was able to use this procedure, which provided him with new cognitive labels for his physiological cues. (p. 166)

Although there are various intrapersonal and interpersonal ways to divert attention in order to avoid or reduce pain, the data already reviewed indicate that no one type of coping strategy or attention-diversion technique has proved to be most effective. Thus the therapist provides patients with descriptions of and training in the use of a variety of different techniques.

The therapist describes the role of attention as a major factor in perceptual activity and therefore a primary concern in examining and changing behavior. Attention has been described as having both selective and amplifying functions, and McCaffery (1979) has suggested that diverting attention may be viewed as a "sensory shielding" from pain. When chronic pain patients withdraw from most activities and external stimulation, they tend to restrict the focus of attention to bodily processes, which may, in turn, exacerbate the perception of pain. Thus, by having patients both increase activity and refocus their attention, perception of pain can be modified.

Individual Tailoring

In conveying the role of attention to the patient, the therapist must be sensitive to the patient's background and resources. This is nicely illustrated in a laboratory study by Ischlondsky (1949), who reported a case in which a classical musician raised his pain threshold by 26% while listening to a Bach fugue, but raised his threshold only one-third as much while listening to a popular song. We have found that encouraging some patients to engage in such diverting mental activities as arithmetic exercises may lack face validity and not prove effective. On the other hand, one of our pain patients was an engineer who found engaging in calculus proofs to be an effective means of distracting himself.

Another patient, however, provided a different note of caution. This patient, who worked as an accountant, initially suggested imagining the overhaul of a highly sophisticated electronics device he had observed at his job. He thought his interest in the field of electronics would make this a useful distracting technique. Further exploration revealed that this patient would have preferred to imagine playing golf, but because he felt a need to impress the therapist with a demonstration of varied talents and interests, he had suggested the electronics image. Golf was settled on, much to the patient's satisfaction.

This last patient illustrates the need to assess adequately the reasons that a particular procedure does not work. At first, the patient was disposed to attribute failure to inadequacies in himself, with an accompanying sense of hopelessness that nothing would work. An examination of what was going on indicated the need to tailor the procedure to the specific patient. Moreover, the therapist was able to use, in a situational analysis, the patient's sense of having to impress him. Perhaps the patient felt that he had to impress people outside of therapy as well. What kind of stress might this "need" impose, and how did it affect the patient's pain experience? This inquiry provided the basis for a cognitive restructuring intervention. Quite often, the concerns surrounding the implementation of specific skills or homework assignments become the focus of treatment. In the context of teaching specific techniques and procedures, themes or recurrent patterns may emerge that in themselves may become the focus of intervention.

Techniques

As we shift our focus to other specific attention-diversion techniques and accompanying rationales, it is important to appreciate the general treatment strategy being employed. The therapist combines both rationale and example, with the patient engaging in experiential exercises. Then the therapist can sensitively examine the patient's experience and reactions to the exercises and use these as the basis for the next set of examples and rationale, and so on. The rationales are constantly punctuated by the patient's *trying out* specific procedures. Throughout, the therapist is conveying the purpose and function of the attention-diversion procedures. For example, consider the next therapist script as a way to introduce the attention-diversion coping skills.

What you are paying attention to at a particular time will influence the pain you feel. The less you focus on pain, the less pain you will feel. Of course, that's easier said than done. But it *can* be done. Let's illustrate why your attention is so important and how it can be controlled.

Your attention is naturally drawn to things in your environment that are most obvious at the moment. If there is a sudden loud noise or bright light in the room, you are almost certain to pay attention to it. In the same way that you tend to focus on this kind of event, normally you are strongly drawn to attend to other intense stimulations, including painful ones. In short, your awareness and attention are like a searchlight. Things on which you focus your attention are pretty clear, but other things and events tend momentarily to fade out of awareness. [The notion of the searchlight was suggested by J. Stevens, 1971, and by William James well before that.]

For example, sit back in your chair, close your eyes, and just take a few moments to relax. . . . Now take some time to pay attention to your awareness and notice where it goes. Say to yourself, "Now I am aware of . . . ," and finish the sentence with what you are aware of at that moment. Notice whether this is something inside, a thought, or outside, some sound. . . . Where does your awareness go? . . . Are you mostly aware of things outside your body or of sensations inside your skin? . . . Now direct your attention to what you were least aware of inside or outside your body and become aware of this, focusing your attention on these sensations. As you focus your attention on one source, either inside or outside, begin to notice how the other source begins to fade.

Continue experimenting with your awareness and realize that your attention is indeed like a searchlight: Whatever you focus your attention on is pretty clear, but other things and events tend to fade out of awareness. If you right now direct your attention to your own breathing . . . the sounds, the feelings, the movement of your chest and stomach . . . you are mostly unaware of the sensations in your hands. . . . As you think about your hands, your attention probably moves there, and you become aware of the sensations there, and the awareness of your breathing has probably faded away. As you can see, your awareness can shift from one thing to another quite rapidly, *but you can only be fully aware of whatever is the focus of your attention at the moment.*

You can control the direction of the searchlight yourself. To illustrate this, let's try another little exercise. While you are sitting back and relaxing for a minute, notice where your awareness goes now. Be aware of what thoughts or images come into your mind . . . pay attention to these thoughts, and notice that it is not easy just to stop them and think about nothing at all. As you have probably experienced before, telling yourself "Don't think about it" often does not help, unless you intentionally think about something else.

Instead of just trying to stop your thoughts then, simply focus your attention on your breathing. Whenever you realize your attention has wandered to thoughts or images, just refocus your attention on the physical sensations of your breathing. Don't struggle or battle. Just notice when you become preoccupied with words and images and then return your attention to your breathing. Do this for a minute or so. . . . Good. Now that we have been able to appreciate the way we can control our attention, you can sit up, eyes open, but relaxed, as we continue to consider the role attention plays in the reduction of pain.

The attention direction that you just tried is commonly used as a means of coping with pain or other kinds of stress. You probably can recall at some time trying to "think about something else" in order to get rid of an unwanted thought or feeling. "Thinking about something else" is easier than just trying to "stop thinking" about the unpleasant thing. You cannot completely focus your attention on more than one thing at a time, so if you consciously direct your attention to something involving, then you cannot attend fully to anything else.

To borrow a metaphor from Neisser (1967), attention can be likened to the chisel of the sculptor. It is a tool through which reality is carved, just as the chisel is the instrument through which the stone is sculpted. Kahneman (1973) has noted that momentary intentions of the individual are capable of guiding both the direction and the quantity of attentional allocation.

Cameron (1978) reported that he was able to have pain patients use a set of distraction techniques to cope with pain. At first, some patients were somewhat resistant, not quite understanding the potential viability of such an attention-diversion coping mechanism. Given this resistance, Cameron suggested a metaphor:

> First, I ask the patient to be aware of the sensations in his thighs as he sits in his chair. I note that those sensations are real, and they have a physical basis, but they are not normally experienced because other things occupy his attention. Then I suggest that he think of a TV set: he could block out the channel 9 signal by tuning in channel 11; the channel 9 signal is still there, but not being tuned in. I suggest that while his pain signals are real, he can learn to "tune them out." Tying the conceptualization to an image not only facilitates communication of the conceptualization, but often serves a "bell ringer" function as well. A number of pain patients have reported that they frequently think of the TV metaphor when experiencing pain and take appropriate action to "tune out." (1978, p. 244)

Such examples go a long way toward making the therapeutic suggestions that are offered more plausible and useful.

SOME STRATEGIES TO DIRECT ATTENTION

As noted previously, before the therapist initiates descriptions of various strategies, he or she should determine whether the patient has used any such techniques. If the answer is yes, then the therapist will want to ask about the patient's experience with it before initiating training. If the patient has used the technique with some success, the therapist will want to build upon the patient's experience. If the patient has not used the technique, the therapist may spend more time preparing the patient for the intervention. The therapist should attempt to ascertain whether the patient has any concerns about the use of the technique (e.g., fear of losing control, fear of the pain's getting worse, fear that medication will be withdrawn) and to address each of them. These concerns must be considered when introducing the various procedures that can be used to direct and control attention.

Specific means of attentional control may be suggested by the therapist as follows:

Although you may do some things to divert your attention already, it will probably be helpful to outline and practice several sorts of such activities. Then you will be able to pick and choose from a wider assortment and to change from one to another when you find it necessary.

Imagery

One of the most commonly used means of diverting attention from an unpleasant stimulus is imagining a pleasant scene. "Think about something nice," the mother tells her child who is receiving an injection. Emergency room doctors have learned the very useful technique of attention diversion. Talking with adults about something that interests them or asking children to pretend they are watching a favorite TV program and then to describe what is happening are two such strategies used routinely in performing painful emergency procedures when it is not possible to use an anesthetic. *The more involving the image is,* the less attention you can give to other events, and therefore *the less pain you will experience.* Perhaps you sometimes have daydreamed about an incident so vividly or have become so involved in reading a book or watching a movie that you completely forgot what you were doing.

The therapist may ask the patient to describe a particularly absorbing movie or book, noting the impact of such an absorbing experience on what he or she attended to. The therapist attempts to use the patient's experience to illustrate the potential usefulness of the techniques to be employed, thus increasing their plausibility and credibility. The therapist continues:

Although you may not frequently experience such an image, it is possible for everyone to do so, with some practice. In research studies it has been shown that peoples' imagination can be so powerful that their muscles actually respond, although to a somewhat lesser degree, while the person images a scene. For example, when people were asked to imagine running in a long race, the measurements of their leg muscles showed that they responded in a manner similar to the leg-muscle responses that they would have had when actually running the race.

Try involving yourself in the following image right now and see just how vivid you can make it. Once again, just sit back and relax in your chair, close your eyes, and let's try to imagine some scenes to illustrate how you can control your attention. [These images were suggested by Horan & Dellinger, 1974; Kroger & Fezler, 1976; and Phillips, 1971.]

Imagine a pure white plate with a lemon on it, resting on a table. See the glossy yellow of the lemon's skin against the whiteness of the china plate. Notice the texture of the lemon. It looks clean and fresh. There is a knife on the table, next to the plate. Now imagine that you're picking up the knife. You hold the lemon on the plate with one hand, and with the other, using the knife, you cut the lemon in two, hearing the knife cut through the lemon and hit the plate. As the keen edge slices into the lemon, the juice runs out onto your fingers and onto the plate. The citrus odor immediately hits your nose: sharp, clean, pungent, delicious, invigorating.

Now you pick up one of the lemon halves, with the juice still dripping onto your fingers and onto the plate. Using the knife again, you cut a wedge from the lemon half, raise the wedge to your mouth, and touch your tongue against it gently. Every taste bud in your tongue is drenched with the tangy lemon juice as your mouth puckers instinctively. A shiver goes up and down your spine, and your shoulders shake. Picture for a moment the lemon, the cutting, the tasting, the smells. . . . Whenever you are ready, you can bring this image to a close. Good.

Notice that in this image the therapist stimulated visual, auditory, tactile, olfactory, and gustatory senses. The inclusion of the various senses enhances the vividness of the image and facilitates the imagery process. The therapist continues:

Was your image vivid? It does take practice to develop imagery skills, but everyone has the potential to imagine a vivid scene, given the right subject matter. Before we try another image, I want you to realize that the way you imagine these scenes can be important. Try to get *inside* your body and actually *feel* yourself doing the things I describe. I want you to create a mental picture in your head. Try to see things in as much detail as possible and—now this is important—try to see them from inside your body. That is, instead of watching yourself almost like you were on a home movie or videotape or watching yourself as another person would, try to see things through your own eyes. Try to be *in* your imaginary scene as much as possible. I want you to involve all of your senses. See and hear, feel and smell. As you use the imagery, you will be able to really feel your way through the scene. In fact, you will be able to be *in* the scene as if it were real.

This will become easier with practice, and it is important now only that you realize that your goal is to experience, as vividly as possible, the scenes I will describe. Like any other skill, it will come more easily with practice.

Now, picture yourself standing by the shore of a large lake, looking out across an expanse of blue water and beyond, to the far shore. Immediately in front of you stretches a small beach, and behind you a grassy meadow. The sun is fierce and very hot, bathing the landscape in a shimmering brightness. It is a gorgeous summer day. The sky is pale blue, with clouds drifting by. The wind is blowing gently, just enough to make the trees sway and make ripples in the grass. Feel the wind on your cheeks. It is a perfect day, and you have it entirely to yourself, with nothing to do, nowhere to go.

You have a blanket and a towel, and you walk off through the meadow. You find a spot, spread the blanket, and lie down on it. It is so warm and quiet. It's such a treat to have the day to yourself to just relax and take it easy. Think about that warm, beautiful day.

You walk toward the water, feeling the soft, lush grass under your feet. You reach the beach and start across it. Now you can feel the hot sand underfoot. It is almost too hot to stand on, but not quite. It's very warm and very nice. Now visualize yourself walking out into the water slowly, up to your ankles, up to your knees. The water is so warm it's almost like a bath. The water is so warm, so comfortable, as the wind continues to blow. You gently splash the water up around you and feel the wind, now cooling on your wet skin. Look around. You are still all alone. You still have this lovely spot all to yourself.

Far across the lake you can see a sailboat, tiny in the distance. It is so far away you can just make out the white sail jutting up from the blue water. You take another look around and decide to return to your spot to lie down and enjoy the sun. Across that warm sand to the grass. You can feel the hot sun warming your skin. It must be 90°, but it is clear and dry. The heat isn't too much to take; it's just nice and warm and comfortable.

You lie down on the blanket, partly in the sun and partly in the shade, and feel the deep, soft grass under your head. You're looking up at the sky, seeing those great billowy clouds floating by, far, far above. In the distance you can hear the rustle of the water against the beach. You can hear the sound of a bird gently singing in a tree nearby. You can even smell the sweet grass around you. You can feel the gentle breeze in your hair and on your skin. You are very comfortable, quite at ease, and totally relaxed. Take a minute or two to sit back and continue the image on your own, enjoying the positive feelings you have been able to bring forth.

How do you feel? Was this image involving for you? Such an image can be very useful in an unpleasant situation. Focusing your attention in detail, involving all of your senses on some images like these, can take your mind away from unpleasant sensations, for example, any pain that you are experiencing.

Pleasant Images

The last image we worked on included only pleasant things and excluded any unpleasant feelings that you might be experiencing while imagining the pleasant things. You can probably think of many more examples of these (e.g., imagining yourself at an enjoyable party or thinking of spending a good time with someone).

At this point the therapist queries the patient about what pleasant image he or she might use. The therapist has the patient share some details and sequences of the pleasant image, including the various senses involved.

If you *focused* your attention on a pleasant scene in some detail, you would likely experience any ongoing unpleasant stimulus differently. You would tend to notice the pain less, it would bother you less, and you would feel more control over your own sensations.

Recall that you can focus your attention fully on only one thing at a time. And *you can choose* what you will focus upon. Your attention may wander from time to time, and you may, for example, occasionally find yourself dwelling upon unpleasant sensations. But you can voluntarily *bring your attention back to an image* when you notice that it has wandered. You can begin to take command of your pain experience.

The therapist conveys to the patient that he or she is in control and is not passive or helpless.

Imagining a Change of Situation

On the other hand, you could use an image that actually involved feeling an unpleasant sensation, but in a far different situation. For example, one patient reported that, when he had experienced his pain, he imagined that he was James Bond, agent 007, and that he had been shot and was being chased by some counteragents. He was fleeing from them in his car down an incredibly dangerous, winding mountain road and was concentrating intensely on keeping the car on the road and on traveling as fast as he possibly could. [This example was suggested by a subject in Knox's 1973 study.]

Under these circumstances, the pain from the imagined bullet was the least of his worries, and it faded into the background, although it was still there. At times you can act almost *as if* you're not in pain. Could you actually fool other people into thinking you are not hurting? Could you fool yourself? A good actor could use the pain as part of the character. How does the actor transform the pain into something useful?

To cope with the pain from a throbbing headache, one woman patient imagined that she was in a beauty parlor, sitting under a hair drier. She could picture several of her friends sitting beside her, and one of her friends asked if she could think of her earliest memory. She became very involved with this image, thus reducing and shifting her attention from her pain.

The particular image that you use in coping with painful stimulation is *not* the most important thing. More important is that you be *involved* in the image, so that you have little attention left to pay to the discomfort. You may still be somewhat aware of the uncomfortable or painful feelings, but these are more in the background as your attention is primarily focused on something else.

Changing Images

Something to keep in mind when you use such images is that there is no reason for you to feel "locked in" to any one image. If you find the scene that you are using to be ineffective, or find that it becomes less vivid after a while, you can easily switch to another scene. Beef up your images; there is no limit to what you can include. Any sensations will be useful—you can include eating, dancing, arguing, sex, running, skydiving—anything that will occupy your attention. They may include fantasies—throw in unexpected things that will keep your attention. Experiment, and with the experimentation you can discard things that don't work and switch to things that are more effective.

Sometimes you may find that you can maintain one, very detailed or involving image for a long time, and at other times, you may jump around from one image to another and back again constantly, or you may find images merging and blending into one another. Plan ahead, so that you have choices readily available, but don't feel locked into your plans. Use as many senses as possible—smell, taste, touch, and so on, as in the example.

Numerous examples of images and imagery techniques are available (e.g., Bresler, 1979; Kroger & Fezler, 1976; McCaffery, 1979; Samuels & Samuels, 1975). The therapist should be familiar with the variety of these imagery procedures, but at the same time keep in mind that there is little evidence that one of these is any better in reducing pain than any other. Rather, we believe that more important than the content of the image is the manner in which it is presented and the involvement of the patient. McCaffery (1979) provides an excellent summary of points that the therapist should keep in mind when using imagery procedures. This summary is reproduced in Table 12-1.

The set that is conveyed to the patient is that he or she is being taught a variety of different coping strategies so that he or she can pick and choose what works best at different times. Sometimes it may be relaxation, other times it may be attention-diversion imagery, and so on. Patients collaborate in generating personally relevant strategies for each coping category. This is further illustrated in the next coping category, mental activities.

TABLE 12-1. *Guidelines for Using Imagery*[a]

---

1. Determine the extent to which the patient already uses his or her imagination, especially in dealing with pain or producing relaxation. There are several characteristics that indicate a person may be a good candidate for imagery, but with both children and adults, it is almost essential that the person:
   • Be able to concentrate.
   • Be able to follow directions.
   • Be willing to respond to suggestions of images.
2. Explain imagery to the patient. Teaching the patient (and family members when appropriate) usually includes:
   • Simple definition of imagery as the deliberate use of a normal way of thinking, that is, imagining.
   • The fact that imagery can affect the body's physiological functioning.
   • The examples of possible effects of imagery upon pain.
   • Brief description of two or more imagery techniques as examples of what may be useful in this situation.
3. Involve the patient in making decisions about the use of imagery techniques. Emphasis is placed upon the patient being in control of:
   • Whether or not he or she will use imagery at any given moment.
   • The situations in which he or she will use imagery.
   • Which specific imagery techniques will be used.
   • Changing the imagery (caution the patient to discuss changes with the nurse).
4. Utilize images the patient has already actually experienced.
5. Employ all five senses in the imagery.
6. Sneak up on the image. (Precede the desired image with descriptions of how the patient arrived at the particular scene.)
7. Use one total image at a time.
8. Consider whether the image is oriented toward or away from the body.
9. Use permissive directions and suggestions when you direct (guide) the imagery.
10. Use soothing and positive descriptions.
11. Utilize periods of minimal or no pain for teaching imagery and for initial practice with it.

TABLE 12-1. (*Continued*)

---

12. Identify and discuss the patient's concerns. In response to the patient's concerns, placing emphasis upon one or more of the following may be helpful:
    - Imagery requires alertness and concentration; it is not like sleep or unconsciousness, although it may be used to go to sleep.
    - Imagery involves a willingness to respond to certain images, not gullibility or giving up control.
    - The patient is in control of the use and type of imagery; the patient does not lose control, nor is it likely that he or she will act in any way he or she does not wish to act.
    - Because of the limitations of imagery and certain precautions that are observed, pain and sensitivity are almost always sufficiently present to act as a protective mechanism.
    - Unwanted prolongation of the so-called trancelike state can be avoided in a number of ways, such as simply determining in advance the approximate duration of the imagery.
    - The ability to use imagery to relieve pain absolutely does not mean the pain is imaginary or not real.
    - The use of a pleasant mental image to relieve pain is not likely to decrease the enjoyment of that experience when it occurs in external reality.
13. Precede imagery with a relaxation technique.
14. Practice the imagery.
15. Teach the patient a technique for ending the imagery.

---

[a]From McCaffery, M. *Nursing management of the patient with pain* (2nd ed.). Philadelphia: J. B. Lippincott Co., 1979, p. 173. Copyright 1979, J. B. Lippincott Co. Reprinted by permission.

MENTAL ACTIVITIES

There are other means of diverting your attention besides imagery. We can divide these into three main classes. Let me describe each of these, and as I do, we will be able to discuss each of them in turn, with your examples and reactions, before we go on to the next way of diverting your attention.

Focusing Attention Outside of Yourself

To occupy your thoughts with something other than unpleasant stimulation, you can attend carefully to your physical surroundings or focus on events, tasks, or objects around you. You can engage in such activities as counting floor or ceiling tiles, examining the construction of a piece of furniture in the room, carefully examining a garment you are wearing, reading a book, or watching television and keeping track of some aspect of the program such as the number of times a commercial tries to sell a product by using "negative thinking" (i.e., if the person doesn't use the product, then others will reject the person or the person will have failed in some way).

Focusing on a Train of Thoughts

You can engage in mental activities other than images. Making a list of things to do before the weekend or planning a day's activities are things that some people have previously used to control attention. Remembering or singing the words to a song, a prayer, or a hymn are other examples. Mental arithmetic, such as counting backward from 100 by sevens, is also attention demanding.

Focusing on Sensations in Your Body

Analyzing the sensations in one part of your body and perhaps comparing them to another part; analyzing the intense stimulation as if you were preparing to write a medical or biology report regarding the sensations experienced (e.g., heat or cold, pressure, tingling); comparing the sensations to feelings you have experienced before—all these are means of directing your attention away from the unpleasant feelings themselves. You may allow yourself to experience discomfort, so that it is no longer simply pain, but rather is of some "scientific" interest—you are more "objective" about it, not so much experiencing the sensations as observing them.

You could rate your pain on the 0-to-5 scale and watch how the pain changes. Notice that pain does not always remain at the same level. On the other hand, you may focus on another part of your body exclusively, so that the painful portion is not in the forefront. Find what works best for you at the moment. Feel free to shift as needed.

Patients are urged to withhold skepticism at this point and to entertain the notion that some of the coping strategies *may* be useful for them. They are reminded that the task is to find the personally most useful strategies and that each procedure is only one of several alternatives.

Summing Up

The first methods of controlling pain that we considered were relaxation and attention-directing imagery. The last methods of controlling attention might be thought of as *mental activities*, but ones that do not involve a mental picture or image. Thus we have dealt with (1) relaxation as a means of actually reducing physical sensations and also as an attention-control exercise, (2) diverting images, and (3) mental activities not involving images.

Following some discussion of these procedures, the patient is offered a summary of the attention-diversion procedures to take home and use as a reminder of the training and as a guide for homework. Homework assignments may consist of generating lists of different strategies, trying different strategies out and rating how effective they were, and recording events and situations that successfully and spontaneously led to diversion of attention.

Note that the particular strategies and examples that we have provided constitute but one set of many possible ways of organizing strategies that might be used. These particular ones were developed for use with outpatients with pain problems. Modifications may be desirable for other groups (e.g., those trying to lose weight, stop smoking, or cut down on alcohol). The important thing to keep in mind is that the coping strategies should be understandable, enthusiastically discussed, and, above all, personally relevant to the patient.

Figure 12-1 provides a summary that might be provided to patients after conducting the discussion just outlined.

Even in the written materials provided to patients, such as the summary sheet shown in Figure 12-1, patients are requested to participate actively, by making lists, thinking of additional examples, and so on. Such active engagement may assist in personalizing materials for patients and may help avoid mindless undertaking of routine tasks.

FIGURE 12-1. *Summary of mental coping skills.*

Besides the RELAXATION that we discussed before, the SENSORY-INPUT and ATTENTIONAL components of pain may be dealt with by attention-control techniques. Attention-control techniques help you to direct and occupy your awareness with things other than painful sensations.

(In the blank spaces below, write down examples you could use for each category.)

Attention-control techniques—some possibilities:
Imagery (involving all your senses in a vividly imagined scene)
1. A pleasant image (such as a beach scene, skiing, or a party) _____

2. A change of situation (such as a football game or a James Bond adventure) _____

Mental strategies
1. Attending to physical surroundings (such as counting ceiling tiles or examining something in the room) _____

2. Focusing on a train of thoughts (such as making a list of things you have to do or engaging in mental arithmetic) _____

3. Focusing on bodily sensations (such as analyzing sensations in your arm or noticing how your pain changes on a rating scale) _____

INTERPRETATION OF SENSATIONS

Whereas the initial phase of the cognitive–behavioral treatment focused on the sensation of pain and its possible reduction by means of relaxation and attention-diversion techniques, the second phase focuses on how the patient can influence the pain experience by altering his or her interpretation of the sensations. As in the previous section, we will describe this mode of treatment by sharing the therapist's comments to the patient. These comments are offered as general guidelines, and thus the exact wording and the examples should be tailored to specific patients in terms of their education, cultural background, socioeconomic status, and presenting problem.

An example of the role of interpretation as a contributor to the pain experience was given earlier, when we contrasted someone cutting himself during an active game, such as hockey or football, with his cutting himself while he is home doing some relatively uninvolving task, such as shaving or reading a newspaper. Although the physical injury may be the same, in the active game he is likely to ignore the cut, perhaps even be completely unaware of it, but at home, during a more leisurely pursuit, he is likely to react more strongly, washing it and applying a Band-Aid, perhaps some first-aid cream, and so on. Most important, in the second situation he is almost certain to find the injury *more painful*. Why should just the setting have such an influence if the degree of injury is exactly the same? Let us take a few moments to explore this problem, for it can lead to another very potent means of controlling pain.

As powerful as pain can be, it is actually a delicate sensation. Pain intensity is very susceptible to change, as we considered before. One of the most powerful influences on pain is emotion. A few examples will help illustrate.

Consider a man who one evening develops an intense and persistent pain in the chest. "Indigestion" may be his first thought. When the discomfort is stronger and lasts longer than he has experienced before, he will probably become more upset and start thinking about the possibility of a heart attack.

At this point the pain serves a useful function. It acts as a signal that something is wrong with the body and encourages a person to take precautions. In this instance he will probably seek a doctor's diagnosis. Until he has that diagnosis, however, the uncertainty about what is wrong will increase his anxiety and cause the pain to feel even worse. He will probably attend directly to the painful sensations. His uncertainty and fear of the worst contribute to the painfulness.

The patient is told by his doctor that he is experiencing a mild attack of food poisoning. The removal of uncertainty will likely then cause the pain to decrease somewhat. His relief at the news that he has a much less serious problem than a heart disorder and the new interpretation of the sensations in his chest make the discomfort less intense and less bothersome, even if it lasts for a few days more.

This example demonstrates the effects that *attitude toward a pain-inducing situation may have* on the experience of pain. Sometimes the effects of attitude on pain may be more complex than in this example, but they are usually no less important. Have you had any instances such as this yourself?

Each time an example is presented, the therapist attends to the patient's nonverbal and verbal reactions to see if the example "took." One means of assessing this is to solicit similar examples from the patient. It is in such instances as this that the full potential of group intervention is evident, as the group members support each other in providing examples and in fostering discussion.

The therapist continues:

Another example that we mentioned earlier, showing how one's reactions to sensations determine pain intensity, is a study done during World War II. Soldiers seriously wounded in battle were compared with civilians who had surgical operations that resulted in *less tissue injury* than the soldiers suffered from their wounds. Only *one-quarter of the soldiers* (who had not received any medication for pain) requested pain-relieving drugs. On the other hand, *83% of the civilians* with similar physical damage asked for pain relievers. What do you think accounts for the differences between the two groups? Why did one group require fewer drugs? . . . Yes, the difference between the two groups lies in their view of physical sensations. The soldiers had been in constant battle, under severe fire, with their lives in danger for weeks. As a result, they saw their injuries positively, as a chance for relief, as an honorable means of saving their lives. For the civilians, however, the surgery was generally a depressing, traumatic experience, filled with worry and anxiety about the future.

Clearly, the physical stimulus is not the only, or even the major, cause of the amount of pain one feels. How one *appraises* or interprets the pain, what his or her attitude toward it is, how he or she interprets the sensations—all these play a major role in the experience of pain.

VOLUNTARY CONTROL OF APPRAISAL

The procedures described in this section focus on the appraisal process, which is particularly relevant to a host of problems falling under the general rubric of behavioral medicine, as noted in Chapters 2 and 3. The thoughts and feelings of individuals and patients who have problems with obesity, alcoholism, smoking, or stress disorders, or who have to cope with acute or chronic illness, are central to any prevention or intervention approach. The techniques described here for pain are analogous to those employed with any of the problems reviewed in Chapter 3.

Although the treatment strategy at this point can be stated in a straightforward manner, there is a danger of oversimplifying complex clinical interactions. The danger is the possible *loss of the patient* by making issues too complex, by talking over the head of the patient, or by translating the sensitive patient–therapist interaction into a didactic lecture. The treatment strategy entails having patients first appreciate that their pain experience can be broken into several phases or stages: preparation, confrontation, critical moments, and the period of self-reflection on performance. Second, patients are guided to reconsider the nature of any pain-engendering thoughts, images, or feelings they may have during each of these phases. In a collaborative manner, the therapist and the patient consider the impact of such negative thoughts on the pain experience. Third, the therapist enlists patients to consider what incompatible pain-reducing and pain-avoiding thoughts and feelings they might use during each of the phases. Fourth, a list of cognitive coping strategies is developed, and a discussion follows as to how the patients can use such strategies to reduce and avoid pain. Once again, the therapist attempts to make the cognitive strategies personally relevant to the patients' experience and needs. In this way, patients develop a more differentiated view of their pain experience and can come to view their pain as a problem to be solved rather than as an occasion for further negative feelings and thoughts, thus contributing to further pain, and so on.

In other words, one task of the intervention is to have patients become aware of the ways in which they may unintentionally exacerbate the unpleasantness they are experiencing and then to provide some means of short-circuiting that contribution to the problem. The therapist helps patients to appreciate the role of their thoughts, interpretations, attributions, and so on, in both the instigation of painful episodes and the exacerbation of pain. The next task will be to assist patients in interrupting any maladaptive chain of cognitive and affective events and gradually to introduce new coping patterns, which eventually may become automatic and habitual.

As noted earlier, treatment generalization is built into this intervention. Patients learn to recognize and interrupt their own habitual maladaptive patterns and to use coping methods of their own choice. They provide themselves with cues and responses that are useful on a day-to-day basis, not just in the clinic or laboratory.

    The therapist may introduce this section of the treatment program as follows:

We have already discussed that what a person thinks about a situation and the things he or she says about what is anticipated are important. We have found that when a painful episode is divided into components or stages, people are better able to keep each part of the situation manageable and are less overwhelmed by it. Breaking the painful experience into elements and keeping it manageable can assist you in employing the various coping strategies that you have available.

    One way of breaking any painful event or episode into parts is to think of it in terms of four stages: (1) preparing for the onset of pain, (2) confronting and handling the sensations, (3) coping with your feelings and sensations at critical moments, and (4) thinking about how you handled the situation and praising yourself for your efforts.

    The therapist can follow up this introduction with several queries designed to probe for the patient's understanding of and reactions to the material and to encourage patients to develop the idea on their own. Some possible ways of doing this follow:

Do these four stages make sense to you? Can you think of any other ways in which the situation might be broken down? Can you imagine breaking down a painful (stressful) situation in such a manner? Think of a painful (stressful) situation you have experienced other than one involving pain. OK. Let's see, how could you go about breaking that into four stages? [Situations that might be considered are ones such as being evaluated, waiting for a medical or dental examination, giving a speech, confronting the boss on some important matter, arguing with one's spouse.] In the situation you chose, what kinds of thoughts and feelings do you think an anxious person would have at each of these stages? What about someone who is not anxious?

The therapist can develop this discussion in more detail:

Let's consider how these four stages of preparing, confronting, handling critical moments, and reflection would apply to a person who is afraid to give a speech in front of a large group. The first stage would be preparing for the situation. What might a speech-anxious person be saying to himself or herself? How might a person who is not anxious view the situation differently? Now, how about the second stage, confronting the situation? What would a speech-anxious person say? A person who is not anxious? OK. How about the third stage, coping with feelings and thoughts at critical moments? And what might each of these people, anxious and nonanxious, do during the fourth, reflective stage? [The therapist uses examples of the high-speech-anxious individual using task-irrelevant, maladaptive, anxiety-engendering thoughts at each of these phases.]

Let's try the same thing for a person who is to undergo intense, unpleasant physical sensations. What might he or she say to himself or herself during each of the four stages? . . .

This is not a lecture or a list of strategies, but a discussion between therapist and patient.

We have been discussing the pain you experience and that it seems to vary and go through different phases. [Here the therapist reviews the various phases of the pain, engaging the patient in a discussion of his or her thoughts and feelings at each phase.] What are the types of thoughts and feelings you had at the phase of preparing for possible pain? At the phase of dealing with intense pain? [and so on] . . . What effect do these feelings and thoughts have on your pain?

Now that we have discussed your thoughts and feelings, I am wondering what different thoughts and feelings you *might* have at each of these phases. . . . You've noted how certain thoughts and feelings may actually make the pain experience worse. Are there thoughts and feelings, are there things you can do at each of these phases to reduce or even avoid your pain?

In a subsequent session, the therapist can incorporate the patient's suggestions in the following ways:

I thought it might be helpful if I summarized what we were talking about last week in terms of the ways you can work to reduce and avoid pain. I thought it would be useful to review them today. I have taken the liberty of having typed up a summary of our discussion, and I also included some suggestions that have been offered by other patients like yourself, as well as some things we have found to work in the past. I would like us to look at these and find out which fit your situation. Let's go over these one at a time, so that we can evaluate each in order to determine the best set of things you can choose to do. [A summary sheet of these various procedures, as shown in Figure 12-2, is given to the patient.]

Remember that each person is different, and we have a number of approaches that have been shown to be successful for various problems. We may have to try out several before we find the ones that best fit you. Thus, if one method is not particularly helpful, it will provide us with valuable information regarding which method is likely to succeed.

In this situation the therapist is *not* merely saying to the patient "Here is a list of things to say to yourself" or "Here is a set of things to

1. Be alert to negative thoughts.
2. Use negative thoughts as signals that it is time to change.
3. Deliberately "say to yourself" helpful things, and use other coping strategies.

Preparation (preparing for the intense stimulation before it becomes too strong)

1. *Reject a helpless attitude. Work at coping; develop a plan.* For example:
   • I can deal with this task. Let me actively prepare.
   • I must just think about what I can do to deal with this. Think about a plan for future events.
   Add here any others that you can think of that will help you to begin using coping techniques when you need them. _____

2. *Keep a positive attitude: Stop negative thoughts and redirect your attention to positive ideas.* Some self-statements you could use:
   • Stop worrying. Worrying won't help anything.
   • What are some of the things I can do instead?
   • I'm feeling anxious—that's natural. But that's no reason to give up. Let me just breathe deeply and relax.
   Add examples here. _____

Confrontation (confronting and handling the intense stimulation)

1. *Make use of the general coping strategies. Switch strategies as necessary, and use self-statements to direct your attention to as many or as few coping strategies as you need.*
   • All right, I'm feeling tense. That lets me know that I should take some slow, deep breaths as I relax more, and switch from the strategy I was using to another one.
   • I won't get overwhelmed. I'll just take one step at a time. Let me just use my skills to handle a bit at a time.
   • STOP these negative thoughts. Let me just concentrate on one of the strategies to do something positive.
   Add examples here. _____

2. *IRMA: Imagery, Relaxation, Mental Activity. Remind yourself of the possibilities in coping techniques.*
   • This pain is getting to me. Wait! Remember IRMA: Imagery, Relaxation, and Mental Activity. OK; let me develop a good Image (or Relax, or use a Mental Activity).
   • Relax. Just breathe deeply and relax.
   • Concentrate *fully* on breathing and relaxation.
   • I won't think about my pain. I will focus my attention on remembering details of the movie I saw last night.
   Take a few moments to review some of the strategies that were covered in both sessions. Then add here any other self-statements that you might use to call these to mind. Develop your own versions of images, relaxation, mental activities, and so on. Add examples here. _____

FIGURE 12-2. (*Continued*)

Critical moments (dealing with the thoughts and feelings that arise at critical moments)

1. *Be realistic in expecting some intense stimulation, but don't magnify* the sensations. Just keep them manageable.
   - When I feel a lot of pain, I should just pause and then focus again on a strategy for dealing with it.
   - I won't attempt to eliminate the pain totally. I just need to keep it manageable.
   - I knew the sensations would rise. But I can keep them under control.
   Add examples here. _____

2. *When you find yourself giving way to unpleasant thoughts or feelings, deliberately STOP them. Substitute coping self-statements to get you back on the right track.* The following are some statements to use in this regard:
   - Things are going pretty badly. I can't take any more—no, wait—just pause. I shouldn't make things worse. I'll review my planned strategies to see what I can switch to.
   - My pain feels terrible. Things are falling apart. No. I'll stop that. Relax. I will focus my attention on something else. That's better, I'm regaining control. Just a slow, deep breath . . . Good.
   - I can't get my mind off the pain. I'll have to stop. *NO!* Wait a minute! I planned for this. Stop the negative thoughts. Let me use a strategy, and I'll get over this difficult time. OK, let me relax, relax, breathe slowly and deeply.
   Add examples here. _____

Once again, remember that the key is to *recognize* negative thoughts and feelings, to *interrupt* them with positive self-statements, and to use these coping self-statements to guide you in the use of *coping strategies.*

Reflecting on how things went (dealing with the feelings and thoughts you had about your ability to cope with, reduce, and eventually avoid the pain)

1. At first you may notice only a little change, but note how you are beginning to gain control. You deserve a pat on the back from yourself for having tried. If you've brought the pain under control even a very little bit, you deserve to feel proud.

FIGURE 12-2. *Cognitive summary sheet.*

do." There is a substantial difference between providing the patient with a verbal palliative or rigid formula and providing the patient with a problem-solving set to encourage active use of one's coping responses. In some instances we have focused on engaging patients in a discussion or providing them with written material on the nature of self-statements and cognitive appraisal. This material is presented in Appendix E. In addition, the therapist's comments are designed to anticipate and subsume the patient's doubts and possible failure with any procedure. Any potential failures by the patient should be anticipated and viewed as valuable information rather than as an occasion for engaging in "catastrophizing" ideation.

There is an element of a paradoxical intention in these therapist messages, for one cannot really fail. The patient is given the set that the reexperience of pain is useful and provides valuable information about which procedures to employ. We should reiterate that a cognitive–behavioral treatment calls for a full set of clinical skills. Although we have provided detailed scripts, the procedures described *should not* be implemented in a mechanical, rote fashion. One must learn and practice how to customize treatment techniques to the specific needs, beliefs, and circumstances of the patient.

Cognitive reappraisal or restructuring continues, with the therapist and the patient considering each of the four phases and the types of pain-engendering thoughts and incompatible thoughts that patients may use.

Phase 1. Preparation

The first stage in a stressful or pain situation is the time before any unpleasant sensations occur, and also the time before the stress becomes very severe. This *preparation* stage gives you the opportunity to prepare yourself for the intense stimulation before it becomes too strong.

Most pain patients we have seen note that there are periods of lesser and greater pain intensity. The patient is encouraged to view the pain as a challenge—as a problem to be solved. That is, the patient is encouraged to see himself or herself as making the decisions and planning ways to deal with the situation—*actively* influencing his or her own sensations. Note that the patient is a collaborator in generating the possible self-statements to be used at each phase.

Let's consider some of the thoughts you may call to mind during this initial phase.

Some Coping Ideas and Self-Statements

The purpose of this phase is to remind yourself that you have a problem to solve, a situation that you have to deal with. The idea is that you *reject a helpless attitude* and instead become determined to *work at coping*, to *develop a plan*. You may need to remind yourself of this if you find yourself feeling helpless and hopeless. Moreover, this phase is designed to make you aware of low-intensity cues, the beginning signs of the onset of your pain, so that you can begin to do something about it. It is easier to do something early than when the pain becomes very intense.

At this point the therapist reviews with the patient various illustrations of the preparatory phase taken from the patient's own experience and then considers possible incompatible cognitive strategies that could be used.

What sorts of statements to yourself could be used to reduce your pain, could act as reminders to cope more effectively? . . . Let's consider some self-statements you can use. We can alter their wording and add to the list so that they fit your own needs. Let's consider some things you might tell yourself when you expect to feel pain.

- Sitting and worrying about pain doesn't help.
- I'll make plans to control it.
- What is it I have to do? I can deal with this task. Let me actively prepare.
- I must just think about what I can do to deal with this. Think about a plan for future events.
- I'm not hurting much now. By thinking of other things, I can make this good feeling last longer. I'll make the pain less severe when it comes.

The point is that you will be aiming to maintain a positive attitude. Discouragement and anxiety *may* occur. But when you keep alert to such feelings, you can counteract them if they crop up.

Catch yourself when you are thinking negative thoughts. STOP them, and *redirect your attention* to coping ideas. Some examples of these thoughts are:

- STOP worrying. Worrying won't help anything. What are some of the helpful things I can do instead?
- I'm feeling anxious—that's natural. But that's no reason to give up. Let me just breathe deeply and relax.

At each point the therapist solicits the patient's reactions to these suggested self-statements and asks the patient if he or she can think of other coping responses to use. This type of discussion is facilitated when treatment is conducted on a group basis, since patients mutually support and encourage each other in generating examples.

Phase 2. Confrontation

Now that we have considered some of the coping things that you can say to yourself during the preparation stage of a painful (stressful) situation, let us proceed to the second stage. As the unpleasant sensations begin to increase in severity, you are directly faced with the intense stimulation and have the challenge of dealing with it. This *confrontation* stage is the one in which you may begin to employ the strategies that you have planned to use. Let's consider some coping ideas and self-statements you may choose to use when you are experiencing pain or find yourself becoming upset.

Now you will want to make full use of the coping strategies available to you. When you feel the need, you should call to mind the things that you can do. A general self-statement can serve to remind you to use a strategy when you need one. Some examples follow. Remember, you aren't locked into any strategies and can switch whenever necessary. You can change details and add to the list to suit yourself.

- All right, I'm feeling tense. That lets me know that I should take some slow, deep breaths as I relax more and switch from the strategy I was using to another one.
- I'm hurting. Instead of letting the pain push me around, I'm going to try to reduce its effects.
- I won't get overwhelmed. I'll just take one step at a time.
- It doesn't help to lie here and hurt. Perhaps if I use this pain as a chance to control my reactions, I won't hurt as bad.
- STOP these negative thoughts. Let me just concentrate on one of the strategies to do something positive.

You can use self-statements to call to mind the various possible strategies. Some patients have found it useful to employ a *cue word or reminder* to remember the kinds of techniques that we have been discussing. One word used is "IRMA." It stands for Imagery, Relaxation, and Mental Activity. Of course there are many possible specific techniques in each of these categories, and later you will be given a chance to work up some particular ones for your own use. The following statements, and similar ones, can serve as reminders of ways that you can cope with unpleasant feelings and sensations.

- This pain is getting to me. Wait! Remember IRMA: Imagery, Relaxation, and Mental Activity. OK; let me develop a good Image (or Relax, or use a Mental Activity) and reduce the amount of pain.
- Relax. Just breathe deeply and relax. Concentrate *fully* on breathing and relaxation.
- I won't think about my pain. I will focus my attention on remembering the movie I saw last night.

A number of other possible self-statements that have been offered by patients at this point include the following:

- You can meet the challenge.
- One step at a time; you can handle the situation.
- Do things even though I have pain.
- Just relax, breathe deeply, and use one of the strategies.
- Don't think about the pain, just about what you have to do.
- This tenseness can be an ally, a cue to cope. Relax. You're in control; take a slow, deep breath. Ah . . . good.
- You have a lot of different strategies you can call upon.
- It's there, but I don't notice it as much when I'm concentrating on doing something.

This is a good place to pause for a moment and review some of the strategies that we have covered. Let's look back over the summary to remind us of the possibilities.

It is important to remind patients that they are not learning formulas by rote. It is also necessary to avoid the perception that the patient's freedom of choice is being limited or that the method is appropriate only to *some* patients for whom those particular self-statements are familiar or appealing. Resistance is best dealt with by preemption, by incorporating possible objections before they occur and have a chance to develop or "inoculate" patients against the proposed intervention strategy.

Remember that these lists are *not* intended to *limit the choice of what you can say to yourself.* Instead, they are examples of the sorts of positive, helpful things that people have used in the past in similar situations and that you might find helpful. In fact, a number of patients have reported that they have used these self-statements, as well as some of the other techniques we have discussed, in stressful situations other than those related to pain. One time was when a patient was in a heated argument with her husband, and in another when a patient was in a bad car accident. I'll be curious to see if you find them similarly useful.

Keep in mind that these self-statements are useful only in that they contain ideas that you find helpful. The lists, plus your additions to them, can serve as a cafeteria-style offering from which you can choose the most helpful things as you prepare for and experience a stressful, painful situation.

Phase 3. Critical Moments

During a stressful or painful situation, there are times when you find that the sensations seem particularly bad or that you feel you can't go on anymore. At such critical moments, you are particularly prone to negative thoughts, which worsen the situation and can lead to your feeling the sensations much more acutely and perhaps to your giving up. You may remember such times from stressful situations in the past. You need to recognize these times and, during them, actively direct your thoughts to coping skills.

It would be unreasonable to expect to totally eliminate feelings of pain in a severe situation. Rather, you can attempt to keep the pain manageable, to stop yourself from overreacting and increasing the unpleasantness.

Coping Ideas and Self-Statements

You know that you will feel some intense sensations. It is only *realistic to expect some discomfort*. But at the same time, you *do not* want to *magnify* the intensity of the sensations—just keep them manageable. You can use such statements as the following to represent this "realistically manageable" idea:

- When I feel a lot of pain, I should just pause, then focus again on a strategy for dealing with it.
- I won't attempt to eliminate the pain totally. I just need to keep it manageable.
- I knew the sensations would rise. But I can keep them under control.

Critical moments often involve the wavering of your attempts to cope. At the time, you may feel you are overwhelmed by unpleasant thoughts or feelings. You may think you "can't go on" or "can't cope anymore." Since these thoughts in themselves worsen the situation, your task is to stop them whenever they occur and to substitute coping thoughts so that you can deal with the situation more effectively. Unpleasant thoughts won't help; pleasant or coping ones may.

Some of the possible ways of stopping the unhelpful thoughts and changing to prearranged techniques are indicated in the examples that follow. Change the wordings to suit yourself, and take the time to add to the list the ways you would find most useful.

- Things are going pretty bad. I can't take it anymore—no, wait—just pause. I shouldn't make things worse. I'll review my planned strategies to see what I can switch to.
- My pain is terrible. Things are falling apart. STOP! Stop that. Relax. I will focus my attention on something else. That's better, I'm regaining control. Just a slow, deep breath. . . . Good.
- I can't get my mind off this pain. The image won't work. I'm going to have to stop. NO! Wait a minute! I planned for this. Stop the negative thoughts.

Let me use a strategy, and I'll get over this difficult time. OK; let me relax, relax, breathe slowly and deeply. Let's reduce that pain again. IRMA, where are you?

At this point the patient is encouraged to add other critical-moment self-statements, ideas to help cope with thoughts that are headed in the wrong direction.

Phase 4. Reflections on How One Did

The patient is reminded not to forget to provide a pat on the back for one's efforts.

It can help to say to yourself that you tried, that you used a strategy well, or that you handled a rough spot successfully, or otherwise to praise yourself for having put forth the effort. In thinking about how it went, consider how you handled the situation relative to past attempts or relative to how you handled your pain prior to beginning this treatment program. Many patients focus only on how much more they have to do rather than on how far they have come. Some patients have set such high personal standards that they feel they rarely deserve a pat on the back. The result of this attitude is that they become frustrated and give up. Slow and steady wins the race! Each effort, each personal experiment, each attempt to cope with the pain deserves careful reflection on what you learned, whether it worked or not and why, and also some praise for having tried.

Patients have offered such reinforcing self-statements as the following:

- I'm handling my pain better. With more work, I'll be able to keep it from messing up my life so much.
- I remembered IRMA. I'm learning how to beat the pain.
- That wasn't as bad as I thought it would be. I handled it pretty well, but I'll do even better next time.
- Wait until I tell the therapist about which procedure worked best.
- Good, I did it. Next time I'll do even better.

Dealing with appraisals by means of self-instructions may be summarized for patients as follows:

To review briefly, what you say to yourself about your pain can make it more or less intense. We have been concerned with a means of influencing your own appraisal or what you say to yourself, your interpretation of the sensations and feelings you experience. By that influence you can change how you feel about the whole situation—you can help make it less unpleasant rather than more unpleasant.

We have divided a painful (stressful) experience into four parts (although they may overlap): preparation, confrontation, critical moments, and reflection. This breakdown helps prevent you from feeling overwhelmed and makes the situation more manageable. Your pain experience may now be viewed as consisting of four phases, and you have specific self-statements and things that you can use in each phase. You don't have to worry about what is to come because you have things to do at each stage. You can keep yourself occupied "right now" by using the self-statements to direct your attention to the positive techniques you have.

One other point should be noted here. At various levels of pain, or at different stages, you may find some coping strategies more effective than others (both self-statements and the techniques we discussed earlier). For example, early in the painful situation, relaxation and imagery may be very useful. As the sensations mount, the more "active" mental strategies, such as mental arithmetic, humming a tune, and thought stopping, may be more useful. The rhythmical nature of some techniques such as relaxation helps to hold your attention. Or just carefully focusing on your slow breathing may be best for you at this more intense stage. Once again, there is no reason that you shouldn't try anything at any time. But you may find that not all strategies are uniformly effective during the whole painful (stressful) situation. Let me encourage you to experiment to find out what works best for you.

Patients have advised us that, when their pain is very intense, rated 5, or most debilitating, on the 0-to-5 scale, they have had difficulty in maintaining a sustained image to divert attention from their pain. It is as if the pain has a prior call on their attention, thus interfering with the use of an imagery-based coping technique. At these extreme points, coping procedures that demand little attentional control, such as relaxing or focusing attention on something rhythmical (e.g., breathing), seem to work best. If these clinical findings are borne out by research, then the strategy of having patients learn what coping techniques work best by means of trial and error can be altered, so that the therapist can describe the possible techniques that seem indicated at each level of experienced pain intensity.

Patients are given a variety of homework assignments designed to help them become aware of their own thoughts and feelings and how they influence pain onset and intensity. Patients may be asked to record thoughts and feelings that precede, accompany, and follow painful (stressful) episodes. We have also asked patients to keep similar records during periods when their pain has been at a low level. The point we try to emphasize is that, although thoughts can make pain worse, they can make things better. Homework assignments may include asking patients to record episodes of pain or stress and to break these down into the four components we outlined, noting whether they can identify the different phases. Practice in using all of the strategies we have discussed in this chapter is also included as a homework task.

The patient may be given a summary sheet (Figure 12-2) describing the procedures discussed in this section. The therapist reviews this summary sheet with the patient and, in particular, carefully considers how the patient will use each of these coping skills in the natural environment to handle his or her pain. As with the other coping skills, the issue of transfer is considered explicitly.

SUMMARY

In this chapter we have reviewed a number of cognitive and behavioral techniques and concepts. The material covered will require a number of sessions to complete with patients. Four to six sessions, or more, may be required, depending on the patient. It probably goes without saying, but the pace of presentation should be dictated to some extent by the needs of the patient rather than by a rigid prescription.

Although a variety of coping skills is presented, one encourages patients *not* to choose the immediately "easiest" procedures rather than those that would help them the most in the long run. The next chapter deals with this issue and extends treatment to the third phase, application training.

CHAPTER 13

APPLICATION AND
FOLLOW-THROUGH PHASE

In addition to delineating overt reinforcement patterns that maintain chronic pain behavior, consideration also must be given to the patient's total psychological and environmental situation, including for example, the nature and quality of interpersonal relationships, particularly within the family network, self-statements about the private meaning of pain and suffering, compensation factors, and particularly important in rehabilitation medicine, the impact of physical disability on the patient's identity.—*Roy Grzesiak (1981)*

In some ways the title of this chapter is a misnomer, since the patient has been encouraged to utilize either already existing or newly developed coping skills during both the initial phase and the second, skills-acquisition and consolidation phase of treatment. This chapter highlights the application of coping skills in the patient's natural environment. *The chapter describes how a variety of cognitive-behavioral procedures is incorporated in treatment and, most important, highlights the anticipatory measures to prevent relapse and prepare for follow-up.*

The focus of the intervention thus far has been on helping the patient to change his or her view of pain (the reconceptualization process) and to develop specific coping skills to handle the pain experience. By the time the third phase of intervention is initiated, the treatment of the pain patient more closely approximates treatment for other types of patients. Interpersonal problems of communication, marital conflict, stress, depression, and vocational choices become the focus of attention. The quote from Grzesiak that introduces this chapter indicates the complexity of the problem and the need for a comprehensive treatment approach. We shall consider the several elements that make up the application phase of treatment.

As in prior phases of treatment, the health care professional should provide a brief description of what will occur when treatment moves into the application phase. It is important that patients and significant others understand the additional demands the program will put upon them and the likely impact their efforts will have on home and social life.

EXERCISE AND ACTIVITIES

Exercise is a very important ingredient in a pain management program. This is because exercise for the pain patient has both physiological and psychological impact. People feel better, pain may decrease, and other people will respond differently to patients when they increase physical activity. Grzesiak (1981) pointed out the following:

> Exercises should be chosen because they are pain relevant, related to func-
> tional weakness, good for general conditioning. The types of exercises chosen
> should be quantifiable in terms of units or numbers of repetitions; time is not
> a reliable unit of measure for exercises. (p. 277)

Most exercise programs begin by having patients work to tolerance (i.e., patients perform each exercise until they are forced to stop because of pain, fatigue, or weakness). After initial measurable baselines or tolerance levels are recorded, quota systems are established to lead to gradually more demanding exercise schedules. An important feature of this exercise program is that patients build up tolerance by exercising at least twice each day. Termination of each exercise session is to occur following the established amount of exercise rather than following the experience or expression of pain (Fordyce & Steger, 1979).

This recommendation is made for two reasons. First, exercises can be more easily completed and increased as muscle tone and strength improves. Many chronic pain patients reduce physical activity and engage in protective behaviors such as sitting in a rigid manner or immobilizing a part of the body in an attempt to prevent exacerbations of pain or to inhibit further tissue damage. The potentially detrimental effects of such behaviors and the misconceptions of anatomy and pain upon which they are based need to be addressed directly with patients and families.

A second reason for the graded increase in physical activity is to enhance the sense of self-efficacy. Directly observable demonstrations of increased physical activity should be reinforcing and should add to a sense of competence and control as well as enhancing motivation to continue working with the treatment regimen. The goals should be attainable, given the patient's physical condition, age, and sex. Activity levels can be charted in order to gauge progress, to provide an index of daily and weekly changes, and to serve as a direct reinforcer of progress to the patient. Many of our patients have pointed with great pride and enthusiasm to their charts, noting progress after several days or weeks in the program.

A cautionary note: Some patients may reach a plateau or may fail to meet specific activity goals. We have found it useful to discuss this with patients early in the treatment program, before it becomes a major problem. We note with patients and significant others that such plateaus or failure to achieve specific goals are not unusual, nor should they be viewed as a failure or lack of "willpower." Instead, they present opportunities to identify factors that might have contributed to the problem and should be incentives to continue working. In a sense, to be forewarned is to be forearmed. We have found it useful, when such plateaus occur, to review with patients their own earlier charts in order to demonstrate concretely how much progress they have already made. This is particularly important to ensuring that setbacks are not viewed as failures of the program or of the patient. We will have more to say about maintenance, relapse, and relapse prevention later in this chapter.

For a program to be successful, patients must be motivated to participate and maintain involvement. A technique used by Karol *et al.* (1981) is to highlight for both patient and significant other the pervasive influence of pain on their lives. Karol *et al.* asked patients and significant others what areas of their lives had been *unaffected* by the pain. Usually the patient's life is full of free time and idleness (especially if pain results in the patient's being unemployed). Karol *et al.* comment, "Using 12 hours per day as an estimate of free time available, there are approximately 130,000 hours of free time in a 30-year period" (p. 13). The starkness of these numbers may be used as a catalyst in having patients and significant others consider the need to begin exercise and activity programs.

Once again, clinical acumen and sensitivity are needed before using such statements. One can well imagine reinforcing a depressed state if information and materials are presented at the wrong time or are over-emphasized. Perhaps what is most important is not the words per se that the therapist uses, but the attitude and general message that the effort is worthwhile, that the therapist has not given up on the patient. It is impossible to separate the import of the "treatment atmosphere" from specific words and techniques. We mention this issue in order to encourage the reader to consider exactly what it is about such psychologically based interventions that may contribute to change. We will continue to describe the specifics of the treatment, since these specifics may help to create an atmosphere that contributes to the change process. The therapeutic atmosphere and rapport may be the oil necessary to keep the gears (specific techniques) running smoothly, and without which the treatment would grind to a halt.

As noted before, the therapist attempts to anticipate possible changes in the patient's level of pain intensity and frequency. For example, in the case of a patient's undertaking certain exercises, or in the case of a patient's returning home from the hospital, the therapist can forewarn the patient and the significant other that there may be a temporary increase in pain, but that this is to be expected, is normal, and should not cause undue alarm. As Fordyce (1976) stated:

> When you do the exercises we've planned, you have a perfect right to expect that several things are going to happen. First of all, you are going to be able to do more and second, you won't make yourself worse. Along with this, though, you have to remember that your activity level will go up faster than the pain level goes down. So don't worry if you find you're doing more but you don't have less pain. The pain will probably fade at a much slower rate— but eventually you'll feel better once your activity level is up. (p. 163)

Recently, Fordyce and his colleagues (Fordyce, McMahon, Rainwater, Jackins, Questad, Murphy, & DeLateur, 1981) provided evidence that pain complaints do not necessarily increase isomorphically with increased physical activity, as might be expected by patients and health care providers. Melzack and Dennis (1978) proposed that the mechanism by which physical activity may reduce chronic pain is through prevention of abnormally reverberatory neural activity that seems to maintain pain even when no other nociceptive stimulus is present. Along with the views of Melzack and Dennis, the therapist can refer to the concept of reducing pain by means of "closing the gate" through physical activity.

In short, patients are encouraged to focus attention on discovering what they can do in spite of pain and not on what they cannot do. Therefore each patient will be expected to work toward individual treatment goals throughout the program, goals that are defined collaboratively by the therapist, patient, and significant others, in behavioral (observable and measurable) terms.

At the same time, it is important to assist patients and significant others in appreciating that they are not going to change everything right away, but can begin the process by establishing realistic daily and weekly goals. Malec et al. (1977) have the patient (1) list activities to change (e.g., play guitar, attend occupational therapy, take walks), (2) indicate current rate of involvement in each of these activities in terms of time and effort, and (3) specify a goal for the coming week. Turk and Kerns (1980) collaborate with patients to establish daily, weekly, and long-term goals in several domains (e.g., physical, social, marital, vocational).

Current Concerns

When we discussed the cognitive–behavioral perspective of therapy in Chapter 1, we proposed that an important objective of treatment was to influence not only the patient's behavior and the consequences of behavior, but also the patient's thoughts and feelings. We referred to both cognitive processes (automatic self-statements and images) and cognitive structures (implicit, guiding current concerns, attitudes, beliefs, and hidden agendas). The exercise and activities programs will help alter cognitive structures related to pain and to the patient's sense of self-efficacy.

In our experience the major preoccupation for the pain patient and his or her family is "pain." Each physical sensation, every situational demand, is appraised in terms of its significance for the patient's pain state. Will this request cause more or less pain? Does this sensation or feeling mean that the pain will increase or decrease? One objective of the exercise and activities programs is to encourage the patient to begin to refocus on other current concerns. The discussion with the therapist conveys to both the patient and the significant other that, as others continue to do things for the patient, he or she becomes less involved with activities. This leads to an investigation of what aspects of the patient's behavior may contribute to other people's doing more and more for the patient.

To provide another example, with the treatment of a smoker, one would have the same concern with the *smoking* as a central focus for the smoker. In this instance the treatment would need to attend not only to having the patient curtail smoking, but also to the smoker's current concerns once smoking is terminated. Though the patient may abstain from smoking, he or she may still view situations as "temptations" to smoke. Is the patient preoccupied with the urge to smoke or the necessity not to smoke? Is the patient worried about gaining weight following the cessation of smoking? It may be helpful to refocus attention away from the current concerns of temptation, the pleasure of smoking, and weight gain and toward the patient's increasing self-control, coping ability, and ability to focus on other tasks, as demonstrated by abstinence over time.

MEDICATION

An issue closely related to activities and exercises is medication. Grzesiak (1981) noted that most physicians do not hope to cure pain with medication, but merely to relieve suffering. Fordyce (1976) estimated that addiction or habituation to pain-relieving medication occurs in more than 50%

of chronic pain patients. One factor that may contribute to these figures is the practice of prescribing medication on a PRN basis. The PRN schedules tend to reinforce pain and pain behaviors by making medication (and thereby relief) contingent upon the patient's expressing suffering to someone administering the medication or to himself or herself as justification for taking the drug.

Fordyce (1976) suggested that patients receive what he called a "pain cocktail"—analgesic medication in a liquid medium. He suggested the systematic reduction of the proportion of active ingredients over time, under the control of the treatment manager (usually a decrease of 20% to 25% per week). The pain cocktail is given at specific times instead of PRN. These arrangements are discussed with the patient, but he or she is not told exactly when the dosages will be reduced. Obviously, such an arrangement requires close cooperation with the medical staff because reduction of some medication is known to be accompanied by serious side effects. Fordyce (1976) suggested quantifying medication use by intake, expressed in terms of unit potency, based on average effective dosage of morphine. (Details on methods and conversion tables describing equivalencies of medications can be found in Halpern, 1974a.)

Self-control and responsibility in medication use may be further enhanced by an alternative approach to specific-interval medication. The therapist may encourage the patient to reduce his or her own medication systematically, may help design the procedure by which this will be accomplished (this may include the use of the "pain cocktail"), and may give major responsibility for medication control to the patient, with, of course, guidance and monitoring. The patient may be asked to record the quantity and time of ingestion. If the patient does not appear to be following the guidelines and reducing the dosage, this may become the focus of discussion (Gottlieb et al., 1977).

One problem with this approach is that patients may not accurately report their medication use (e.g., Taylor et al., 1980). This possibility should be openly discussed with the patient, noting that failure to report accurately will not hurt the therapist, but may greatly hinder progress and may lead to additional complications. Compliance with the program remains, however, the patient's responsibility. Once the patient completes the program, medication will be almost completely under the patient's control, since analgesic medications are readily available from sympathetic physicians who may not be completely familiar with the patient's history. Anticipated success in medication reduction can enhance the generalization of a sense of responsibility.

Turner (1979) provided an example of discussing medication effects in a forthright manner:

You may be surprised to find out how Valium works. It does have a direct muscle relaxant effect in large doses. However, in lower doses such as you have taken, the direct muscle relaxant effect is minimal. Valium does not do anything to correct the underlying problem with your back. Most of the Valium's effect is in the brain. It acts on the feelings and the judgment centers. It makes you feel less anxious, tense, upset; it takes the edge off things for you. (pp. 106–107)

Following an introduction such as this, the therapist can check to see if the patient has indeed experienced these effects and then discuss possible side effects, such as blunted emotional state, decrease in ability to think clearly, and decrease in response time. The therapist may also mention that scientists have recently discovered that natural morphine-like substances, called "endorphins," are produced in the brain, and may then share the speculation that such techniques as acupuncture, hypnosis, and various psychological treatments may relieve pain by causing these substances to be released. The therapist can raise the possibility that the proposed therapeutic tasks, such as relaxation, may be doing the same thing. In this manner, the therapist engages the patient in a discussion of current and past medication practices, tries to have the patient reconceptualize why these drugs work when they do so, considers the side effects of such medication, and provides the basis for recognizing that the proposed training procedures may be a more effective means to achieving similar goals.

Comparisons of alternative treatments to medication require caution, however, lest the patient be offered unrealistic hope for dramatic change or overly optimistic expectancies for recovery of lost functioning. Untempered enthusiasm may create difficulties for the patient, just as can providing the bleakest details about the patient's condition. In certain circumstances uncertainty about the facts may be of value in maintaining a basis for hope. The absence of hope can have devastating effects (Frank, 1974; Weisman, 1976), and some balance must be achieved between realistic expectancies and ambiguity, when little that is constructive can be done.

Finally, resistance to reducing medication is often due to the patient's fear and concerns about losing analgesic relief from pain, fear of the pain itself, and misunderstanding of the physical consequences of the withdrawal. These concerns should be anticipated and subsumed into the discussion by the health care provider, even if not raised by the patient. It may be, however, that the patient is so interested in medication as to subvert any attempt to change, by withdrawing from treatment if necessary. In such instances even the therapist's sincerest attempts to facilitate change may be fruitless.

SOCIAL SUPPORTS

Increasing attention has been given to the importance of social networks and supports in influencing adaptive coping processes. Viewing the patient apart from his or her social context results in an incomplete picture (Cassel, 1974a, 1974b; Christopherson & Lunde, 1971; Kaplan, Cassel, & Gore, 1977). Simply having a number of supportive individuals or groups available will not necessarily, however, prove to be beneficial. For example, social supports may prove to be detrimental when they result in a usurping of activities that the patient is capable of performing. It is important for the maintenance of self-esteem and sometimes for physical rehabilitation that patients perform activities they are capable of performing. Well-meaning significant others who cater to the patient may hinder recuperation.

Many self-help groups are available for chronically ill patients (e.g., Reach for Recovery for mastectomy patients, diabetes clubs, ostomy and hemophilia associations). Such organizations are unlikely to be of equal utility for all patients. One of the ostomy patients interviewed by Follick and Turk (1978) was quite dissatisfied with his local ostomy association: "They always talk about ostomies. I don't consider myself an 'ostomate,' but just a guy who has had this kind of surgery. My entire life does not focus on the ostomy." Of course this patient may be denying his concerns, but at this point he appears unlikely to attend an ostomy support group or to benefit from it.

Again, one can note the importance of tailoring treatment recommendations to the individual. These comments harken back to our comments about the role of the patient's current concerns and self-identity. One wonders about the degree to which such self-help organizations may implicitly reinforce, at least for some patients, current preoccupation with medical problems instead of nurturing alternative competing interests.

At the level of the patient–spouse interaction, this same concern has been raised by Fordyce (1976), who says to the spouse:

> When your wife talks about her pain, she's going to feel worse and you're going to feel worse if you just sit there and ruminate with her about it. If you help her stop talking about her pain all the time, she's going to feel better and you're going to feel better. (p. 141)

But such a statement should not be offered until the therapist has collected the evidence that such a pain-reinforcing interaction exists. The therapist works with both patient and significant other to help them recognize patterns of implicit reinforcement that characterize their interactions. The therapist can use the patient's and the significant other's diaries and pain intensity ratings to raise these issues in a Socratic-type exchange. Once the significant other's reactions are reasonably well defined, the therapist asks the patient about the impact of such reactions— how do the significant other's reactions make the patient feel? The significant other, in turn, is asked whether he or she knew that this was the patient's reaction and whether this was the intent. In this back-and-forth manner, the therapist sets the stage for considering in what other ways the significant other might response to the patient's pain complaints.

Instead of merely telling the patient what these other alternatives might be, the therapist can use his or her own befuddlement and make the solution a mutual effort, engendering a problem-solving set in the patient and the significant other. Obviously, the precise alternatives developed will depend largely on the nature of the patient–significant other interaction. The therapist guides the discussion into a consideration of how "well behaviors" (alternative responses incompatible with pain behaviors) can also be nurtured and supported.

A variety of techniques are used to help the patient cope with the host of stressful life events that accompany changes in the pain condition. We will deal with these techniques only in general terms, since they have been discussed in more detail elsewhere (see Cormier & Cormier, 1979; Meichenbaum & Jaremko, 1982). These techniques include role playing, imagery rehearsal, and graduated *in vivo* exposure, among others.

ROLE PLAYING

We have used role playing and behavioral rehearsal in two ways. One is to help the patient consolidate and integrate the components of the training program. To achieve this, the patient is asked to role-play a situation in which the therapist and the patient reverse roles. The patient is asked to act as the therapist, and the therapist will be a novice patient who has not yet begun the training. This exercise is consistent with attitude research (e.g., Janis & King, 1954; McGuire, 1964) indicating that, when people have to improvise in a role-playing situation, they tend to generate exactly the kinds of arguments, illustrations, and motivating appeals that they regard as most convincing. The therapist can use such role playing diagnostically to assess the patient's motivation and ability to implement the training regimen and to assess understanding of treatment components.

The therapist may introduce this role playing by reminding the patient that he or she has learned a number of ways to control pain, including such means as mental or physical relaxation, attention diversion, cognitive reappraisal or the use of self-talk, and increased activities.

It is important for the patient to feel that there is a variety of possible alternatives to sample. The patient is told that it is important to know a variety of pain management techniques because what proves helpful in one situation or at one time may not be most effective in another situation or at another time; moreover, techniques that at first do not appear useful may turn out to work in some situations or activities that cause pain, and then the patient can be encouraged to plan ahead for such occasions.

An analogy that has proved helpful in conveying this coping strategy to patients is the way athletic teams develop game plans. This anticipatory planning is viewed as the appropriate time to develop strategies to cope more effectively with intense nociceptive sensations. Preplanning lowers the risk of becoming overwhelmed at times of severest pain, while implicitly fostering an expectation that episodes of severe pain will pass. Table 13-1 is a sample summary sheet of various treatment procedures. The patient may be given a review sheet such as this prior to role playing.

The second way in which role playing has been used is to have the patient describe a conflict situation involving another person that contributes to or exacerbates the patient's pain. This situation may be re-enacted, with the patient now acting as the adversary and the therapist acting (or coping) as the patient. As the therapist plays the patient role, his or her *modeling* includes not only desirable coping *behaviors*, but also coping *strategies* (i.e., dealing, by use of coping self-statements, with whatever negative thoughts, images, and feelings the patient is likely to have in that situation). Both patient and significant other may also participate in such role reversals and behavioral rehearsals.

TABLE 13-1. *Skills Training: Summary of Training for Role Playing*

I. *Conceptualization of the "pain experience" as susceptible to personal, intentional influence.* (Elaboration of specific conceptualization elements that have been developed, such as gate-control theory, and of different components of pain, such as sensory input and reactions of the individual to that sensory input.)

II. *Relaxation* can be employed to reduce the sensory input. Focus on:
   A. *Tensing and relaxing various muscles* that receive the intense stimulation.
   B. *Slow, deep breathing,* with 3 seconds to 5 seconds inhaling, 3 seconds to 5 seconds holding, and 5 seconds exhaling.
   C. *Thinking of pleasant or relaxing words or pictures while exhaling* (e.g., the word "calm" or a picture of a feather gently floating).

III. *Attention-diverting coping strategies.*
   A. One cannot focus on more than one thing fully at any one time.
   B. A person can select what he or she will focus attention upon and what will be excluded from attention.

TABLE 13-1. (*Continued*)

C. A variety of different coping strategies is available. These can be employed at various times in a stressful situation. A person can switch from one strategy to another as often as he or she wishes.

D. Sample coping strategies:

1. *Focusing attention on physical characteristics of the environment* (e.g., counting the ceiling tiles, studying the construction of something in the room, studying articles of clothing that are worn).

2. *Focusing attention on various thoughts* (e.g., doing mental arithmetic, making a list of all the things you have to do over the weekend, thinking of and singing the words of various songs you recall).

3. *Focusing attention on the part of the body experiencing intense sensations* (e.g., analyzing the sensations in one part of the body and comparing them to another part or analyzing the intense stimulation as if preparing to write a biology report regarding the sensations experienced).

4. *Imaginative inattention.* Ignoring the intense sensations by engaging in mental imagery that, if real, would be incompatible with the experience of pain (e.g., imagining yourself enjoying a pleasant day on the beach or a pleasant party, or spending an enjoyable afternoon with your girl friend, boy friend, spouse, or family).

5. *Imaginative transformation of pain.* Interpreting the sensations you are receiving as something other than pain or minimizing those sensations as trivial or unreal (e.g., visualizing and thinking about the part of the body in which the intense sensation occurs as having been filled with Novocain, and feeling the numbness produced; seeing or picturing yourself as the Six Million Dollar Man, whose limbs are mechanical and capable of great feats of strength, but incapable of experiencing pain; imagining the part of the body as being made of rubber and thus unable to feel pain, considering all the implications of what it would be like to have a rubber limb).

6. *Imaginative transformation of context.* Picturing an image or mental scene in which the situation in which the intense sensations are being experienced is different from the actual situation that you are in. That is, you are aware of the sensations, but you picture them arising in a different context (e.g., picturing yourself as James Bond having been shot in a limb and driving a standard transmission car while being chased by enemy agents; picturing yourself receiving an injury in a hockey or football game, but continuing to play despite the injury; visualizing yourself receiving an injury while on a date and not wanting to let your girl friend or boy friend know that you are hurt).

E. Coping strategies that employ visual images are like mental pictures that can be related to a wide variety of situations. The greater the degree of involvement, absorption, and vividness of the image, the more effective such strategies will be in effectively coping with a stress. Sample coping strategies 4, 5, and 6 are strategies that employ such imagery.

(Continued)

TABLE 13-1. (*Continued*)

IV. *Self-instructional training.* Self-instructional training involves dividing a stressful situation into three phases, with self-reflection throughout the situation. The phases are:
A. *Preparing for the intense stimulation before it becomes too strong.* Self-instructions and statements that can be made at this phase include:
  1. What is it I have to do? (*Viewing the situation as a problem that you can do something about.*)
  2. I can develop a plan to deal with it. (*Prepare yourself by making a plan or mental outline of how you will deal with the sensations when they arise.*)
  3. Just think about what I have to do. (*Focus on what the situation requires.*)
  4. Think of the things that I can use to help cope. (*Review all the strategies that you know of and that may be helpful.*)
  5. Don't worry; worrying won't help anything. (*Use any anxiety or worry as a cue to remind you to focus on what you have to do.*)
  6. Remember, I can shift my attention to anything I want to. (*Reassure yourself about your ability to employ various coping strategies.*)
  7. When I use mental imagery, I'll see how vivid I can make the scene. (*Review various aspects of the different images and strategies that can be used.*)
B. *Confronting and handling the intense stimulation.* Self-instructions and statements that can be made at this phase include:
  1. I can meet this challenge. (*View the situation as a challenge that you deal with.*)
  2. One step at a time, I can handle the situation. (*Don't do everything at once and don't be overwhelmed, but use each of the skills you have learned.*)
  3. Just relax, breathe deeply, and use one of the strategies. (*Review and use any of the strategies that you have outlined in your plan for coping.*)
  4. Don't think about the pain, just about what I have to do. (*Focus your attention on the task at hand and what you can do right now to help you cope.*)
  5. I'm feeling tense; that can be an ally, a cue to switch strategies and to take some slow, deep breaths. (*Expect to feel tense at times; that's not unusual. But use tension as a cue to relax and to review which strategy to employ next.*)
  6. Remember, I can switch back to some strategies that I used before. (*There is no reason why you can't return to some strategies already used.*)
C. *Coping with thoughts and feelings that arise at critical moments* (when you notice that the intensity of the sensations seems to be increasing or you think you can't go on anymore). Self-instructions or statements that can be made at this phase include:
  1. When I feel any pain, just pause and keep focusing on what I have to do. (*Keep in mind the task at hand and what you have to do.*)
  2. Don't try to eliminate the pain totally; just keep it manageable. (*Remember, you expected to feel some intense sensation, but don't overreact and make things worse.*)

TABLE 13-1. (Continued)

3. I knew the sensations would rise; just keep them under control. (Don't magnify the intensity of the sensations you experience.)
4. Remember, there are a lot of things I can do; I can keep things under control. (You have been taught a number of different strategies that will help you keep the intense stimulation under control.)
5. Things are going pretty bad; I can't take anymore—just pause, don't make things worse, review your plan of strategies to see which you can switch to. (Sometimes you may have unpleasant thoughts or feelings; use those as cues to review the strategies available for you to use.)
6. I feel terrible; things are falling apart. Stop—relax; I can focus my attention on something else, keep things under control. (If you find yourself focusing on unpleasant sensations or thoughts, remember that you can choose what you will focus your attention upon.)

D. Self-reflection and positive self-statements. Throughout the preceding three phases, you might evaluate your performance (e.g., how am I doing?, that worked pretty well). Remember, people frequently criticize themselves, but rarely praise their behavior. Throughout a stress situation, once you evaluate how you are doing, if you think you should be doing better, you can use that as a cue to try different strategies; if you are doing well, you should give yourself a "pat on the back." Self-reflective statements that might be used throughout a stressful situation include:

1. That's it! I've outlined what I have to do and when I will use each strategy.
2. I'm doing pretty well! It's not as hard as I thought.
3. I'm doing better at this all the time.
4. Don't let negative thoughts interfere with using my plan.
5. Wait till I tell the therapist what things worked best.
6. I knew I could handle it! I'm doing pretty well.
7. I'm doing better than I expected; wait till I tell my wife (husband, therapist, etc.).

V. The attention-diverting coping strategies and self-instructional training can help you deal with reactive components of the pain experience. Using relaxation to deal with the sensory input, and using the coping and self-instructional strategies, you will be able to enhance your pain tolerance and alter your perception of intense sensations.

IMAGERY REHEARSAL

Another means of providing patients with an opportunity to rehearse coping skills is to use imagery rehearsal or to engage in what is known as the "work of worrying" (Breznitz, 1971; Janis, 1958; Marmor, 1958). As in the procedure of systematic desensitization (Wolpe, 1959), the patient is asked, while relaxed, to imagine himself or herself in various pain-engendering and stressful situations that vary in intensity.

In systematic desensitization the patient is asked to imagine scenes from a graded hierarchy. If the patient experiences any stress (anxiety, pain), he or she signals the therapist, who then instructs the patient to terminate the image and continue relaxing. These procedural steps follow from the concept of counterconditioning as outlined by Wolpe (1959). In recent years, however, the explanation of desensitization has been subjected to much theoretical and empirical criticism. (See the review by Davison & Wilson, 1972, for a summary of these arguments.) An alternative view of the desensitization process suggests that imagery rehearsal is a useful way of teaching the patient a set of coping skills, or fostering self-control (Goldfried, 1977).

This view attends more to the fact that, when desensitization patients are instructed to imagine hierarchy scenes, they are in fact providing themselves with a model for their own behavior. The closer the imagery comes to representing real experiences, the greater the likelihood of generalization. Through imagery, patients may mentally rehearse the specific thoughts, feelings, and behaviors they will use to cope with stress and pain.

To maximize the similarity between the images used in desensitization and real-life experiences, a cognitive–behavioral approach to desensitization adds *coping* images to the *mastery* images that have been commonly used. *Mastery* imagery involves patients' viewing themselves successfully handling the problem situation. There is no suggestion in these images that the patient will experience stress or pain in the real-life situation. *Coping* imagery, in contrast, involves patients' imagining themselves becoming anxious, beginning to experience pain, or having maladaptive thoughts, and then coping with these difficulties, using approaches they have already developed to deal with the situation. Kazdin (1973), Meichenbaum (1971), and Sarason (1975) have provided evidence of the therapeutic value of coping over mastery modeling in the change process. The patients' images can be seen as providing some of the same functions in this instance as a model might.

Types of Imagery Use

The inclusion of coping imagery means that the three different types of images are presented. First, patients are instructed to imagine scenes from a graded hierarchy in the traditional way employed in desensitization procedures as described by Paul (1966). The patient imagines the scene presented by the therapist. At this point there is *no* suggestion that the patient will experience any stress or pain.

The second type of imagery in the cognitive–behavioral approach is employed when the patient signals that a particular scene is causing him or her to become tense. In standard desensitization this signal would cause the therapist to instruct the patient to stop the image and just go on relaxing. Instead, under a coping-imagery procedure, the therapist would state:

> See yourself coping with this stress by use of the procedures that we have practiced. For example, see yourself taking a slow, deep breath, slowly filling your chest cavity. Good. Now slowly exhale. As you exhale, note the feeling of relaxation and control settling in. Good. Now stop the image and just relax.

The therapist is including in the imagery scene ways of coping with the stress and pain the patient is experiencing.

Other coping imagery that the therapist can use if the patient signals stress or pain is the following:

> See yourself coping with your pain. Relax. Good. Now hear yourself saying, "What is the problem? What is it I have to do? Just use my plan. IRMA" [covered in Chapter 12: Imagery, Relaxation, and Mental Activity].

The patient is encouraged to use any personally generated self-statements and images that would facilitate coping and inhibit pain-engendering thoughts and feelings. If the coping imagery techniques do not reduce the patient's stress or pain, then he or she should signal the therapist by raising a finger, terminating the image on the instruction of the therapist and then relaxing. The therapist would then reintroduce the same image, with the coping technique included. If the patient still experienced stress or pain, then the therapist has likely made too large a jump in the hierarchy steps and, following the standard desensitization procedure, should introduce an intermediate scene.

In the third set of images, the therapist can directly suggest that the patient may experience stress or pain and then can include in the image ways in which the patient may cope with his or her stress or pain. For example, in the case of a patient suffering from headaches related to evaluation, the following scene was offered:

> See yourself taking an important exam, and as you are thumbing through the exam booklet, you feel some tenseness in the back of your neck. Your eyes begin to wander about the room, your thoughts wander, and so on. . . .
> [The therapist can employ specific examples tailored to the patient's experi-

ence.] Notice what you have been feeling and doing. These are the reminders, the cues to cope. [Therapist pauses.] Good. See yourself taking a slow breath; hold, hold. See yourself parting your lips, and as you are breathing out, you are reminding yourself how to handle the stress.

When treatment is conducted on a group basis, each patient is encouraged to use the specific set of self-statements and images that work for him or her. The therapist's use of the generic instruction "reminding yourself" or "self-instructing" provides sufficient individual choice. Following the imagery exercise, the group can discuss the specific techniques each patient chose to employ. The therapist should be flexible in implementing the coping imagery. For example, he or she may wish to offer specific self-statements and coping techniques that the group has discussed in previous sessions or may wish to provide a general guideline.

When we began our initial work on coping imagery, there was a concern that the inclusion of such scenes might raise the likelihood that the patient would indeed reexperience his or her maladaptive behaviors. We wondered whether we might be doing our patients a disservice by suggesting that following treatment they might reexperience their presenting problems. Our clinical and research experience, however, has suggested that this is *not* the case. Rather, we were closer to the productive process of the "work of worrying." We believe that patients are likely to have setbacks and problems following training, and the use of imagery rehearsal has proved an important component in the enhancement of maintenance of therapeutic gains. Patients who successfully undergo desensitization treatment likely experience anxiety, stress, and pain following treatment; the cognitive–behavioral treatment approach can influence how patients view this stress, what they say to themselves about it, and how they will cope with it.

In summary, three different types of imagery are used in the cognitive–behavioral approach: (1) mastery imagery, as in desensitization; (2) coping imagery in response to the patient signaling stress or pain; and (3) coping imagery offered directly by the therapist.

A hierarchy of between 10 and 16 items of pain-engendering situations is usually used. The imagery procedures are presented in the following manner: Items 1 through 8 in the hierarchy are presented in a standard mastery manner. On items 1 through 3, if patients signal any stress or pain, the therapist merely has the patient terminate the image and go on relaxing. The scenes are then re-presented in the standard desensitization manner. This initial phase of treatment is designed to familiarize patients with the imagery procedures. On the remaining scenes, 4 through 16, if the patient signals stress, then the therapist suggests that the patient imagine himself or herself coping with the stress or pain. Following a scene in which the patient signals stress or pain, the therapist would re-present the scene, but this time include the coping activities.

On the last 8 scenes of the hierarchy (scenes 9 through 16), the therapist varies between mastery and coping imagery. On some occasions the therapist presents a scene that involves the patient's becoming stressed or experiencing pain and then coping with the stress and pain; for other scenes the therapist makes no initial suggestion of the patient's becoming stressed or experiencing pain, with coping employed only in response to signaled stress.

This imagery sequence is based on our clinical experience with the procedure. Research is needed to further assess the therapeutic value of these changes. Once one views the desensitization process in terms of a coping and a self-control training paradigm, then the specific parameters of the imagery process, such as length and sequence, seem less critical. The length of the coping images ranges from 30 seconds to 3 minutes. Clinical experience and sensitivity are required in reading patients' reactions to the presentation of the imagery scenes. The major guideline concerning this phase of treatment is to have patients mentally rehearse behavioral and cognitive coping skills that they will employ in stressful and pain-engendering situations.

Hierarchy Development

Another important therapeutic feature of the imagery rehearsal stage is the development of the hierarchy of scenes that will be imagined. We have found it quite therapeutic and educational to discuss with the pain patient the variety of situations in which he or she becomes stressed and experiences pain and how the patient and others respond when the patient is in pain. These various situations can be ascertained from the pain diary, pain intensity ratings, pain questionnaires, and interviews with the patient and the significant other. These situations are arranged in a hierarchy along a dimension of pain-engendering situations.

One arranges the hierarchy from least painful to most painful situations. In setting up the hierarchy, the lowest item (the least pain engendering) focuses on a scene in which the patient is preoccupied with pleasant activities, enjoying himself or herself. The patient may occasionally notice the pain, but would rate it at a low intensity. The top hierarchy scene reflects the patient's total preoccupation with pain. The intensity is so severe that the patient cannot think about anything else. A sense of despair, even fear, is evident: The patient feels that he or she will not be able to stand the pain for even 1 second longer. Scenes intermediate to these two extremes are used to develop the hierarchy. The discussion of the hierarchy scenes can prove an important aspect of treatment as the patient and therapist consider how the various situations vary along several dimensions.

Following is a sample hierarchy developed with one patient. The items will be different for each individual patient, and this example is *not* intended as a general scheme.

1. While lying awake trying to fall asleep, you feel a slight twinge of pain—a rating of 1 on the pain intensity rating.
2. Tossing in bed in the middle of the night worrying about the pain getting worse, you note that the pain is 3 on your 0-to-5 scale.
3. You are seeing your spouse and thinking of waking him because of the pain bothering you. You feel the tensing of your muscles.
4. You lie there quietly thinking that the pain will continue to get worse and worse. You begin to cry.
5. As the time drags on and the pain increases, you now rate it as a 4. You note a feeling of helplessness. No one understands how bad it gets. Your sense of anxiety and fear increases.
6. Feeling that you cannot stand it any longer, trembling, you get off your bed. You begin to pace, changing positions. You rate the pain as a 5, and you fear you will not be able to stand the pain for even 1 second longer.

The patient is asked to imagine himself or herself in each scene and, in particular, to become sensitive to the kinds of thoughts and feelings experienced before, during, and after the pain episode. The following excerpt illustrates the coping imagery procedure. The therapist uses the patient's previous account to generate this image and incorporates coping techniques within it.

Now, as you sit in the chair, relaxed, imagine the scene in which you are waking up in the middle of the night from pain. It is very quiet. You don't wish to disturb anyone, but you are in pain. You have feelings of becoming depressed—"Oh no, not again"—and of hopelessness—"I'll never be able to have a good night's sleep." As you begin to feel the tension building in your body, you first rate the pain on your 6-point scale. It is severe—a 3, maybe a 4. "What can I do about it?" You can hear yourself saying, "Oh yes, my plan for such occasions—don't make the pain worse." See yourself taking a slow breath. Breathing easily and evenly, helping reduce the pain. "Now to shift my attention. . . . Good."

The therapist continues in this fashion, including the patient's reactions as cues, as reminders to use the coping procedures that have been discussed in treatment. Following such scenes (and several may be covered in one session), the therapist checks with the patient about his or her re-actions to the imagery content and how the patient can implement the coping procedures in a natural environment. The transfer of such coping techniques from imagery to real life is unlikely to occur unless this process is nurtured and reinforced.

The patient is encouraged to recognize and interrupt low-intensity prodromal signs of problems. The therapist may suggest that, as the patient learns to moderate the intensity of experiences, they may, in turn, become less frequent.

Kroger and Fezler (1976), Meichenbaum (1978), and Singer and Pope (1978) consider further the potential of imagery in the reduction of stress and pain.

GRADED EXPOSURE TO PAIN-INDUCTION PROCEDURES

Another way to consolidate coping skills besides role playing and imagery rehearsal is graded exposure both in the clinic (or lab) and in real-life settings. In Chapter 9 we described how one can use pain-induction procedures such as muscle ischemia and the cold-pressor task for assessment purposes. These same procedures can be used during the application phase of treatment to facilitate training skills and to maximize the patient's feelings of control and self-efficacy. We view this exposure to pain as optional because we do not have enough data on its unique contribution to the overall cognitive–behavioral treatment regimen. It holds sufficient promise, nevertheless, to bear description.

Prior to the actual exposure to the pain-induction procedure, patients may be asked to listen to a tape describing the muscle-ischemia task and to plan how they could control the pain experience. For example, the therapist might say the following:

One of the best ways to determine how helpful various techniques are in control-ling pain is to try them out in a controlled situation. We can do this by inducing some pain, using a means that is completely harmless and that can be stopped when you want. You recall from undergoing it earlier [during assessment] that this involves inflating a blood-pressure cuff around your arm, which depletes oxygen. The result is a slowly intensifying, dull, aching type of pain that many patients have told us is similar to their own pain. [A similar description of the cold-pressor test might also be employed, depending upon the apparatus available.]

Before undertaking the task, though, let's take some time to prepare for it. Review some of the strategies that we have discussed and prepare a mental "game plan" for yourself to use. You can then try out the plan and the strategies in an imagined practice task.

This cassette tape contains a description of the blood-pressure experience. While listening to the tape, let your imagination vividly recapture your experience during the first time you underwent this task. As you mentally relive that session, imagine yourself now using your planned strategies to deal with the sensations and your reactions. Allow yourself to experience all of the feelings you previously had, but this time you are able to deal with these by use of the techniques that you have reviewed. The tape will not cue you to use the strategies. Rather, call them forth yourself as you need them: relaxation, breathing, images, mental activities, self-statements at each of the stages—use whatever tools are at your disposal, as you would use them were you in a real-life experience. When you are ready, turn on the tape on the cassette recorder. But first, please take some time to review the strategies and prepare a game plan, if you have not already done so.

Keep in mind that, at various levels of pain, or at different stages, you may find particular coping strategies more effective than others. For example, sometimes at moderate pain levels, relaxation and imagery may be very useful. As the sensations mount, more active mental strategies, such as mental arithmetic, humming a tune, or thought stopping, may be more useful. The rhythmical nature of some techniques helps you to hold your attention. Or just carefully focusing on your slow breathing may be best with the most intense pain. Once again, there is no reason that you shouldn't try anything at any time. But you may find that not all strategies are uniformly effective during the whole stressful situation.

The intent is to have the patient view the various techniques as tools to be tried and experiments to be engaged in and then to be discussed and modified. Since the various coping techniques had been taught in a cafeteria-type manner, the patient is encouraged to pick and choose what works best for him or her.

Following this imagery preparation, the patient is exposed to the muscle-ischemia task (see Appendix A). This exposure is followed by a review of what the patient did to control the pain. This discussion focuses on having the patient compare the pain experience now that he or she has a host of ways to control pain with the experience during prior exposure(s). Additional exposures to the cold-pressure or muscle-ischemia tasks may be employed to consolidate further the skills and the patient's perception of competence. The therapist can manipulate the time of exposure or, in the case of the cold-pressor task, the temperature of the water ($10°C$, $5°C$; Hilgard et al., 1967) in order to alter, to some extent, the intensity of the nociceptive stimulus. To enhance the patient's perception of self-efficacy, the therapist may modify the time or temperature over repeated trials in a graded, inoculation fashion.

The objective of this graded exposure in the clinic is to provide the patient with evidence that he or she can affect the nature (intensity and frequency) of pain. The exposure should lead to detailing how the patient can use the same procedures to control clinical pain.

GRADED EXPOSURE *IN VIVO*

This sense of resourcefulness is nurtured by means of graded homework assignments for the patient to engage in more challenging pain-incompatible activities *in vivo*. Since we described the nature and importance of homework assignments in Chapters 9 and 10, we will briefly reiterate some important points here.

Homework assignments are employed throughout treatment for several reasons: (1) to enhance patients' perceptions of self-confidence and control; (2) to break the cycle of withdrawal, increased debilitation, and dysphoric affect; (3) to assist the therapist in learning about difficulties patients may encounter in their natural environment; and (4) to facilitate the transfer of behavior from the therapy sessions to the natural environment. To accomplish each of these purposes, it is important to include homework assignments that are relevant for the individual needs, age, sex, and physical condition of the patient. Homework assignments should be concrete, measurable, and observable and should increase in difficulty over the course of training.

Each homework assignment should contain a *do* statement and a *quantity* statement (Shelton & Ackerman, 1974). The do statement specifies what the patient will accomplish (e.g., attend a movie, walk, talk with children about schoolwork), and the quantity statement tells the patient how often tasks are to be completed (e.g., twice a week, once a day) or how many repetitions are to be done (e.g., ten leg raises, five sit-ups). Furthermore, the therapist should establish specific homework assignments in conjunction with the patient and, at times, the significant other. Setting up *ideal*, but unrealistic, homework assignments with minimal relevance to the patient's interests or situation is likely to foster nonadherence.

To clarify any misunderstandings regarding homework assignments, and to increase their likelihood of successful completion, we employ several strategies. We ask patients (when feasible) to write down the homework assignments that they agree to complete. We ask them to repeat back to us what they are supposed to do and how frequently and, most important, to note any concerns they have or impediments they foresee in successfully completing the assignments. The importance of asking about concerns was dramatically pointed out to us by one of our patients who agreed to carry out some physical exercises, but then expressed great concern that the exercise "might break my spinal fusion." With this patient it was important to clarify his misconception regarding spinal fusions and to reassure him that his physician and physical therapist had approved of the specific exercises.

We believe that self-efficacy and resourcefulness are enhanced by independent practicing of skills and successful completion of homework because patients are more likely to attribute success to their own efforts and capabilities rather than to external supports. This may be a particular concern with inpatient treatments that control much of the patient's activity, but that often fail to prepare patients for maintenance and generalization outside of the hospital or clinic. The importance of incorporating outpatient sessions and homework with inpatient programs will be discussed later in this chapter.

An additional important point is what happens and what the therapist does when homework assignments are not successfully completed. We have found that it is important to address this possibility with patients before they begin assignments and to emphasize the importance of cooperation and responsibility. Failures may arise for a number of reasons, and these must be considered and treated in somewhat different manners. We attempt to establish whether the cause of the failure was (1) a misunderstanding, (2) resistance, (3) memory failure, (4) an unsupportive environment, (5) excessive demands, or (6) either fear of failure or, in some cases, fear of succeeding. Each of these must be considered and discussed with the patient. At times we have had to reassess the nature of the task demands and modify them. The point to underscore is collaboration. The therapist must work with the patient to foster self-competence and resourcefulness that can be maintained after treatment.

The therapist must be sensitive to how patients view homework assignments. In one instance a depressed patient who had a history of headaches and back pain reacted negatively to the suggestion of homework since she had been the only child of a set of parents who were schoolteachers. In this case the patient's resistance grew out of her resentment that she was being checked up on by her therapist, as she had been by her parents and by her husband. The treatment focused on this perception and its impact on her pain disorder. In this case the patient's resistance concerning homework became the focus of intervention. Once the homework assignments were characterized as "personal experiments" and described as an opportunity to find out what works and what still needs to be done, the patient responded in a more accepting and collaborative fashion.

There is a need to ensure that the therapy does *not* translate into a didactic, tutorial interchange. In fact, the therapist may wish to be cautious about using the term "homework assignment." The patient's self-statements or metacognitions about each intervention must be carefully assessed. The goal is to establish a collaborative working relationship, and the therapist must be cautious about interacting with patients as if they were students in a lecture class.

When the reason for resistance or noncompliance with the homework assignment is primarily a "paralysis of will" or a general depressed condition, the thought processes that contribute to this affective experience become the focus of attention. Like depressed patients, pain patients often make erroneous conclusions about themselves (Lefebvre, 1981), especially after growing depressed as a result of their chronic pain condition.

Chronic pain often leads to completely one-sided views of life—its being hopeless, worthless, full of pain, devoid of pleasure, incapacitating. Even though pain may persist, patients generally are able to increase activity levels and sources of pleasure, with some help.

One means of assisting in this process is through the assignment of homework in a graded sequence. This homework has two goals: (1) through increasing activity and encouraging attention to be directed externally, it can help lower pain perception and boost positive feelings; (2) it provides an occasion for patients to collect personal data that can be used in therapy sessions to combat one-sided views of themselves. Patients' information on successful experiences can be used to help them revise their hopeless and helpless attitudes, to appreciate the pleasure they do experience, and to maximize occasions for future pleasure instead of sabotaging any such possibilities.

A. Beck *et al.*'s (1979) summary of key features of graded assignments is applicable to patients with a variety of problems:

1. Problem definition—for example, the patient's belief that he is not capable of attaining goals that are important to him.
2. Formulation of a project. Stepwise assignment of tasks (or activities) from simpler to more complex.
3. Immediate and direct observation by the patient that he is successful in reaching a specific objective (carrying out an assigned task). The continual concrete feedback provides the patient with new corrective information regarding his functional capacity.
4. Ventilation of the patient's doubts, cynical reactions, and belittling of his achievement.
5. Encouragement of realistic evaluation by the patient of his actual performance.

6. Emphasis on the fact that the patient reached the goal as a result of his own effort and skill.
7. Devising new, more complex assignments in collaboration with the patient. (p. 132)

Essential is the use of modest goals, sometimes involving small steps. Giving up is well ingrained for most patients and will be elicited by even slight difficulty with initial tasks. Only following several successes should demands be increased. Failure is likely to lead to confirmation of the patient's hopeless views and thus needs to be avoided. This can sometimes be accomplished by reinterpreting, as a partial success, what the patient identifies as failure. An attempted walk around the block that goes only one-quarter of the way and back, for example, can be seen not as a "failed walk," but as a successful first attempt to increase exercise. The total half-block distance now sets the patient a goal for the next day, and if he or she travels half of the block every day for the next week, it will amount to more than three blocks' distance that was not covered last week.

Rehearsal of homework exercises in the session and careful attention to the patients' evaluation of their likelihood of success can also assist patients in avoiding failure experiences. It is generally unwise to ignore a patient's reluctance to attempt a task by suggesting that he or she "just try it out." Failure may, in fact, be built into such attempts. Instead, it is better to attempt to uncover the source of the reluctance and modify the task accordingly. The cognitive restructuring procedures offered by A. Beck *et al.* (1979) provide further examples of ways of dealing with homework assignments.

LIFE-STYLE CHANGES

To appreciate the impact that pain can have on patients' life-styles, consider the following case study: Ruby was a 42-year-old woman who experienced 3 years of severe pain following a whiplash sustained in a car accident. Her pain was severe enough to disrupt all aspects of her life. Ruby reported that her pain did not allow her to get a good night's sleep. Consequently, she was fatigued most of the time. She neglected her husband, children, friends, and home.

Her husband, Jack, was fed up with her complaints. The expense of Ruby's medication and medical treatments drained the family's finances and curtailed vacations and other pleasures. Ruby had no interest in any previously enjoyed activities, including sex. She wanted to be left alone.

Ruby's teenage children, Jennifer and Roy, were equally troubled by her behavior. They felt she had become a different person since the accident and were demoralized by her unpredictable behavior. She would belittle them for no apparent reason, and they felt they could not please her. Confused and angry, the children began staying away from home as much as possible. Ruby then became angry because they stayed away and accused them of lack of caring. She was depressed and guilty about her behavior.

Jack, who was a salesman, also spent more and more time away from home, often volunteering for extended selling trips. His inaccessibility led to more anger on Ruby's part. The continual conflicts served to drive Jack further away.

Jack and Ruby's former friends no longer visited them because Ruby constantly talked about her pain and suffering and complained that no one understood her condition. Friends stopped inviting the couple out because Ruby's pain was unpredictable, and she often had to back out of plans at the last moment.

Ruby's life had "collapsed" (to use her word). She spent her time lying down, in bed, or seeking new medical treatments. The boundaries of her existence were restricted to home and physicians' offices or hospitals.

Unfortunately, Ruby's case is not atypical of patients we have treated. Chronic pain can and does devastate patients' lives and the lives of the entire family. Thus the treatment of patients with chronic pain requires major changes in their pain-dominated life-style. The goals of treatment include altering pain-engendering environments, in addition to learning self-control techniques.

The discussion at the beginning of therapy may provide avenues for life-style intervention approaches for the patient. In the course of treatment, it may be noted, for example, that a patient evidences a life-style devoid of any stimulation unrelated to illness or pain. Lack of activity and external stimulation often leads to preoccupation with oneself, one's plight, and one's symptoms, as in the case of Ruby. Such self-directed attentional focus is likely to increase dysphoric affect, which in turn may result in increased pain perception. Failure to engage in physical activity may lead to muscle atrophy and increased weakness, pain, and debilitation and may interfere with the natural healing processes of the body (e.g., Melzack & Dennis, 1978). Thus a vicious circle may be created.

Gottlieb *et al.* (1977), Sternbach (1974b), and Turner (1979) have reported on the potential contribution of group therapy (group support and pressure) in helping patients begin to alter their life-styles. Sternbach states the following:

> Group support makes less difficult the ability of patients to become aware of
> how they use their pain to receive payoffs such as sympathy, narcotics,

financial compensation, or admiration for bravery. Such payoffs are usually not consciously conceived by the patients, and when this is presented in didactic fashion, the group tends to rally and protest their good intentions. However, once an individual patient has his pain game described to him by other patients who have had similar games, he is more inclined to accept it and analyze his behavior. This is more effective than when feedback is provided by the staff. Patients may deceive themselves and the staff, but they cannot long deceive the other patients with whom they are living, and feedback from the others, given supportively, soon stops the game playing. (pp. 103–104)

The group may consider how such patterns of activities develop and, with the therapist's assistance, may come to initiate a plan for change. Resistant patients may be goaded by the observation that, if nothing seems to have much effect on the level of pain, then they might as well be active as inactive. Inactivity has not helped; perhaps in the long run increased activity will (Melzack & Dennis, 1978). Fordyce (1976), Gottlieb *et al.* (1977), Khatami and Rush (1978), Mitchell and Mitchell (1971), Swanson *et al.* (1976), and Sternbach (1974b) all provide examples of how life-style changes may be used in therapy for chronic pain.

In such interventions an attempt is made (1) to manipulate the social system in which patients find themselves so that they are less rewarded by pain behaviors and more rewarded for a normal life-style and (2) to alter how patients view their life situation in relation to pain. Families may be involved, and in the course of group and/or individual therapeutic sessions, patients can plan how to alter environments gradually, setting significant, but realistic, goals. These goals are generally activity-oriented and life-style-oriented rather than pain-centered (e.g., Greenhoot & Sternbach, 1974). A reduction in the level of pain may result from such changes and thereby reduce the *importance* of pain for patients.

COGNITIVE RESTRUCTURING

Cognitive restructuring is a summary label that describes a host of procedures, including rational–emotive therapy (Ellis, 1962), cognitive therapy, (A. Beck *et al.*, 1979), problem-solving training (Goldfried & Davison, 1976), and stress-inoculation training (Meichenbaum & Jaremko, 1982). Since each of these treatment approaches has been described in detail elsewhere, we will not reiterate this material here (see especially Cormier & Cormier, 1979; Mahoney & Arnkoff, 1978; Turk, 1982). In fact, the topic of cognitive restructuring could constitute a book itself.

Briefly, cognitive restructuring is designed to help patients (1) to appreciate that there is a relationship between their thoughts and feelings and their behaviors and (2) to identify faulty, self-defeating, pain-engendering thoughts, and then to replace these cognitions with coping thoughts, feelings, and behaviors. For example, patients who report thoughts that they are incompetent and helpless in controlling the pain they experience would be guided to appreciate how such thoughts may exacerbate the intensity and increase the duration of their pain, thus acting as self-fulfilling prophecies.

The general therapeutic strategy is to have patients discuss their pain experience, monitor their reactions to pain, and then consider the impact of such reactions on the maintenance and intensification of pain and on the onset of the next pain episode. The therapist helps the patient to consider how such reactions (thoughts, feelings, and behaviors) prevent the patient from initiating and pursuing more adaptive coping behaviors. The therapist tries to have the patient view such thoughts and feelings as hypotheses worthy of testing in the form of personal experiments rather than as given truths. The cognitive restructuring focuses on what the patient perceives the consequences of such personal experiments to be and on the implications this holds for the patient's prior expectations, appraisals, attributions, and current concerns. This continual therapeutic effort is designed to help the patient (1) to identify patterns of maladaptive coping behavior involving negative, pain-engendering thoughts, images, feelings, and behaviors; (2) to use positive coping resources in both pain-related experiences and nonpain areas; and (3) to engage significant others in the intervention process.

SKILLS TRAINING

Before one begins any skills-training program, it is necessary to ensure that a deficit does, in fact, exist. A careful cognitive–behavioral analysis will determine whether patients have the knowledge of what is required and the ability to implement this knowledge or whether the patients' thoughts and feelings (expectations, sense of self-efficacy, etc.) interfere with such knowledge and performance. For example, R. Schwartz and Gottman (1976) found that nonassertive people actively inhibited appropriate assertive behaviors that were within their repertoires with ongoing cognitive concerns about possible negative social consequences. In our clinical practice, we have asked patients what advice they would have for someone else who had their problems (e.g., coping with chronic pain). Quite often, patients offer potentially useful coping strategies. The questions then become whether patients have the component skills with which to implement their proposed advice, and, if they do have such skills, what may interfere with implementation.

The answers to these questions will result in individualized prescriptions concerning skills, although the training of problem-solving heuristics will be common. This problem-solving training involves teaching patients how to (1) define the problem or stressor; (2) set realistic goals; (3) examine alternatives; (4) consider others' perspectives and motives; (5) select an appropriate strategy; (6) delineate necessary steps to reach a goal; (7) rehearse by means of imagery, role playing, and *in vivo* practice; and (8) reward themselves for having tried.

In a related vein, Gottman, Notarius, Gonso, and Markman (1976) have trained the expression of feelings to improve communication. They teach patients and significant others an *XYZ* method, in which they are encouraged to state, "When *you* do *X* in situation *Y, I* feel *Z*"; for example, "When you ask me if I would like to go out when I am really sick, I feel irritated and then worthless." This exercise permits the patient and the significant other to develop listening skills and to begin to formulate interventions. The goal is for both parties to see such exchanges as problems to be solved rather than as personal attacks or provocations.

In addition, patients and significant others may be taught communication skills to employ with health care providers. Failure to obtain information concerning medication or other treatments because of inhibitions in making requests may increase a sense of passivity, a lack of control, and reduced adherence.

PREPARING FOR POSTTREATMENT

It is suggested that, during the final treatment session, all aspects of training be reviewed. The patient may be provided with another set of pain intensity rating cards and a pain questionnaire (described in Chapter 9). Two weeks following treatment termination, the patient and the significant other can return with these materials to review progress and maintenance skills. At the 3-month, 6-month, and 1-year follow-up appointments, the patient, significant other, and therapist can consider any difficulties that have arisen and can assess pain behavior. Patients may be encouraged, however, to make appointments between specific follow-up dates if they deem it necessary.

We have found it advisable, especially with chronic pain patients, *not* to have the treatment terminate abruptly, but instead to build in a transition period. It is important to have posttreatment plans defined and agreed upon. Grzesiak (1981) suggests that for inpatient treatment programs it is helpful to provide a week of formal outpatient treatment before the patient assumes activities at home. This transition is necessary because the inpatient setting is unnatural, with many of the patients' activities under the control of health care providers. The addition of outpatient treatment should increase the generalization of therapeutic gains. A number of explicit assignments can be implemented once on an outpatient basis. For example, the patient can be asked to report on pain behavior by means of a diary, pain intensity ratings, and exercise records. Some steady contact with the health care provider is advisable.

Although we do not have data on exactly what type of contact (i.e., follow-through or booster sessions) would prove most effective with what type of pain patient, nor exactly when such contact sessions should be conducted, we believe this contact is important. To enhance both transfer and maintenance of treatment effects, we recommend that the therapist gradually increase the time interval between sessions from weekly or twice weekly, to every other week, to once a month for 4 months to 6 months and that the therapist include at least a 1-year follow-up. Obviously, the frequency and timing of such follow-through sessions will vary from case to case.

Follow-through sessions cannot be mere extensions or repetitions of the original treatment program. With the patients' improvements, even small changes are likely to elicit expectations in others that may result in emotionally charged demands on the patients. As pain patients improve, the treatment concerns change from pain control to other stressed aspects of life (vocational concerns, marital conflict, etc.).

One concern that is discussed with the therapist is how the health care system will be used in the future. As Karol *et al.* (1981) noted, the chronic pain patient should consider a number of factors when deciding to use the health care system.

1. *Severity*: How severe is the pain? Is it about the same as before, or is it much worse? Are there other indicators (e.g., spitting up blood) to suggest that medical attention is necessary?
2. *Similarity*: How similar is the new pain to the previous pain? Is it in the same part of the body? (For example, pain in the calf muscle instead of the thigh muscle may not be a different pain problem.)
3. *Self-help*: Does the pain decrease when you use techniques covered in this program? Can the pain be decreased by using some self-help strategies (e.g., progressive relaxation)?

4. *Risk of being wrong*: What is the risk if you do not use the health
   care system and you are wrong? What is the danger if you decide
   that the pain is chronic and it really is an acute problem? (For
   example, the risk may be much greater if the pain is in the area of
   the chest rather than in the calf.)
5. *Acute results*: If you decide that the problem is acute and use the
   health care system, do the acute methods work? If they don't
   work, there is a good chance that the problem is chronic.

In addition to these questions, the therapist can convey to the patient
that there are likely to be times in the future when the patient's pain may,
in fact, increase. If this occurs, the therapist notes, the patient is encouraged not to panic or "catastrophize." Instead, the therapist encourages
the patient to use the variety of skills that have been worked on in
treatment or even to create new ways to cope. The door is always left open
for future treatment if necessary.

As we noted in Chapter 3, Marlatt and Gordon (1980) developed a
similar approach that they call *relapse prevention*. In their case they were
working with patients who were addicted to alcohol and other drugs, and
they considered what could be done to help patients appreciate the factors
that contribute to relapse. For example, they focus upon what may
constitute high-risk situations for the individual to drink again and what
are the interpersonal and intrapersonal skills needed to cope with these
demands. They also focus upon what alcoholic patients might say or
imagine to themselves if they should take a drink following a period of
abstinence: "Once an alcoholic, always an alcoholic." "I knew this program
wouldn't work for me. What's the use?" Pain patients have similar thoughts
and feelings that accompany pain episodes, especially if a period of pain-
free behavior has been experienced. The therapist should consider with
the pain patient possible ways of avoiding and dealing with relapses.

Discussion of relapse must be done in a delicate fashion. On the one
hand, the therapist does not wish to convey an expectancy of treatment
failure, but on the other hand, the therapist wishes to anticipate and
subsume into treatment the patient's possible reactions to the likely
recurrence of pain. Two clinical techniques could be used at this point.
First, the therapist can reanalyze with the patient previous reactions that
have followed relapses. Second, the therapist can call upon imaginary
pain patients and suggest to the patient the types of thoughts and feelings
they had upon the reexperience of pain and what they did to cope with
them. The therapist can mention that he or she does not know if the
patient will have such feelings and thoughts, but that it is worthwhile to
determine the patient's possible reactions to similar situations.

Such discussions help the patient plan for the posttreatment period. As Malec *et al.* (1977) emphasized, it is important for the patient not to think of the treatment program as ending, but rather as switching into a different phase.

A review with patients of what they have learned from treatment and how they have changed from the pretreatment phase can encourage recognition of how the patients' own efforts contributed to this change. Discussion can enhance patients' sense of competence and mastery. In this way, patients can discuss current and anticipated life events that may be problematic. The goal is to help patients realize that they have plans and abilities to cope with these events. By this type of discourse, the therapist conveys the expectation and conviction that the changes that have been achieved will be maintained.

FUTURE DIRECTIONS

CHAPTER 14

AFTERTHOUGHTS AND IMPLICATIONS

The increasing interest in behavioral medicine opens up significant opportunities for research and applications. But there is a danger that overoptimistic claims or widespread application without an adequate scientific base and sufficient evaluation by pilot testing can lead to failure and disillusionment.—*Neal Miller (1979)*

WHERE WE HAVE BEEN

Behavioral medicine is a rapidly growing field covering a diversity of topics and populations, which can be viewed both longitudinally, along a continuum from health through terminal illness and death, and cross-sectionally, from the patient to the family, health care provider, health care system, and the broader social–cultural environment. Because of this diversity, we have chosen to examine briefly the breadth of the field, with examples along the health–disease–illness continuum, and depth of coverage restricted to pain and pain management. We have focused cross-sectionally on the level of the patient, family, and health care provider, mentioning only in passing the health care and social systems.

We have neglected almost completely such important subareas in behavioral medicine as the development and maintenance of health beliefs, pediatrics, geriatrics, sexuality, medical decision making, education of health care providers, and death and dying. Several recent compendiums have provided coverage of these areas (e.g., Doleys, Meredith, & Ciminero, 1982; Ferguson & Taylor, 1980; McNamara, 1979; Melamed & Siegel, 1980; Pomerleau & Brady, 1979; Prokop & Bradley, 1981; G. Stone, Cohen, & Adler, 1979).

We have given the greatest amount of attention to pain and pain management because of the seriousness of the problem, the complexity of the phenomenon, and the extensive literature in this area. Furthermore, many of the conceptual and treatment issues surrounding pain management are equally relevant to other diseases and illnesses, and the topics we discussed can be generalized to them.

In the first section of the book, we provided a general orientation to the cognitive–behavioral perspective, emphasizing several major characteristics, namely, the importance of information selection and processing by the individual, reciprocal determinism of the individual and the environment, collaboration between therapist and patient, and potential modifiability of maladaptive thoughts and feelings. We then provided an overview of the application of this perspective to a sample of subareas along the health–disease continuum, noting the promising, yet rudimentary, nature of the research on cognitive factors in these areas. Next we examined the research on psychological factors in pain perception, the pain experience, and pain management. We reviewed the major psychologically based treatment approaches for pain management and, in the final section, provided a detailed cognitive–behavioral treatment guide for pain management.

At the outset of this book, we quoted Neal Miller's dictum that "we should be bold in what we attempt and cautious in what we claim." At this point we would like to modify that dictum to read, "We should be cautious both in what we attempt and in what we claim," for all too often, treatments are employed prematurely, without systematic research and understanding of the psychological and physiological underpinnings of diseases. Overly enthusiastic claims are unsubstantiated by controlled treatment outcome studies or adequate follow-up. Throughout this book we have emphasized collaboration between the therapist and the patient; at this point we would like to emphasize collaboration among workers in the field who come from different disciplines.

The overwhelming discovery for us in writing this book has been in recognizing the breadth of the field of behavioral medicine and the complexity of the cognitive–behavioral perspective and treatment regimen. We were both surprised and dismayed by the amount of detail involved. We do not, however, feel that our intervention is unique in being so complex. A consideration of other treatment programs, such as those offered by Fordyce and Sternbach, as well as the host of pain-management programs reviewed in Chapters 6 and 7, indicates that all treatments are multifaceted. Clinical problems are much more complex than is suggested in the treatment literature, and they require comprehensive interventions. Moreover, there are several aspects of treatment that require even more consideration than offered in this book. For example, we noted that the cognitive–behavioral treatment approach could be adapted for children, but did not describe how (Meichenbaum, 1977).

WHERE WE NEED TO GO

Given the nature of cognitive–behavioral interventions and the present state of the art, the question that now arises is where to focus research efforts. Our proposed agenda has several items that we would like the reader to consider. Our priorities are, first, to develop psychometrically sound assessment procedures; second, to examine the intricacies of cognitive and affective processes at all points along the health–disease–illness continuum; and third, to demonstrate a robust treatment effect for the cognitive–behavioral treatment approach in order to ensure that the effort is worthwhile. Although we have reviewed a host of studies providing encouraging clinical data with a wide variety of behavioral medicine problems, a convincing set of data has not been forthcoming. Note that this conclusion could be directed at almost all other treatment approaches as well. For "convincing data," we require the inclusion of adequate control groups matched for credibility (see Kazdin & Wilcoxon, 1976, for discussion of necessary controls) and adequate follow-up assessments of clinical populations.

We believe that cognitive–behavioral treatment has reached the stage at which such comparative outcome studies are warranted. Interestingly, the National Institute of Mental Health and the United States Veterans Administration concur at least in the areas of depression and pain management, respectively, in which they are sponsoring comparative outcome research in the evaluation of cognitive therapy of depression and the evaluation of cognitive-behavior modification, operant conditioning, and biofeedback in pain management. This is particularly important, for despite all the attention given to pain management, Fordyce and Steger (1979) observe: "*It is important to note that a systematic, controlled study of alternative approaches to similar pain problems has yet to be attempted*" (p. 138, original emphasis).

An important feature of such outcome work is the need to consider individual differences of patients' responses to treatment (e.g., Bradley *et al.*, 1978; Fordyce, 1976; Sternbach, 1974b). To do away with a uniformity myth concerning patients, it is necessary to consider carefully those who do and those who do *not* respond to treatment; it is also important to identify which components of multifaceted treatments are of benefit to which subset of patients and which components are of use to other patients. A related issue is our concern about the inadequacy of our dependent measures and the lack of consistency across classes of measures. For example, pain is not a unitary process, whether we are considering patients with headaches or with chronic low back pain. We have described some innovative cognitive and affective assessment procedures that may be of use in helping us better understand such individual differences. In short, there is a great need to better understand the nature of the problems we attempt to treat.

We must be cautious in developing our understanding of the pathophysiology of problems that come under the purview of behavioral medicine before we begin implementing specific intervention procedures. Application of psychologically based treatments without consideration of basic physiological processes can lead to negative results, which may impede the development of behavioral medicine. (See Seeburg & DeBoer, 1980, for an example of the potentially devastating results following from the misapplication of a behavioral technique.) Moreover, traditional assessment procedures that are based on psychiatric populations are often employed with medical populations for which little normative data have been produced. Generalizations from psychiatric patients to medical patients may lead to misdiagnosis and inappropriate intervention (Bradley & Prokop, 1981).

Disillusionment with traditional assessment devices has led to the development and use of new techniques that, unfortunately, often fail to establish reliability and validity (Keefe, 1979; Russo, Bird, & Masek, 1980; Turk & Kerns, 1980). See, for example, the work by Bakal and his colleagues (Bakal et al., 1981) and by Philips (1978) on headache patients in which the nature of migraine- and tension-headache patients is being reconsidered. A similar effort is needed with other disorders.

The assessment research strategy that was discussed in Chapter 2 is a useful way to study patients' adjustive demands and adaptive responses. Such an analysis will permit us to predict better the course of adaptation, to identify individuals at risk for less satisfactory adjustive responding, to design therapeutic interventions, and to instigate institutional change. To reiterate, the approach includes an examination of the predominant concerns and variations in adjustive demands throughout the course of illness. This problem-identification phase may include such techniques as self-report questionnaires, diaries, interviews, role playing, and behavioral observation. In addition to patients, other relevant groups such as significant others and health care providers are included to help generate lists of problem areas and specific demands that emerge over the course of the illness. A related concern is to enumerate response options or identify coping responses. In this second phase, the investigator conducts research to enumerate the interpersonal and intrapersonal (i.e., sense of self-efficacy, metacognitions, etc.) coping response that patients use to cope with their illness. The third stage consists of the assessment of the relative efficacy of each of the response options. This evaluation is made by relevant patient groups as well as health care providers.

Follick and Turk (1978) have described how this process can be used in the study of chronic illness, such as in the case of ostomy patients. We believe that such a sequential research strategy is needed before the widespread application of techniques with diverse populations. Comprehensive, disease-specific analyses are required if we are to develop more effective treatment interventions.

Once we have meaningful treatment effects, we can foresee some efforts at dismantling the cognitive–behavioral treatment approach. We have, however, some reservations about this dismantling research strategy, given the complexity of the package and the need to individually tailor treatment intervention. (The sensitive customizing of the treatment is one of the strengths of a cognitive–behavioral approach.) But we can foresee studies that ask such questions as the following: Does one lose or gain anything by including significant others or by conducting treatment on a group basis? When and how should booster sessions be conducted? How much improvement accrues from the comprehensive assessment per se (diary, pain ratings, questionnaires, imagery reconstructions, etc.)? What types of patients benefit from specific treatment components?

WHAT MEDIATES THE EFFICACY
OF COGNITIVE-BEHAVIOR MODIFICATION

Perhaps one of the most interesting and important questions has to do with the issue of what mediates the efficacy of the cognitive–behavioral interventions. If treatment procedures reduce the pain or stress experience, as we have argued, what are the mechanisms that could mediate such change?

Throughout the preceding chapters, we have focused on the role of cognitive and affective factors at all points along the health–disease–illness continuum from health promotion and symptom perception through treatment and rehabilitation. We have proposed that psychological factors related to the processing of information will likely influence the individual's response. Recent work on stress and coping tends to support this assertion.

The earliest work on stress focused on the characteristics of the physical stimuli per se (e.g., heat, cold, virus; Selye, 1956). Mason (1975c) pointed out that, despite the fact that a number of agents had been employed to produce a stress response, these diverse stimuli shared one important characteristic: exposure to a novel, strange, or unfamiliar environment. Frankenhaeuser (1980) suggested that, in addition to novelty, anticipation and lack of control also characterized many of the situations in which stress responses were induced. Thus the common thread that may explain the organisms' responses seems to be the psychological relevance of the stimulus rather than the physical stress to which they are exposed. Stress researchers have become much more aware of the importance of how the individual perceives (appraises) a given event and of his or her coping resources in determining how stressful it is rather than attending exclusively to the characteristics of the situation or environmental task (e.g., Frankenhaeuser, 1980; R. Lazarus, 1966; Mason, 1975c). It has been suggested that physical stressors may even fail to elicit physiological stress responses if the emotional distress that typically accompanies their administration is eliminated (Mason, 1971, 1975a).

The concept of coping, in particular, has received increasing attention. As we discussed in Chapter 2, the ways in which individuals cope with symptoms, their life situations, and diseases will influence their health maintenance behaviors, the course of their disease, and the medical treatment they receive. The individual may minimize his or her risk of developing a disease, minimize the seriousness of symptoms, persist in or reinitiate maladaptive attempts to cope with disability, and so on. Such behaviors may be viewed as exerting indirect influences on health and illness, but psychological factors may also have direct effects on physiological functioning.

Several authors have suggested that psychological events processed by the central nervous system can be transduced into functional and structural changes (e.g., Amkraut & Solomon, 1975; Bowers, 1977; Frankenhaeuser, 1980; Triesman, 1968; Weiner, 1977). How might this direct effect come about?

A substantial body of research has demonstrated that anticipation of physical or psychological stimuli may produce physiological responses (e.g., autonomic arousal, hormonal secretions) equal to the responses that are present during the actual experience. (See reviews of this literature by Mason, 1971, and Rose, 1980.) Furthermore, the ways in which individuals cope with environmental demands also appears to shape hormonal responses to stress (e.g., Glass, 1977; Katz, Weiner, Gallagher, & Hellman, 1970; G. Wolff, Friedman, Hofer, & Mason, 1964). Frankenhaeuser (1980) has suggested that psychological factors related to appraisal may be the triggers of both the sympathetic–adrenomedullary response and the pituitary–adrenocortical systems. Thus psychological factors may influence secretion of stress-related hormones such as cortisol and the catecholamines.

Catecholamines are neurotransmitters involved in the regulation of blood pressure, heart rate, and cardiac output; the shunting of blood from the viscera to brain and muscle; the mobilizing of blood glucose; and so on. It has been apparent for some time that increases in catecholamines accompanying emotional stress not only have important effects on blood-pressure regulation, but also may serve a crucial role in the pathophysiology of a number of diseases (e.g., Glass, 1977; Rose, 1980).

Although direct evidence of a causal relationship between catecholamine secretion and disease is still lacking, data from several sources suggest that, if periods of high secretion are prolonged or repeated frequently, the cardiovascular system may be adversely affected (Frankenhaeuser, 1980; Glass, 1977). There is some indication, for example, that the Type A coronary-prone individual may be characterized by low flexibility in physical arousal related to situational demands. This rigid pattern of response may account for the increased risk of CHD among individuals with this behavior pattern (Frankenhaeuser, Lundberg, & Forsman, cited in Frankenhaeuser, 1979). Glass (1977), for example, has argued that fluctuations in catecholamines sufficiently dramatic to influence the pathogenesis of CHD are elicited by a coping style that alternates between initial efforts to control stressful transactions and helplessness when coping efforts fail. He further notes that this coping pattern is characteristic of individuals with the Type A behavioral pattern and may account for the increased susceptibility of these individuals to CHD.

Another way in which psychological factors may contribute to physiological changes is through the immune system. The immune system has a fundamental role in the maintenance of body homeostasis and health (Rogers, Dubey, & Reich, 1979). Stress appears to have an immunosuppressive effect. Solomon and his colleagues have argued that T cells, B cells, and macrophages (immunological defenders) are all susceptible to destruction by stress-response hormones such as corticosteroids (Solomon, Amkraut, & Kasper, 1974). Moreover, it is argued that the changes in the immune balance need only be slight in order to increase dramatically a person's susceptibility to pathogens generally present in the body or environment (Amkraut & Solomon, 1975; Cassel, 1976). So, when a situation is perceived as threatening, and/or when psychological defenses are unable to contain the emotional reactions to the perceived stress, the person's biological defenses may diminish, making him or her potentially more vulnerable to infections as well as to cancer. (Through suppression of the immunological surveillance system, cancer cells are more apt to escape detection until it is too late.)

The clinical literature has repeatedly emphasized the importance of psychological factors in both the onset and the course of a variety of diseases known to be at least partly influenced by disturbances in the immune system, including cancer (e.g., Bahnson, 1969), infectious diseases (e.g., Day, 1951; Imboden, Canter, & Cluff, 1961), autoimmune diseases (e.g., Engel, 1955; Rimon, 1969), and allergies (e.g., Engels & Wittkower, 1975). In at least two studies, one of patients with breast cancer (Pettingale, Greer, & Tee, 1977) and another of patients with rheumatoid arthritis (Hendrie, Paraskevas, Baragar, & Adamson, 1971), there have been specific correlations between immunoglobulin levels and emotional state.

Thus it appears that psychological factors may influence health, disease, and illness both indirectly through the individuals' appraisals and more directly through the autonomic and immune systems.

HOW PSYCHOLOGICAL FACTORS MIGHT MEDIATE THE PHYSIOLOGY OF PAIN

In Chapters 5 and 6 we presented data describing the relative efficacy of cognitive and behavioral coping strategies in the mediation of pain and suffering. These data tend to support the importance of cognitive and affective factors in pain perception and response to nociceptive stimuli. These psychological variables may modulate pain perception directly by "closing the gate" postulated by Melzack and his colleagues (Melzack, 1973; Melzack & Casey, 1968; Melzack & Wall, 1965). Another way in which cognitive and behavioral factors might reduce pain is through prevention or blockage of abnormal reverberatory neural activity, which has been hypothesized as underlying prolonged pain (e.g., Melzack & Dennis, 1978). That is, even moderate reductions in pain produced by psychological techniques (e.g., through relaxation, distraction, increased sense of control) may enable patients to become more physically active, thereby interfering with the hypothesized reverberatory neural activity.

Many patients, especially those with musculoskeletal pain, resort to pain-induced immobilization. Immobilization may result in muscle weakness surrounding the painful area and increased discomfort beyond the initial pain problem. A further mechanism to explain the efficacy of the approach we have suggested is that it may provide the opportunity and incentive for patients to increase therapeutic activities that subsequently improve strength and range of motion. The result may be improved ambulatory status and general activity level, thereby reducing the additional pain associated with immobility (Dietrich, 1976).

Additional data have been presented that individuals' appraisals (beliefs, attributions, internal dialogues) concerning the relative efficacy of various pain-treatment modalities can potentiate the effectiveness of pain-management approaches. For example, Melzack, Weisz, and Sprague (1963) demonstrated the importance of subjects' beliefs on the effectiveness of audio analgesia. Melzack, Ofiesh, and Mount (1976) also reported that patients' beliefs in the efficacy of the Brompton mixture increased the analgesic properties of this medium. It has also been suggested that the analgesic effect of morphine can be facilitated in patients who are overly anxious or experiencing acute stress (e.g., Beecher, 1959). And, recently, Chen (1980) has reported that subjects' appraisals could potentiate or reverse the efficacy of nitrous oxide (N_2O) with dental pain. From data such as these, it appears that appraisals and other cognitive processes may have a synergistic effect with physical pain-management procedures.

Psychological methods of reducing stress and pain share a common feature—they decrease anxiety, depression, tension, and perceived lack of control. Anxiety, tension, depression, and perceived incontrollability appear to exacerbate a variety of somatic symptoms and the perception of pain. These psychological variables have been shown to modulate the production of stress hormones, neurotransmitters, and automatic arousal, including increased muscle tension. Consequently, modification of anxiety, depression, tension, and perceived lack of control may lead to decreased production of ACTH, catecholamines, and cortisol, decreased muscle tension, and increased availability of neurotransmitters (e.g., serotonin), thereby directly modifying pain perception, pain response, and suffering (Benedetti, 1979; Johansson & von Knorring, 1979).

Although a discussion of the neurochemical nature of pain is beyond the scope of this book, we cannot help but speculate about the potential importance of some recent findings. Snyder (1977) suggested that there may be a neuropharmacological mechanism mediating pain behavior. Thus, when behavioral expressions are modified, corresponding changes may occur in the neuropharmacological substrate. For example, the recent biochemical research that indicates an association between endogenous opiate-like substances (endorphins and enkephalins) and analgesics suggests that similar processes may be operating in both morphine- and stimulation-induced analgesia (Hughes, Smith, Kosterlitz, Fothergill, Morgan, & Morris, 1975; Simon, Hiller, & Edelman, 1975).

Several investigators (e.g., Almay, Johansson, von Knorring, Terenius, & Wahlstrom, 1978; Sjolund, Terenius, & Eriksson, 1977) have found that endorphins are decreased in patients suffering from chronic, intractable, benign pain and cancer pain. Weisenberg (1980) suggested that "ultimately, it might be possible to achieve the ideal nonaddicting pain-control strategy, with the fewest side effects and complications when we will be capable of behaviorally unlocking the body's own endogenous pain-control system" (p. 86), and E. Hilgard (1975) suggested that biobehavioral mechanisms may be involved with various psychologically based interventions.

That such a suggestion may not be so farfetched is indicated by the findings that, simultaneous with the secretion, under stress, of ACTH by the pituitary gland, another hormone is also secreted called endorphin-B (Guillemin, Vargo, Rossier, Minick, Ling, Rivier, Vale, & Bloom, 1977). The ACTH stimulates secretion of corticosteroids by the adrenals, whereas endorphin-B seems to affect morphine-sensitive brain tissue, presumably acting like an analgesic. This may explain why Beecher and others have observed reduced amounts of pain in wounded soldiers; how psychological stress may influence the immune system, leading to the development of a number of diseases; and why psychologically based interventions may be effective. Obviously, considerable empirical work is needed before such speculations are supported, but the linkage between neurochemical researchers and treatment investigators is an exciting future direction (e.g., Amkraut & Solomon, 1975; Benedetti, 1979; Bowers & Kelly, 1979; Varni, 1981a, 1981b). While we are *not* endorsing a reductionistic view of psychological phenomena, we welcome and encourage interdisciplinary collaboration in both treatment and research.

In summary, this book has been an organizer and a heuristic device for the authors in identifying the needed new research directions, the present state of the art, and the clinical sensitivity required. We hope that it has served a similar function for the reader.

INSTRUCTIONS FOR BEHAVIORAL TRIALS

COLD-PRESSOR TEST PROCEDURE

A number of studies (e.g., Lovallo, 1975; Scott & Barber, 1977a; Turk, 1977) have shown that immersion of a limb in circulating ice water maintained at 2°C or lower produces a continuing aching or crushing pain. The apparatus (see Figure A-1) we have employed in the cold-pressor test consists of a standard ice chest divided into two parts by wire mesh, with ice confined to one-third of the tank. A cradle is provided for the patient's arm that allows the hand and arm to be immersed in the ice water approximately 30 cm from the fingertip to mid-forearm. The water in the ice chest is circulated vigorously by a submerged bilge pump, to avoid local warming of the water. The cradle consists of plastic webbing on an aluminum frame that is hinged to the top of the ice chest to support the arm before immersion and to permit removal of the arm as quickly as possible. The cradle is attached to an automatic timer that engages upon the cradle's entry into the ice chest and disengages rapidly upon removal.

The instructions provided to patients vary, depending upon how the apparatus is being used. If the cold-pressor test is being employed as an assessment procedure, the patients are asked to indicate when the pain reaches a level that is equivalent to their pain and to remove their arms when the pain intensity reaches an "intolerable level." With this information, the therapist can determine a pain ratio score (Sternbach, 1974b) consisting of the patient's matching of his or her clinical pain to the pain produced by the cold pressor (timed in seconds) divided by the maximum tolerance of the cold-pressor test (timed in seconds) multiplied by 100. Sternbach suggests that the difference between patients' matching of the induced pain to their experienced pain and the maximum tolerance for the cold-pressor task serves a valuable diagnostic function. As Sternbach notes, "when the former [patient's matched pain rating] is much higher and it is often very much higher—we assume the patient is exaggerating the severity of his pain and we discuss the difference with him. If the pain estimate is much lower, as occasionally happens, we assume the patient is unusually stoical for some reason, and we

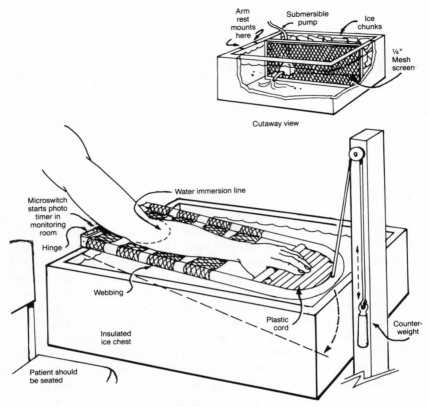

FIGURE A-1. *Apparatus employed in cold-pressor test.*

discuss that with him" (1974a, p. 287). Although we consider Sternbach's assessment approach interesting and potentially quite useful, much more research is needed to appreciate the clinical significance of his measures.

The cold-pressor task may also be used to help the patient consolidate skills learned during the training, thus providing an opportunity for the patient to try newly acquired skills in a controlled pain situation. The patients are encouraged to use their pain intensity ratings that are offered at various times during the cold-pressor assessment as occasions to examine how well they are coping and what their thoughts and feelings are. The therapist can manipulate the temperature of the water in the cold pressor, raising it to increase tolerance, and thereby increasing the patient's sense of self-efficacy. Temperature may be decreased as the patient has success with coping. Thus graded mastery may be fostered. If the therapist wishes to vary the temperature in small increments, he or she may use a refrigeration unit to maintain various water temperatures.

The basic procedure in using the cold-pressor test, whether used for assessment or training, is as follows:

1. Explain the purpose of the task, either to assist in establishing the level of pain intensity or as an opportunity to practice various skills acquired and to learn what is most effective.
2. Patient sits in a straight-back chair at the level of the ice chest.
3. Identify which is the nondominant arm and ask patient if there is anything wrong with it. If there is any problem with the nondominant arm, or if the patient's pain is located in the nondominant arm, then the dominant arm is used.
4. Patient removes any jewelry from the arm to be immersed.
5. Explain the basic procedure and mention that questions may be asked. Mention that some discoloration is common and that this will rapidly decrease after removal of the arm.
6. Place the arm to be immersed in a bucket of room-temperature water for 1 minute prior to immersion in the ice chest.
7. Place arm on the cradle and ask patient to push gently down so that the cradle enters the ice water.
8. Upon removal of arm from the water, assure the patient that the discomfort he or she feels will decrease rapidly. Note that many patients report that the discomfort is worse immediately upon removal of the arm from the water.
9. Give patient a towel to dry arm.

MUSCLE-ISCHEMIA PROCEDURE

Patients are asked to raise their nondominant arm over their head for 1 minute to drain excess venous blood. In the original development of the procedure, an Esmark bandage was wrapped about the subjects' arms at this point; however, we found that this was unnecessary. After the arm is lowered, the sphygmomanometer (blood-pressure) cuff is inflated about the arm to a pressure of 240 mm Hg. Following the inflation of the cuff, a hand dynamometer (Lafayette Instrument #205), blocked at 8 kg of force (below maximum effort for a population of healthy males), is squeezed 20 times for a duration of 2 seconds each, with a rest of 2 seconds between squeezes. The squeeze–relax–squeeze cycle can be presented by a taped message. The purpose of the exercise is to deplete the amount of oxygen in the arm muscles, thus increasing the rate at which ischemia will occur.

There is a tendency for the pressure to decrease slightly over time, but with it raised to 240 mm Hg, sufficient pressure remains to occlude the blood flow up to 46 minutes following the inflation of the cuff. The range of an individual's tolerance is from 3.3 minutes to 56 minutes. We use 50 minutes as the safety ceiling.

The patients are told that the ischemia procedure has been widely used by physicians and that no permanent injury or damage will result from its application. We emphasize that the procedure is "perfectly safe and harmless." We also tell the patients that they may experience any or all of a number of sensations, including pressure, numbness, throbbing, discoloration of the arm and hand, some bluing around the fingernails, changes in temperature (either warmth or coolness), and feelings of discomfort and pain. The procedure is described in detail so that the patient understands what to expect and will not overreact to the uncertainty of the situation.

Following the removal of the cuff, patients are told to raise their nondominant arm over their heads in order to reduce the return of the blood flow to the arm, since rapid return can be discomforting. Usually, it is necessary for patients to use their dominant arm to support the arm that has received the muscle-ischemia procedure. Complete return of blood flow to the arm takes from 3 minutes to 5 minutes following removal of the blood-pressure cuff. When the cuff is being removed, patients are informed that at first the sensations they experience may be as intense as when the cuff was still inflated, but that those sensations will pass rapidly. This last instruction is provided because it has been noted that some patients may become upset when the discomfort is not immediately terminated following removal of the cuff.

The following references provide further details about the muscle-ischemia procedure: Smith *et al.* (1966) and Sternbach (1974a).

APPENDIX B

INFORMATION TO REFERRAL SOURCES

The Pain Management Program is interdisciplinary in nature, involving physicians, physical therapists, health psychologists, social workers, and vocational counselors. The program emphasizes the responsibility of the patient and his or her family in the treatment program. The patient will be asked to practice various skills and exercises at home. The treatment program is flexible, with an individual treatment plan tailored to the needs and desires of the patient and his or her family.

Typically, the program lasts 12 weeks, with weekly meetings in group, couple, family, or individual format. During the evaluation sessions, information is obtained regarding the nature of the patient's medical condition and its impact on all aspects of his or her life, as well as how it has affected the family. Information is obtained regarding occupational, recreational, social, marital, and physical spheres of the patient's and the family's lives as they have been influenced by the presence of the patient's pain. Spouses and significant others living with the patient attend the evaluation sessions. Treatment is based on the information obtained during these sessions and from questionnaires and other assessment procedures, as well as from consultations with physicians and physical therapists. In this collaborative manner, treatment goals are established for the patient.

Although the specific details of the treatment program are individualized, some common features include:

1. Graded exercises to increase muscle strength and tone. The number and nature of the exercises will be determined on the basis of the patient's current medical condition, age, and sex. Exercises will begin at a level *below* what the patient is capable of during the initial evaluation and will be increased gradually until an appropriate level is reached. Consultation with physicians and physical therapists will determine the nature of the exercise program.
2. Medication reduction. An evaluation of the patient's drug intake will be conducted with the patient's physician, and if it is determined that the intake should be reduced, then the patient will be encouraged to reduce

gradually the intake of drugs. Continuous use of analgesic medications often results in habituation to the analgesic effects and extended use can lead to deleterious side effects. That is, analgesics for acute pain of brief duration are often beneficial, but with chronic pain such drugs often prove less effective, if not harmful.

3. Relaxation training to help in removing muscle tension and emotional arousal that often accompany long-standing pain.
4. Enhancement of marital and family communications, since pain of long duration often interferes with effective and appropriate patterns of communication. Marital and/or family conflict can be stressful, resulting in increased tension and exacerbations of pain.
5. Stress-management training designed to help patients learn to deal more effectively with those aspects of their lives that may exacerbate pain.
6. Coping skills training that includes training in the utilization of specific techniques designed to help the patient cope with levels of discomfort that are particularly severe.
7. Particular homework tasks related to all of the preceding items.
8. Follow-up evaluations at 3 months, 6 months, and 12 months after termination of the Pain Management Program.

To be eligible for the Pain Management Program, patients should:

1. Have pain of 4 months' duration or longer.
2. Be capable of participating in some physical therapy program.
3. Have no additional medical or surgical procedures being planned.
4. Have no significant psychiatric problem (e.g., schizophrenia).

For further information about the program, contact _____.

PATIENT PAIN QUESTIONNAIRE[1]

For us to better understand the nature of your pain, the factors that are causing you to experience it, and what may be done to help you, please fill out this questionnaire as carefully as possible.

This will take some thought and time. It is most important, however, that you answer each item completely. You may be tempted to give only one-word answers, such as "yes" or "no." For the information to be of greatest value, it is essential that you answer each question in as much detail as possible.

We will have a chance to go over your answers together. Thank you for your cooperation.

Date: _____

Patient's full name: _____

Age: _____ Marital status: _____

Occupation: _____ Education: _____

Mailing address: _____ Phone: _____

Religion: _____ Nationality: _____

With whom are you currently living? (Indicate relationship; e.g., husband, wife, two children [ages], mother.) _____

Do you smoke? _____ How frequently? (pack(s)/day) _____

Do you drink alcoholic beverages? _____ How much? _____

How often? _____ When? _____

How long have you had the pain you are currently experiencing? _____

Are you currently taking medication? _____ What kind (the name, type, and amount—include aspirin, sedatives, sleeping pills, etc.)? _____

How often do you take them? _____

1. On the actual pain questionnaire, additional space is provided for patients' responses.

How long have you been taking medication? _____
Have you had any surgery in the past for problems other than your current pain?
_____ If yes, describe the problem(s) and the surgical procedure(s) if you
are aware of it (them).

Have you been involved in any accidents prior to the development of your current
pain? (Describe.)

Do you have any physical ailment other than your present problem? _____
(Describe.)

What treatments have you received for this (these) problem(s)? (Describe.)

Does the pain come and go, or is it constant? (Describe.)

Does the pain come on suddenly or over a span of days or weeks? (Describe.)

Does the pain impair or interfere with: appetite _____ sleeping _____
urination _____ sexual activity _____ working _____ doing
housework _____ bowel movement _____? If yes, describe.

Does the pain ever wake you up from sleep? _____ If so, how often?
_____ What do you do when awakened?

Does the pain ever become severe enough to make you cry? _____ If so,
how frequently? _____ Alone or in the presence of others?
(That is, who is present?)

Pain usually varies in intensity. When is it worst? (Describe.)

Describe when the pain is least severe.

Is there anything common about the situations when the pain is the *worst*?
(Explain.)

Is there anything common about the situations when the pain is the *least*?
(Explain.)

If the pain is due to an accident, is litigation or an insurance settlement pending? If
yes, describe current state of litigation or settlement.

Is your weight increasing, decreasing, or remaining steady? _____

How much (loss or gain)? _____

Describe any previous treatments you have undergone for your pain (medication, surgery, acupuncture, hypnosis, nerve block, etc.). List the physicians or practitioners who administered the treatment(s).

Have any of these treatments proved effective? _____ If yes, which one(s) and for how long was your pain relieved?

Has your latest pain caused you to miss any days at work or prevented you from conducting housework? _____ How frequently? _____

Have you ever experienced periods of pain in the past? _____ When?

How many times?

When did the pain first start?

How long did the period(s) last?

What led to the pain's stopping? (Describe.)

Was your pain during these past times similar to or different from your present pain?

How serious is your present pain problem as far as you are concerned?

How would you describe the pain you are currently experiencing? (Be specific. Provide as many details as possible.)

What is your understanding of the cause of the pain?

If you are aware of the nature or the cause of the pain, describe how you obtained this information (doctors, friends, books, etc.).

What do you think should be done to help you with your present pain (e.g., treatments you have heard of)?

Suppose that you did not have the pain; what would you do differently from what you are currently doing?

How would your life be different? (Describe.)

Are there any situations or objects of thought that make you particularly distressed? (Describe.)

Does your pain ever seem to make you angry, irritable, or hard to live with? (Describe.)

People agree that the following five words represent pain of increasing intensity[2]:

1	2	3	4	5
mild	discomforting	distressing	horrible	excruciating

To answer each question below, write the *number* of the most appropriate word in the space beside the question.

1. Which word describes your pain right now? _____
2. Which word describes it at its worst? _____
3. Which word describes it when it is least? _____

Some of the following words describe your present pain. Circle the words that best describe it. Leave out any word group that is not suitable. Use only a single word in each appropriate group—the one that applies *best*.

1	2	3	4
Flickering	Jumping	Pricking	Sharp
Quivering	Flashing	Boring	Cutting
Pulsing	Shooting	Drilling	Lacerating
Throbbing		Stabbing	
Beating		Lancinating	
Pounding			

5	6	7	8
Pinching	Tugging	Hot	Tingling
Pressing	Pulling	Burning	Itchy
Gnawing	Wrenching	Scalding	Smarting
Cramping		Searing	Stinging
Crushing		Scarring	

9	10	11	12
Dull	Tender	Tiring	Sickening
Sore	Taut	Exhausting	Suffocating
Hurting	Rasping		
Aching	Splitting		
Heavy			

2. These three questions and the list of adjectives that follows them are from Melzack, R. The McGill Pain Questionnaire: Major properties and scoring methods. *Pain*, 1975, *1*, 277–299. Copyright 1975, Elsevier Biomedical Press B.V. Reprinted by permission.

13	14	15	16
Fearful	Punishing	Wretched	Annoying
Frightful	Grueling	Blinding	Troublesome
Terrifying	Cruel		Miserable
	Vicious		Intense
	Killing		Unbearable

17	18	19	20
Spreading	Tight	Cool	Nagging
Radiating	Numb	Cold	Nauseating
Penetrating	Drawing	Freezing	Agonizing
Piercing	Squeezing		Dreadful
	Tearing		Torturing

Have any members of your family had problems with pain? (Describe.)

Has there been any recent disharmony/conflict between you and your spouse, your parents or your children? _____ If yes, please describe.

Have you discussed the pain with your family, friends, employees, employer? (With whom?)

What have you told them? (Describe.)

What were their reactions? (Describe.)

When you are experiencing pain, do you share this with others? (Explain.)

Can others tell when you are in pain? _____ How can they tell? (Explain.)

What do others do specifically when you tell them you are in pain or when they discover that you are in pain? Try to be as specific as possible.

What do you do to relieve or manage your pain (e.g., relax, think about something else, lie down)? (Describe the procedures you use in detail.)

Do they work? (Comment on the usefulness of each of the things you do to relieve or manage your pain.)

Have you been able to control, manage, or alleviate the pain in the past? (Explain techniques employed.)

What I am going to ask you to do now is something slightly different. To understand fully how pain affects you, think of a recent incident when pain was particularly bad. Close your eyes for a moment and picture that situation. Relive in your mind that incident. What I would like you to do is to tune into the thoughts, images, and feelings you had in this situation, in as much detail as possible. Please describe these thoughts and feelings in as much detail as possible. What were the feelings and thoughts you had when you first noticed the pain? (Please feel free to use the back of this sheet of paper.)

What were the feelings and thoughts that occurred to you as you tried to cope with the pain? (Be specific.)

Do you have such thoughts and feelings in other situations?

Do you recognize a common theme or link that runs through these thoughts? (Describe.)

Are these thoughts or images disturbing or upsetting to you? (Describe in detail.)

Are the thoughts and images helpful in managing and reducing your pain? (Describe in as much detail as possible.)

Finally, some patients have indicated that the kinds of feelings, thoughts, stressors, and conflicts they experience contribute to their pain. I am wondering in your case whether such factors are also present. Please describe. If such factors do apply in your case, what do you think might be done to change them?

How would you describe yourself? Provide as much detail as possible.

Additional comments:

Place an × on each line to indicate your present feeling or situation.
Example:
How hungry are you right now?
  Not at all ——————×————————————————— Extremely
  hungry   hungry
The placement of the × indicates a mild amount of hunger.

Please try to answer each of the following. Try to be as honest and accurate as you can in marking your answers. Be sure to read each item carefully, including the descriptions on the lines.

1. Rate the level of your pain at the present moment (right now).[3]
   No pain _____ The most intense
   pain I ever experi-
   enced
2. How severe has your pain been during the last week (on the average)?
   Not at all _____ Extremely
   severe severe
3. In general, how much does your pain problem interfere with your day-to-day
   activities?
   Pain doesn't _____ Pain extremely
   interfere at all interferes
4. How much suffering do you experience because of your pain?
   No suffering _____ Extreme amount
   at all of suffering
5. How much has your pain affected your ability to work?
   No change _____ Extreme change
   from before from before pain
   pain
   _____ Mark here if retired for reasons other than your pain problem.

GO BACK OVER YOUR ANSWERS AND MAKE SURE YOU HAVE COM-
PLETED EACH ONE. DO NOT LEAVE ANY BLANK.

6. How much has your pain affected your ability to participate in recreational
   and other social activities?
   No change _____ Extreme change
7. How much has your pain affected your marriage and other family relationships?
   No change _____ Extreme change
8. How much has your pain affected your ability to do household chores?
   No change _____ Extreme change
9. How much has your pain affected your friendships with people other than
   your family?
   No change _____ Extreme change
10. How much has your pain affected the amount of satisfaction or enjoyment
    you get from work?
    No change _____ Extreme change
    _____ Mark here if not currently working.

3. Clarification of the patient's responses are obtained during interviews.

11. How much has your pain affected the amount of satisfaction or enjoyment you get from participation in social and recreational activities?
No change _____ Extreme change

12. How much has your pain affected the amount of satisfaction you get from family-related activities?
No change _____ Extreme change

13. How satisfying is your job at the present time?
Not at all _____ Extremely
satisfying   satisfying

14. How satisfying is your relationship with your spouse (significant other)?
Not at all _____ Extremely
satisfying   satisfying

GO BACK OVER YOUR ANSWERS AND MAKE SURE YOU HAVE COMPLETED EACH ONE. DO NOT LEAVE ANY BLANK.

15. How supportive, helpful, or understanding do you feel that your fellow employees at work are toward you in relation to your pain problem?
Not at all _____ Extremely
supportive   supportive

16. How supportive or helpful is your spouse (significant other) to you in relation to your pain problem?
Not at all _____ Extremely
supportive   supportive

17. How supportive, helpful, or understanding are others in general toward you in relation to your pain?
Not at all _____ Extremely
supportive   supportive

18. How worried is your spouse (significant other) about you in relation to your pain problem?
Not at all _____ Extremely
worried   worried

19. How angry does your spouse (significant other) get with you in relation to your pain problem?
Not at all _____ Extremely
angry   angry

20. How frustrated does your spouse (significant other) become in relation to your pain problem?
Not at all _____ Extremely
frustrated   frustrated

21. How attentive is your spouse (significant other) to your pain problem?
Not at all   _____ Extremely
attentive   attentive

22. How dependent on others do you think your pain has made you?
Not at all   _____ Extremely
dependent   dependent

GO BACK OVER YOUR ANSWERS AND MAKE SURE YOU HAVE COMPLETED EACH ONE. DO NOT LEAVE ANY BLANK.

23. Rate your overall mood during the past week.
Extremely   _____ Extremely
low mood   high mood

24. During the past week, how satisfied have you felt with your life in general?
Not at all   _____ Extremely
satisfied   satisfied

25. During the past week, how much control do you feel that you've had over your life?
Not at all   _____ Extremely in
in control   control

26. During the past week, how much do you feel that you've been able to deal with your problems?
Not at all   _____ Extremely well

27. During the past week, how irritable have you been?
Not at all   _____ Extremely
irritable   irritable

28. During the past week, how tense or anxious have you been?
Not at all   _____ Extremely
tense or   tense and
anxious   anxious

GO BACK OVER YOUR ANSWERS AND MAKE SURE YOU HAVE COMPLETED EACH ONE. DO NOT LEAVE ANY BLANK.

When your spouse or significant other knows you're in pain (or experiencing heightened pain), how is he or she likely to respond? Mark how frequently he or she is likely to do each of the following:

    0 = Never
    1 = Almost never; rarely

2 = Occasionally
3 = Fairly often
4 = Almost always
5 = Always

_____ Asks me what he or she can do to help
_____ Ignores me
_____ Expresses sympathy
_____ Gives me a massage
_____ Acknowledges my pain, but leaves me alone
_____ Leaves the room
_____ Reads to me
_____ Takes over my jobs or duties
_____ Talks to me about something else to take my mind off the pain
_____ Tries to involve me in some activity
_____ Tries to get me to rest
_____ Expresses irritation at me
_____ Gets me some pain medication
_____ Gets me an alcoholic beverage
_____ Gets me something to eat or drink
_____ Tries to comfort me by listening to my complaints
_____ Expresses frustration at me
_____ Tells me not to exert myself
_____ Expresses anger at me
_____ Encourages me to work on a hobby
_____ Turns on the TV to take my mind off my pain
_____ Other (specify) _____
_____   _____

GO BACK OVER YOUR ANSWERS AND MAKE SURE YOU HAVE COM-
PLETED EACH ONE. DO NOT LEAVE ANY BLANK.

Think of the last time you experienced a moderate level of pain—for example, a
3 or 4 on a 6-point scale of pain intensity, where 0 equals no pain and 5 is excruciating pain. What did you try to do to help relieve or cope with the pain? Try to be
as specific as possible. List as many or as few things that come to mind.

In addition to what you have listed, what else do you typically do when your pain
increases in intensity (becomes more severe)?

GO BACK OVER YOUR ANSWERS AND MAKE SURE YOU HAVE COM-
PLETED EACH ONE. DO NOT LEAVE ANY BLANK.

Behavior checklist
Indicate how often you do each of the following:

0 = Never
1 = Almost never; rarely
2 = Occasionally
3 = Fairly often
4 = Almost always
5 = Always
NA = Not applicable

_____ Take out the trash
_____ Wash dishes
_____ Mow the lawn
_____ Work in the garden
_____ Take a short walk
_____ Go grocery shopping
_____ Visit friends
_____ Visit relatives
_____ Go out to eat
_____ Go to a movie
_____ Play cards or other games
_____ Do some physical exercises
_____ Take a ride in a car
_____ Take a trip
_____ Go swimming or play some active sport
_____ Play with children or grandchildren

_____ Work on the car
_____ Wash the car
_____ Go bowling
_____ Go to a sporting event
_____ Go to church
_____ Help with the housecleaning
_____ Prepare a meal
_____ Work on a hobby
_____ Read a book
_____ Work on a needed house repair
_____ Go to a park or beach
_____ Do a load of laundry
_____ Talk to a friend on the phone
_____ Write letters
_____ Other (specify) _____
_____

GO BACK OVER YOUR ANSWERS AND MAKE SURE YOU HAVE COM-
PLETED EACH ONE. DO NOT LEAVE ANY BLANK.

Thank you for completing this rather lengthy questionnaire. Your answers will be most useful in helping us understand your pain. Is there anything else that I should know about you that would be helpful in formulating a treatment plan?

SIGNIFICANT OTHERS
PAIN QUESTIONNAIRE

Place an × on each line to indicate your present feeling or situation.
Example:
How nervous are you about being here for this interview?

Not at all   ————————×————————————   Extremely
nervous   nervous

The placement of the × indicates a mild degree of nervousness.

Please try to answer each of the following. Try to be as honest and accurate as you can in marking your answers. Be sure to read each item carefully, including the descriptions on the lines.

1. How severe was your spouse's pain during the past week?[1]

   Not at all   ————————————————————   Extremely
   severe   severe

2. In general, how much does your spouse's pain interfere with his or her day-to-day activities?

   Pain doesn't ———————————————————— Pain extremely
   interfere at all   interferes

3. How much physical suffering does your spouse experience because of pain?

   No suffering ———————————————————— Extreme amount
   at all   of suffering

4. How much has your spouse's pain affected his or her ability to work?

   Not at all   ———————————————————— Extremely
   affected   affected

GO BACK OVER YOUR ANSWERS AND MAKE SURE YOU HAVE COMPLETED EACH ONE. DO NOT LEAVE ANY BLANK.

5. How much has your spouse's pain affected his or her ability to participate in recreational activities?

   No change   ———————————————————— Extreme reduction

---

1. Detailed explanations of these ratings are obtained during interviews with significant others.

6. How much has your spouse's pain affected his or her ability to do household chores?

No change _____ Extreme reduction

7. How much has your spouse's pain affected his or her friendships with people other than your family?

No change _____ Extreme reduction

8. How much has your spouse's pain affected the amount of satisfaction or enjoyment he or she gets from work?

No change _____ Extreme reduction

_____ Mark here if spouse is retired for reasons other than his or her pain problem.

9. How much has your spouse's pain affected the amount of satisfaction or enjoyment he or she gets from participation in social and recreational activities?

No change _____ Extreme reduction

10. How much has your spouse's pain affected the amount of satisfaction he or she gets from family-related activities?

No change _____ Extreme reduction

11. How much has your spouse's pain affected your ability to work?

Not at all affected _____ Extremely reduced

_____ Mark here if you are retired.

GO BACK OVER YOUR ANSWERS AND MAKE SURE YOU HAVE COMPLETED EACH ONE. DO NOT LEAVE ANY BLANK.

12. How much has your spouse's pain affected your ability to participate in recreational and other social activities?

No change _____ Extreme reduction

13. How much has your spouse's pain affected your marriage and other family relationships?

No change _____ Extremely worse

14. How much has your spouse's pain affected the amount of household chores you do?

No change _____ Extreme increase

15. How much has your spouse's pain affected your friendships with people other than your family?

No change _____ Extreme reduction

16. How much has your spouse's pain affected the amount of satisfaction or enjoyment you get from work?

No change _____ Extreme reduction

_____ Mark here if you are not currently working for reasons other than your spouse's pain problem.

17. How much has your spouse's pain affected the amount of satisfaction or enjoyment you get from participation in social and recreational activities?

    No change _____ Extreme reduction

18. How much has your spouse's pain affected the amount of satisfaction you get from family-related activities?

    No change _____ Extreme reduction

19. How satisfying is your relationship with your spouse?

    Not at all _____ Extremely
    satisfying   satisfying

20. How worried are you about your spouse's pain problem?

    Not at all _____ Extremely
    worried   worried

GO BACK OVER YOUR ANSWERS AND MAKE SURE YOU HAVE COMPLETED EACH ONE. DO NOT LEAVE ANY BLANK.

21. How angry do you get with your spouse about his or her pain problem?

    Not at all _____ Extremely angry
    angry

22. How frustrated do you get with your spouse about his or her pain problem?

    Not at all _____ Extremely
    frustrated   frustrated

23. How attentive are you to your spouse's pain problem?

    Not at all _____ Extremely
    attentive   attentive

24. How dependent on you is your spouse because of his or her pain problem?

    Not at all _____ Extremely
    dependent   dependent

25. Rate your overall mood during the past week.

    Extremely _____ Extremely
    low mood   high mood

26. During the past week, how satisfied have you felt with your life in general?

    Not at all _____ Extremely
    satisfied   satisfied

27. During the past week, how much control do you feel that you've had over your life?

    Not at all _____ Extremely in
    in control   control

28. During the past week, how much do you feel that you've been able to deal with your problems?

    Not at all _____ Extremely well

29. During the past week, how irritable have you been?

Not at all _____ Extremely
irritable   irritable

GO BACK OVER YOUR ANSWERS AND MAKE SURE YOU HAVE COM-
PLETED EACH ONE. DO NOT LEAVE ANY BLANK.

30. During the past week, how tense or anxious have you been?

Not at all _____ Extremely tense
tense or   and anxious
anxious

When you know your spouse or significant other is in pain (or experiencing
heightened pain), how are you likely to respond? Mark how frequently you are
likely to do each of the following:

  0 = Never
  1 = Almost never; rarely
  2 = Occasionally
  3 = Fairly often
  4 = Almost always
  5 = Always

_____ Ask what I can do to help

_____ Ignore him or her

_____ Express sympathy

_____ Give him or her a massage

_____ Acknowledge the pain, but leave him or her alone

_____ Leave the room

_____ Read to him or her

_____ Take over his or her job or duties

_____ Talk to him or her about something else to take his or her mind off
                              the pain

_____ Try to involve him or her in some activity

_____ Express irritation at him or her

_____ Get him or her some pain medication

_____ Get him or her an alcoholic beverage

_____ Get him or her something to eat or drink

_____ Try to comfort him or her by listening to his or her complaints

_____ Express my frustration at him or her

_____ Tell him or her not exert himself or herself

_____ Express anger at him or her

_____ Encourage him or her to work on a hobby

_____ Turn on the TV to take his or her mind off the pain

_____ Other (specify) _____

_____   _____

GO BACK OVER YOUR ANSWERS AND MAKE SURE YOU HAVE COM-
PLETED EACH ONE. DO NOT LEAVE ANY BLANK.

Think of the last time your spouse experienced a moderate level of pain—for
example, a 3 or 4 on a 6-point scale of pain intensity, where 0 equals no pain and 5
is excruciating pain. What, if anything, did you try to do to help him or her relieve
or cope with the pain? Try to be as specific as possible. List as many or as few
things that come to mind.

APPENDIX E

VOLUNTARY CONTROL OF APPRAISAL

The therapist may discuss the role of self-statements with patients or may provide this information in the form of bibliotherapy. For example, the therapist may convey the following (in terms appropriate for the patient):

We have seen how the ways you view your pain may have a very marked effect on how you feel. Let us explore how we can use such appraisal processes to control pain and how we can bring them under our own immediate control. Consider how our thoughts may affect us. If, for example, you fail to get something you very much wanted, your first reaction may be disappointment. You may bemoan your misfortune and become upset and perhaps even depressed. Notice that in this instance you may view your disappointment as something important, perhaps as a sign that you can't succeed or just aren't measuring up to the standards you set for yourself. Such *thoughts* contribute to the bad *feelings* you have, and such *feelings* increase the likelihood you will have further negative *thoughts*. In short, a cycle is set up.

Although this pattern may seem familiar to you, so might a different reaction. On occasion you may have started out with the disappointment and the unhappy appraisal, but then realized that you were just getting more and more upset by such thoughts about your disappointment. It is as if the unpleasant thoughts themselves serve a useful function: They call your attention to the cycle of depressing thoughts, leading to feeling lousy, leading to more dwelling on unpleasantness, leading to more depression or anxiety, and so on.

To stop this cycle of negative thoughts and feelings, it is necessary to become aware of them and then to interrupt them and begin to produce different, incompatible coping thoughts, feelings, and behaviors. As we will see, it will be easier and more effective to interrupt such dysfunctional thoughts and feelings early on, in the bud, as one might say, before they get out of hand. Becoming aware of the early signs of such negative thoughts and feelings will help us learn how to control how we feel as well as the amount of pain we experience.

One way that you may occasionally have tried to stop such negative thoughts is by *changing your thoughts* concerning an event. You might begin telling yourself you just didn't try hard enough and that you will work harder next time, or that for one reason or another you don't really care that much about it. You won't always be successful in this attempt at self-convincing, but often you will at least interrupt the negative cycle and begin to change your interpretation of the event, thereby lessening the unpleasant feelings.

It is possible to *intentionally* change our interpretation of physical sensation sufficiently to reduce or increase our experience of that sensation. We do it all the time, although we are not usually aware of it. Whenever we experience some unpleasant sensation—whether pain or sorrow or disappointment—we often attempt to change our own feelings about it, to lessen its impact. "It's not the end of the world," "Could have been worse," "I suppose it doesn't really matter in the end"—these are some of the most commonly used catch phrases offered. The point is that you can affect your own feelings in a fairly direct, intentional fashion. *You are influencing your thoughts by* an ongoing series of *statements to yourself*, in which you tell yourself what to think and to believe, and even how to act.

We can use such "self-statements" when we are experiencing pain. We can think, for example, "Just relax and keep calm—it will be over soon" (trying to produce the relaxation that we practiced) or "Don't think about it. Think about something else that's pleasant" (using an imagery technique).

It is useful, then, to employ *direct self-statements* to help yourself deal with a painful experience. Such self-statements can alter your thoughts and feelings about the sensations and can thereby *reduce their painfulness*. Moreover, these self-statements act as plans for handling future problems, as when you go over or "practice" in your mind a future event, thinking about how you would react to different events. Just as positive thoughts can influence your feelings in positive ways, so can negative thoughts act negatively: "This is awful. My pain is without control, has no end, no end. I won't be able to take this for long"; or "Oh. It really hurts. Nothing can ever be done. Oh, I wish I weren't alive." Such negative-toned self-statements often are self-fulfilling. When you are telling yourself that something is awful, you are making your experience more and more unpleasant. Whether or not it is awful, you can make the experience better by intentionally changing what you say to yourself.

Unfortunately, the negative things are often as automatic as the positive ones that we discussed earlier. Therefore you have to (1) be alert to the negative thoughts, especially as they begin; (2) use them as signals that it is time to change thoughts; and (3) deliberately "say to yourself" helpful things and use other coping strategies.

You may find that speaking about your thoughts as "self-statements" is somewhat strange. But there is a good reason for using the phrase. Calling a thought a "statement to yourself" emphasizes the deliberateness of that particular thought that it is under your control. Making these deliberate statements to yourself may also seem unusual to you at first. You might think that all that you need to do is to decide to change your train of thoughts. But when you recognize that it *is* time to change your thoughts, it is important that you *actually say to yourself* some *words* to direct that change.

It may, at first, seem like an unusual thing to do, although many people report using this device. Don't be discouraged from using the method just because it seems unfamiliar at first. On the other hand, you may already use some method similar to this, as many people do. For example, the conscious saying to yourself, either silently or aloud, "Just relax; relax; breathe deeply . . . and slowly" or any other of the phrases from the relaxation exercises will help you to concentrate on relaxing and to partly exclude other sensations.

Patients are reminded that the task is to find the most personally useful strategies and that each procedure is only one of several alternatives. In this way, the therapist tries to have the patients appreciate the direct manner by which they can control their appraisal processes and, in turn, their pain.

REFERENCES

Abelson, P. Cost-effective health care: Editorial. *Science*, 1976, *192*, 862.

Abrams, D. B., & Wilson, G. T. Effects of alcohol on social anxiety in women: Cognitive versus physiological processes. *Journal of Abnormal Psychology*, 1979, *88*, 161–173. (a)

Abrams, D. B., & Wilson, G. T. Self-monitoring and reactivity in the modification of ciagarette smoking. *Journal of Consulting and Clinical Psychology*, 1979, *47*, 243–251. (b)

Acharya, A., Michaelson, M. H., & Erickson, D. L. *Use of a problem-solving approach in the treatment of chronic pain.* Paper presented at the Second World Congress on Pain, Montreal, Canada, August 1978.

Ad Hoc Committee on the Classification of Headache, National Institute of Neurological Diseases and Blindness. Classification of headache. *Journal of the American Medical Association*, 1962, *179*, 717–718.

Agnew, D. C., & Merskey, H. Words of chronic pain. *Pain*, 1976, *2*, 73–81.

Ainslie, G. Specious reward: A behavioral theory of impulsiveness and impulse control. *Psychological Bulletin*, 1975, *82*, 463–496.

Aitken-Swan, J. Nursing the later cancer patient at home. The family's impression. *Practitioner*, 1959, *183*, 64–69.

Alioto, J. D., & Cox, B. G. *A didactic–experiential approach to stress management for the relief of pain of psychophysiological etiology.* Paper presented at the Second World Congress on Pain, Montreal, Canada, August 1978.

Almay, B. G. L., Johansson, F., von Knorring, L., Terenius, L., & Wahlstrom, A. Endorphins in chronic pain: I. Differences in CSF endorphin levels between organic and psychogenic pain syndromes. *Pain*, 1978, *5*, 153–162.

American Cancer Society. *Cancer facts and figures.* New York: Author, 1978.

American Pain Society. *Minutes of the new board of directors of the American Pain Society.* Nutley, N.J.: Author, September 1980.

Amkraut, A., & Solomon, G. F. From the symbolic stimulus to the pathophysiologic response: Immune mechanisms. *International Journal of Psychiatry in Medicine*, 1975, *5*, 541–563.

Anderson, J. A. D., Basker, M. A., & Dalton, R. Migraine and hypnotherapy. *International Journal of Clinical and Experimental Hypnosis*, 1975, *23*, 48–58.

Anderson, N. B., Lawrence, P. S., Olson, T. W., & Dick, M. C. *Reactive effects of self-monitoring on muscle-contraction headache pain.* Paper presented at the annual meeting of the Association for Advancement of Behavior Therapy, New York, 1980.

Anderson, T. P., Cole, T. M., Gullickson, G., Hudgens, A., & Roberts, A. H. Behavior

379

modification of chronic pain: A treatment program by a multidisciplinary team. *Journal of Clinical Orthopedics*, 1977, *129*, 96–100.

Andrasik, F., & Holroyd, K. A. A test of specific and nonspecific effects in the biofeedback treatment of tension headache. *Journal of Consulting and Clinical Psychology*, 1980, *48*, 575–586.

Andrew, J. M. Recovery from surgery, with and without preparatory instruction, for three coping styles. *Journal of Personality and Social Psychology*, 1970, *15*, 223–226.

Andreychuk, T., & Skriver, C. Hypnosis and biofeedback in the treatment of migraine headache. *International Journal of Experimental and Clinical Hypnosis*, 1975, *23*, 172–183.

Antonovsky, A. Conceptual and methodological problems in the study of resistance resources and stressful life events. In B. S. Dohrenwend & B. P. Dohrenwend (Eds.), *Stressful life events: Their nature and effects*. New York: Wiley, 1974.

Apgar, V. A. A proposal for a new method of evaluation of the new born infant. *Anesthesia and Analgesia Current Research*, 1953, *32*, 260–267.

Armentrout, D. P. *A holistic approach to treating chronic pain*. Paper presented at the Second World Congress on Pain, Montreal, Canada, August 1978.

Armor, D. J., Polich, J. M., & Stambul, H. B. *Alcoholism and treatment* (R-1739-NIAAA). Santa Monica: The Rand Corporation, 1976.

Arthritis Foundation. *Arthritis, the basic facts*. Atlanta: Author, 1976.

Auerbach, S. M., & Kilmann, P. R. Crisis intervention: A review of outcome research. *Psychological Bulletin*, 1977, *84*, 1189–1217.

Averill, J. R. Personal control over aversive stimuli and its relationship to stress. *Psychological Bulletin*, 1973, *80*, 286–303.

Avia, M. D., & Kanfer, F. H. Coping with aversive stimulation: The effects of training in a self-management context. *Cognitive Therapy and Research*, 1980, *4*, 73–81.

Axelrod, S., Hall, R. V., Weis, L., & Rohrer, S. Use of self-imposed contingencies to reduce the frequency of smoking behavior. In M. J. Mahoney & C. E. Thoresen (Eds.), *Self-control: Power to the person*. Monterey, Calif.: Brooks/Cole, 1974.

Ayalon, O. Coping with terrorism: The Israeli case. In D. H. Meichenbaum & M. E. Jaremko (Eds.), *Stress prevention and management: A cognitive–behavioral approach*. New York: Plenum, 1982.

Baekeland, F., & Lundwall, L. Dropping out of treatment: A critical review. *Psychological Bulletin*, 1975, *82*, 738–783.

Bahnson, C. B. (Ed.). Second conference on the psychophysiological aspects of cancer. *Annals of the New York Academy of Sciences*, 1969, *164*, 307–634.

Bailey, C. A., & Davidson, P. O. The language of pain intensity. *Pain*, 1976, *2*, 319–324.

Bakal, D. A. Headache: A biophysical perspective. *Psychological Bulletin*, 1975, *82*, 369–382.

Bakal, D. A. *Psychology and medicine: Psychobiological dimensions of health and illness*. New York: Springer, 1979.

Bakal, D. A., Demjen, S., & Kaganov, J. A. Cognitive behavioral treatment of chronic headache. *Headache*, 1981, *21*, 81–86.

Bakal, D. A., & Kaganov, J. A. A simple method for self-observation of headache frequency, intensity and location. *Headache*, 1976, *16*, 123–128.

Bakal, D. A., & Kaganov, J. A. Muscle contraction and migraine headache: Psychophysiologic comparison. *Headache*, 1977, *17*, 208–215.

Bandler, R. J., Jr., Madaras, G. R., & Bem, D. J. Self-observation as a source of pain perception. *Journal of Personality and Social Psychology*, 1969, *9*, 205–209.

Bandura, A. Self-efficacy: Toward a unifying theory of behavioral change. *Psychological Review*, 1977, *84*, 191–215.

Bandura, A. The self system in reciprocal determinism. *American Psychologist*, 1978, *33*, 344–359.

Bandura, A. The self and mechanisms of agency. In J. Suls (Ed.), *Social psychological perspectives on the self*. Hillsdale, N.J.: Erlbaum, 1980.

Baranowski, T. *Cognitive–emotional social learning theory aspects of patient compliance*. Paper presented at the annual meeting of the American Psychological Association, New York, September 1979.

Barber, T. X. *Hypnosis: A scientific approach*. New York: Van Nostrand Reinhold, 1969.

Barber, T. X. *Cognitive strategies and cognitive style: Some behavioral implications*. Paper presented at the annual meeting of the American Psychological Association, San Francisco, August 1977.

Barber, T. X. Hypnosuggestive procedures in the treatment of clinical pain: Implications for theories of hypnosis and suggestive therapy. In T. Millon, C. J. Green, & R. B. Meagher, Jr. (Eds.), *Handbook of health care clinical psychology*. New York: Plenum, 1982.

Barber, T. X., & Calverly, D. S. *Effects of hypnotic induction, suggestions of anesthesia, and distraction on subjective and physiological responses to pain*. Paper presented at the annual meeting of the Eastern Psychological Association, Philadelphia, April 1969.

Barber, T. X., & Cooper, B. J. Effects on pain of experimentally induced and spontaneous distraction. *Psychological Reports*, 1972, *31*, 647–651.

Barber, T. X., & Hahn, K. W. Physiological and subjective responses to pain producing stimulation under hypnotically-suggested and waking-imagined "analgesia." *Journal of Abnormal and Social Psychology*, 1962, *65*, 411–418.

Barnes, G. E. Extraversion and pain. *British Journal of Clinical Psychology*, 1975, *14*, 303–308.

Barofsky, I. Sociological and psychological aspects of medication compliance. In I. Barofsky (Ed.), *Medication compliance: A behavioral management approach*. Thorofare, N.J.: Charles B. Slack, 1977.

Basker, M. Hypnosis in migraine. *British Journal of Clinical Hypnosis*, 1970, *2*, 15–18.

Beaser, S. B. Teaching the diabetic patient. *Diabetes*, 1956, *5*, 145–149.

Beck, A. T. *Cognitive therapy and the emotional disorders*. New York: International Universities Press, 1976.

Beck, A. T., & Greenberg, R. L. *Coping with depression* (pamphlet). New York: Institute for Rational Living, 1974.

Beck, A. T., Rush, A. J., Shaw, B. F., & Emery, G. *Cognitive therapy of depression*. New York: Guilford, 1979.

Beck, N. C., Geden, E. A., & Brouder, G. T. Preparation for labor: A historical perspective. *Psychosomatic Medicine*, 1979, *41*, 243–258.

Beck, N. C., & Hall, D. Natural childbirth: A review and analysis. *Obstetrics and Gynecology*, 1978, *52*, 371–379.

Beck, N. C., & Siegel, L. J. Preparation for childbirth and contemporary research on pain, anxiety, and stress reduction: A review and critique. *Psychosomatic Medicine*, 1980, *42*, 429–447.

Beck, N. C., Siegel, L. J., Geden, E. A., & Brouder, G. T. Labor preparation and behavioral medicine. *International Journal of Mental Health*, 1980, *9*, 149–163.

Beecher, H. K. Pain in men wounded in battle. *Annals of Surgery*, 1946, *123*, 96–105.

Beecher, H. K. Pain and some factors that modify it. *Anesthesiology*, 1951, *12*, 633–641.

Beecher, H. K. The powerful placebo. *Journal of the American Medical Association*, 1955, *159*, 1602.

Beecher, H. K. *Measurement of subjective responses: Quantitative effects of drugs.* New York: Oxford University Press, 1959.

Beecher, H. K. Surgery as placebo: Quantitative study of bias. *Journal of the American Medical Association,* 1961, *176,* 1102–1107.

Beecher, H. K. Pain: One mystery solved. *Science,* 1966, *151,* 840–841.

Beers, T. M., & Karoly, P. *Cognitive strategies, expectancy, and coping style in control of pain.* Paper presented at the 11th annual convention of the Association for Advancement of Behavior Therapy, Atlanta, December 1977.

Bellack, A. S., & Hersen, M. Self-report inventories in behavioral assessment. In J. D. Cone & R. P. Hawkins (Eds.), *Behavioral assessment: New directions in clinical psychology.* New York: Brunner/Mazel, 1977.

Benedetti, C. Neuroanatomy and biochemistry of antinociception. In J. J. Bonica & V. Ventafridda (Eds.), *Advances in pain research and therapy* (Vol. 2). New York: Raven, 1979.

Benson, H. *The relaxation response.* New York: Avon Books (paperback edition), 1976.

Benson, H., Greenwood, M. M., & Klemchuk, H. The relaxation response: Psychophysiologic aspects and clinical applications. *International Journal of Psychiatry in Medicine,* 1975, *6,* 87–97.

Berenson, B., & Carkhuff, R. *Sources of gain in counseling and psychotherapy.* New York: Holt, Rinehart & Winston, 1967.

Bergstrom-Whalan, M. Efficacy of education for childbirth. *Journal of Psychosomatic Research,* 1963, *7,* 131–146.

Berlyne, D. E. Attention, perception, and behavior theory. *Psychological Review,* 1951, *58,* 137.

Berne, E. *Games people play.* New York: Grove, 1964.

Bernstein, D. A., & McAlister, A. The modification of smoking behavior: Progress and problems. *Addictive Behaviors,* 1976, *1,* 89–102.

Best, J. A. Mass media, self-management, and smoking modification. In P. O. Davidson & S. M. Davidson (Eds.), *Behavioral medicine: Changing health life styles.* New York: Brunner/Mazel, 1980.

Best, J.A., Bass, F., & Owen, L. E. Mode of service delivery in a smoking cessation programme for public health. *Canadian Journal of Public Health,* 1977, *68,* 469–473.

Best, J. A., & Block, M. Compliance in the control of cigarette smoking. In R. B. Haynes & D. L. Sackett (Eds.), *Compliance with therapeutic and preventive regimens.* Baltimore: The Johns Hopkins University Press, 1979.

Best, J. A., Owen, L. E., & Trentadue, L. Comparison of satiation and rapid smoking. *Addictive Behaviors,* 1978, *3,* 71–78.

Best, J. A., & Steffy, R. A. Smoking modification procedures tailored to subject characteristics. *Behavior Therapy,* 1971, *2,* 177–191.

Bieber, I. The concept of irrational belief systems as primary elements of psychopathology. *Journal of the American Academy of Psychoanalysis,* 1974, *2,* 91–100.

Bieber, I., & Drellich, M. G. Psychological adaptation to serious illness and organ ablation. In H. I. Lief, V. F. Lief, & N. R. Lief (Eds.), *The psychological basis of medical practice.* New York: Hoeber, 1963.

Bing, E. *Six practical lessons for an easier childbirth.* New York: Grosset & Dunlap, 1967.

Black, P. Management of cancer pain: An overview. *Neurosurgery,* 1979, *5,* 507–518.

Black, R. G. Management of pain with nerve blocks. *Minnesota Medicine,* 1974, *57,* 189–194.

Blackwell, B. Treatment adherence. *British Journal of Psychiatry,* 1976, *129,* 512–539.

Blakenship, G. W., & Skyler, J. S. Diabetic retinopathy: A general survey. *Diabetes Care*, 1978, *2*, 127–137.

Blanchard, E. B., Andrasik, F., Ahles, T. A., Teders, S. J., & O'Keefe, D. Migraine and tension headache: A meta-analytic review. *Behavior Therapy*, 1980, *11*, 613–631.

Blank, J. *Nurses' and patients' perceptions of the needs of the advanced cancer patient.* Unpublished manuscript, Yale University School of Nursing, New Haven, Conn., 1979.

Blittner, M., Goldberg, J., & Merbaum, M. Cognitive self-control factors in the reduction of smoking behavior. *Behavior Therapy*, 1978, *9*, 553–561.

Blitz, B., & Dinnerstein, A. J. Effects of different types of instructions on pain parameters. *Journal of Abnormal Psychology*, 1968, *73*, 276–280.

Blitz, B., & Dinnerstein, A. J. Role of attentional focus in pain perception: Manipulation of response to noxious stimulation by instructors. *Journal of Abnormal Psychology*, 1971, *77*, 42–45.

Block, A. R., Kremer, E., & Gaylor, M. Behavioral treatment of chronic pain: Variables affecting treatment efficacy. *Pain*, 1980, *8*, 367–375.

Bloom, J. R. *Psychological aspects of breast cancer* (Annual Report, HEW Contract NO 1-CN-55313). Menlo Park Calif.: Stanford Research Institute, 1977.

Bloom Cerkoney, K. A., & Hart, L. K. The relationship between the health belief model and compliance of persons with diabetes mellitus. *Diabetes Care*, 1980, *3*, 594–598.

Bobey, M. J., & Davidson, P. O. Psychological factors affecting pain tolerance. *Journal of Psychosomatic Research*, 1970, *14*, 371–376.

Bond, M. R. The relation of pain to the Eysenck Personality Inventory, Cornell Medical Index and Witley Index of Hypochondriasis. *British Journal of Psychiatry*, 1971, *119*, 671–678.

Bonica, J. J. *The management of pain.* New York: Lea & Febiger, 1953.

Bonica, J. J. Organization and function of a pain clinic. In J. J. Bonica (Ed.), *Advances in neurology* (Vol. 4). New York: Raven, 1974. (a)

Bonica, J. J. Preface. In J. J. Bonica (Ed.), *Advances in neurology* (Vol. 4). New York: Raven, 1974. (b)

Bonica, J. J. Importance of the problem. In J. J. Bonica & V. Ventafridda (Eds.), *Advances in pain research and therapy* (Vol. 2). New York: Raven, 1979.

Bowen, W. F., & Turk, D. C. *Cognitive–behavioral treatment of three medical conditions.* Paper presented at the annual convention of the Association for Advancement of Behavior Therapy, San Francisco, December 1979.

Bowers, K. S. Pain, anxiety, and perceived control. *Journal of Consulting and Clinical Psychology*, 1968, *32*, 596–602.

Bowers, K. S. Hypnosis: An informational approach. *Annals of the New York Academy of Sciences*, 1977, *296*, 222–237.

Bowers, K. S., & Kelly, P. Stress, disease, psychotherapy, and hypnosis. *Journal of Abnormal Psychology*, 1979, *88*, 490–505.

Bradley, L. A., Prieto, E. J., Hopson, L., & Prokop, C. K. Comment on "Personality organization as an aspect of back pain in a medical setting." *Journal of Personality Assessment*, 1978, *42*, 573–578.

Bradley, L. A., & Prokop, C. K. Research methods in medical psychology. In P. C. Kendall & J. N. Butcher (Eds.), *Handbook of research methods in clinical psychology.* New York: Wiley, 1981.

Bradley, L. A., Prokop, C. K., Gentry, W. D., Hopson, L. A., & Prieto, E. J. Assessment of chronic pain. In C. K. Prokop, & L. A. Bradley (Eds.), *Medical psychology: Contributions to behavioral medicine.* New York: Academic Press, 1981.

Bradley, L. A., Prokop, C. K., Margolis, R., & Gentry, W. D. Multivariate analyses of the MMPI profiles of low back pain patients. *Journal of Behavioral Medicine*, 1978, *1*, 253–272.

Brehm, J. W. *A theory of psychological reactance.* New York: Academic Press, 1966.

Brena, S. F., & Unikel, I. P. Nerve blocks and contingency management in chronic pain states. In J. J. Bonica & D. Albe-Fessard (Eds.), *Advances in pain research and therapy* (Vol. 1). New York: Raven, 1976.

Brengelmann, J. C., & Sedlmayr, E. Experiments in the reduction of smoking behavior. In J. Steinfeld, W. Griffiths, K. Ball, & R. M. Taylor (Eds.), *Smoking and health* (Vol. II: *Health consequences, education, cessation activities, and government action).* Washington, D.C.: U.S. Department of Health, Education & Welfare, 1977.

Bresler, D. E. *Self-control of pain; The use of relaxation and guided imagery in a self-help pain control program.* Paper presented at the Second World Congress on Pain, Montreal, Canada, August 1978.

Bresler, D. E. *Free yourself from pain.* New York: Simon & Schuster, 1979.

Brewer, W. There is no convincing evidence for operant or classical conditioning in adult humans. In W. Weimer & D. Palermo (Eds.), *Cognition and the symbolic processes.* New York: Halstead, 1974.

Breznitz, S. A study of worrying. *British Journal of Social and Clinical Psychology*, 1971, *10*, 271–279.

Brief, A. P., Alday, R. J., Sell, M. V., & Melone, M. Anticipatory socialization and role stress among registered nurses. *Journal of Health and Social Behavior*, 1979, *20*, 161–165.

Brightwell, D. R., & Sloan, C. L. Long-term results of behavior therapy for obesity. *Behavior Therapy*, 1977, *8*, 898–905.

Brooks, G. R., & Richardson, F. C. Emotional skills training: A treatment program for duodenal ulcer. *Behavior Therapy*, 1980, *11*, 198–207.

Brown, J. M. *Cognitive activity, pain perception and hypnotic susceptibility.* Paper presented at the annual meeting of the American Psychological Association, New York, September 1979.

Brown, R. A., Fader, K., & Barber, T. X. Responsiveness to pain: Stimulus-specificity versus generality. *Psychological Record*, 1973, *23*, 1–7.

Brownell, K., & Stunkard, A. *Spouse intervention and drug treatment for obesity.* Paper presented at the annual meeting of the American Psychological Association, New York, September 1979.

Budzynski, T. H., Stoyva, J. M., Adler, C. S., & Mullaney, D. J. EMG biofeedback and tension headache: A controlled outcome study. *Seminars in Psychiatry*, 1973, *5*, 397–410.

Bulpitt, C. J., & Dollery, C. T. Side effects of hypotensive agents evaluated by a self-administered questionnaire. *British Medical Journal*, 1973, *3*, 485–490.

Butler, B. The use of hypnosis in the care of the cancer patient. *Cancer*, 1954, *7*, 1–14.

Byron, R., & Yonemoto, R. Pain associated with malignancy. In B. Crue, Jr. (Ed.), *Pain research and treatment.* New York: Academic Press, 1975.

Cahalan, D., Cisin, I. H., & Crossley, H. *American drinking practices.* New Brunswick, N.J.: Rutgers Center of Alcohol Studies, 1974.

Cahalan, D., & Room, R. *Problem drinking among American men.* New Brunswick, N.J.: Rutgers Center of Alcohol Studies, 1974.

Cairns, D., & Pasino, J. Comparison of verbal reinforcement and feedback in the operant treatment of disability due to chronic low back pain. *Behavior Therapy*, 1977, *8*, 621–630.

Cairns, D., Thomas, L., Mooney, V., & Pace, J. B. A comprehensive treatment approach to chronic low back pain. *Pain*, 1976, *2*, 301–308.

Calsyn, D. A., Louks, J., & Freeman, C. W. The use of the MMPI with chronic low back pain patients with a mixed diagnosis. *Journal of Clinical Psychology*, 1976, *32*, 532–536.

Cameron, R. The clinical implementation of behavior change techniques: A cognitively oriented conceptualization of therapeutic "compliance" and "resistance." In J. P. Foreyt & D. P. Rathjen (Eds.), *Cognitive behavior therapy: Research and application*. New York: Plenum, 1978.

Cameron, R. Behavioral treatments for clinical pain. In R. Roy & E. Tunks (Eds.), *Chronic pain: Psychosocial factors in rehabilitation*. Baltimore: William & Wilkins, 1980.

Cameron, R., & Shepel, L. *A cognitive view of the pain patient and pain team consultation*. Unpublished manuscript, University of Saskatchewan, October 1980.

Campbell, A., & Worthington, E. L., Jr. A comparison of two methods of training husbands to assist their wives with labor and delivery. *Journal of Psychosomatic Research*, 1981, *25*, 557–564.

Campbell, A., & Worthington, E. L., Jr. Teaching expectant fathers how to be better childbirth coaches. *The American Journal of Maternal Child Nursing*, in press.

Cangello, V. W. The use of hypnotic suggestion for relief in malignant disease. *International Journal of Clinical and Experimental Hypnosis*, 1961, *9*, 17–22.

Cangello, V. W. Hypnosis for the patient with cancer. *American Journal of Clinical Hypnosis*, 1962, *4*, 215–226.

Cannon, W. B. *Wisdom of the body*. New York: W. W. Norton, 1932.

Carlin, A., & Armstrong, H. Aversive conditioning: Learning or dissonance reduction? *Journal of Consulting and Clinical Psychology*, 1968, *32*, 674–678.

Carlsson, S. G., & Gale, E. N. Biofeedback in the treatment of long-term temporomandibular joint pain. *Biofeedback and Self-Regulation*, 1977, *2*, 161–171.

Carlsson, S. G., Gale, E. N., & Ohman, A. A treatment of temporomandibular joint syndrome with biofeedback training. *Journal of the American Dental Association*, 1975, *91*, 602–605.

Carr, J. E., Brownsberger, C. N., & Rutherford, R. C. Characteristics of symptom-matched psychogenic and "real" pain patients on the MMPI. *Proceedings of the 74th Annual Convention of the American Psychological Association*, 1966, 215–216.

Cassel, J. An epidemiological perspective of psychosocial factors in disease etiology. *American Journal of Public Health*, 1974, *64*, 1040–1043. (a)

Cassel, J. Psychosocial processes and "stress": Theoretical formulations. *International Journal of Health Services*, 1974, *4*, 471–482. (b)

Cassel, J. The contribution of the social environment to host resistance. *American Journal of Epidemiology*, 1976, *104*, 107–123.

Cassell, S. Effects of brief puppet therapy upon the emotional responses of children undergoing cardiac catheterization. *Journal of Consulting Psychology*, 1965, *29*, 1–8.

Catchlove, R. F. H., & Ramsay, R. A. Psychosocial assessment of chronic pain patients. *Pain Abstracts*, 1978, *1*, 287.

Cautela, J. R. The use of covert conditioning in modifying pain behavior. *Journal of Behavior Therapy and Experimental Psychiatry*, 1977, *8*, 45–52.

Cautela, J. R., & Upper, D. The behavioral inventory battery: The use of self-report measures in behavioral analysis and therapy. In M. Hersen & A. S. Bellack (Eds.), *Behavioral assessment: A practical handbook*. New York: Pergamon, 1976.

Cedercreutz, C., Lahteenmaki, R., & Tulikoura, J. Hypnotic treatment of headache and vertigo in skull injured patients. *International Journal of Clinical and Experimental Hypnosis*, 1976, *24*, 195–201.

Chaney, E., O'Leary, M., & Marlatt, G. A. Skill training with alcoholics. *Journal of Consulting and Clinical Psychology*, 1978, *46*, 1092–1104.

Chapman, C. R. *A behavioral perspective on chronic pain.* Paper presented at the annual convention of the American Psychological Association, Montreal, Canada, August 1973.

Chappell, M. N., Stefano, J. J., Rogerson, J. S., & Pike, F. H. The value of group psychological procedures in the treatment of peptic ulcer. *American Journal of Digestive Diseases*, 1936, *3*, 813–817.

Chappell, M. N., & Stevenson, T. I. Group psychological training in some organic conditions. *Mental Hygiene*, 1936, *30*, 588–597.

Charney, E. Patient–doctor communication: Implications for the clinician. *Pediatric Clinics of North America*, 1972, *19*, 263–279.

Chaves, J. F., & Barber, T. X. Acupuncture analgesia: A six-factor theory. *Psychoenergetic Systems*, 1974, *1*, 11–21. (a)

Chaves, J. F., & Barber, T. X. Cognitive strategies, experimenter modeling, and expectation in the attenuation of pain. *Journal of Abnormal Psychology*, 1974, *83*, 356–363. (b)

Chaves, J. F., & Brown, J. M. *Self-generated strategies for the control of pain and stress.* Paper presented at the annual meeting of the American Psychological Association, Toronto, Canada, August 1978.

Chaves, J. F., & Doney, T. *Cognitive attenuation of pain: The roles of strategy relevance, absorption, and expectation.* Paper presented at the 10th annual convention of the Association for Advancement of Behavior Therapy, New York, December 1976.

Chen, A. C. N. *Behavioral and brain evoked potential (BEP) evaluation of placebo effects: Contrast of cognitive mechanisms and endorphins mechanisms.* Paper presented at the second general meeting of the American Pain Society, New York, September 1980.

Chertok, L. *Motherhood and personality: Psychosomatic aspects of childbirth.* Philadelphia: J. B. Lippincott, 1969.

Christensen, D. B. Drug-taking compliance: A review and synthesis. *Health Services Research*, 1978, *13*, 171–187.

Christopherson, L. K., & Lunde, D. T. Selection of cardiac transplant recipients and their subsequent psycho-social adjustment. *Seminars in Psychiatry*, 1971, *3*, 36–45.

Ciminero, A. R., Calhoun, K. S., & Adams, H. E. (Eds.). *Handbook of behavioral assessment.* New York: Wiley, 1977.

Cinciripini, P. M., & Floreen, A. *An evaluation of an inpatient behavioral program for chronic pain.* Paper presented at the 15th annual convention of the Association for Advancement of Behavior Therapy, New York, November 1980.

Clark, J. W., & Bindra, D. Individual differences in pain thresholds. *Canadian Journal of Psychology*, 1956, *10*, 69–76.

Clark, M., Gosnell, M., & Shapiro, D. The new war on pain. *Newsweek*, 1977 (April 25), *89*, 48–58.

Clark, W. C. Pain sensitivity and the report of pain: An introduction to sensory decision theory. *Anesthesiology*, 1974, *40*, 272–287.

Clark, W. C., & Hunt, H. F. Pain. In J. A. Downey & R. C. Darling (Eds.), *Physiological basis of rehabilitation medicine.* Philadelphia: W. B. Saunders, 1971.

Clawson, T. A., Jr., & Swade, R. H. The hypnotic control of blood flow and pain: The cure of warts and the potential for the use of hypnosis in the treatment of cancer. *American Journal of Clinical Hypnosis*, 1975, *17*, 160–169.

Coates, T. J., & Perry, C. Multifactor risk reduction with children and adolescents taking care of the heart in behavior group therapy. In D. Upper & S. Ross (Eds.), *Behavior group therapy: An annual review* (Vol. 2). Champaign, Ill.: Research Press, 1980.

Coates, T. J., & Thoresen, C. E. Teacher anxiety: A review with recommendations. *Review of Educational Research*, 1976, *46*, 159–184.

Cobb, A. B. (Ed.). *Special problems in rehabilitation*. Springfield, Ill.: Charles C Thomas, 1974.

Cobb, S. Social support and health through the life course. In M. Riley (Ed.), *Aging from birth to death: Interdisciplinary perspectives*. Boulder, Colo.: Westview Press, 1979.

Cogan, R. *Comparison of the effectiveness of fast panting, slow panting, and "he" breathing during labor*. Unpublished manuscript, Texas Tech University, 1976.

Cogan, R. Practice time in prepared childbirth. *Journal of Obstetric, Gynecologic and Neonatal Nursing*. 1978, *7*, 33–38.

Cogan, R., Henneborn, W., & Klopfer, F. Predictors of pain during prepared childbirth. *Journal of Psychosomatic Research*, 1976, *20*, 523–533.

Coger, R., & Werbach, M. Attention, anxiety, and the effects of learned enhancement of EEG in chronic pain: A pilot study in biofeedback. In B. L. Crue, Jr. (Ed.), *Pain: Research and treatment*. New York: Academic Press, 1975.

Cohen, F. Personality, stress, and the development of physical illness. In G. C. Stone, F. Cohen, & N. E. Adler (Eds.), *Health psychology—A handbook. Theories, applications, and challenges of a psychological approach to the health care system*. San Francisco: Jossey-Bass, 1979.

Collins, F. L., Jr., & Thompson, J. K. Reliability and standardization in the assessment of self-reported headache pain. *Journal of Behavioral Assessment*. 1979, *1*, 73–86.

Cone, J. D., & Hawkins, R. P. (Eds.). *Behavioral assessment: New directions in clinical psychology*. New York: Brunner/Mazel, 1977.

Copp, L. A. The spectrum of suffering. *American Journal of Nursing*, 1974, *74*, 491–495.

Coppolino, C. A. *Practice of hypnosis in anesthesiology*. New York: Grune & Stratton, 1965.

Cormier, W. H., & Cormier, L. S. *Interviewing strategies for helpers: A guide to assessment, treatment, and evaluation*. Monterey, Calif.: Brooks/Cole, 1979.

Cousins, N. Anatomy of an illness (as perceived by the patient). *New England Journal of Medicine*, 1976, *295*, 1458–1463.

Cox, G. B., Chapman, C. R., & Black, R. G. The MMPI and chronic pain: The diagnosis of psychogenic pain. *Journal of Behavioral Medicine*, 1978, *1*, 437–443.

Craig, K. D., Best, H., & Reith, G. Social determinants of reports of pain in the absence of painful stimulation. *Canadian Journal of Behavioural Science*, 1974, *6*, 169–177.

Crasilneck, H. B. Hypnosis in the control of chronic low back pain. *American Journal of Clinical Hypnosis*, 1979, *22*, 71–78.

Crasilneck, H. B., & Hall, J. A. Clinical hypnosis in problems of pain. *American Journal of Clinical Hypnosis*, 1973, *15*, 153–161.

Crasilneck, H. B., Stirman, J. A., Wilson, B. J., McCranie, E. J., & Fogelman, M. J. Use of hypnosis in the management of patients with burns. *Journal of the American Medical Association*, 1955, *158*, 103–106.

Creer, T. L., & Burns, K. L. Self-management training for children with chronic bronchial asthma. *Psychotherapy and Psychomatics*, 1978, *32*, 270–278.

Cuevas, J. L., Hamilton, J., Katrandies, M. A., Safranek, R., Gannon, L., & Haynes, S. N. *A psychophysiological investigation of muscle-contraction and migraine headache*. Paper presented at the annual convention of the Association for Advancement of Behavior Therapy, New York, November 1980.

Cullen, J. W., Fox, B. H., & Isom, R. N. (Eds.). *Cancer: The behavioral dimensions*. New York: Raven, 1976.

Dahlstrom, W. G. Prediction of adjustment after neurosurgery. *American Psychologist*, 1954, *9*, 353. (Abstract)

Dalessio, D. J. *Wolff's headache and other head pain*. New York: Oxford University Press, 1972.

Dallenbach, K. M. Pain: History and present status. *American Journal of Psychology*, 1939, *52*, 331–347.

Daniels, L. K. Treatment of migraine headache by hypnosis and behavior therapy: A case study. *American Journal of Clinical Hypnosis*, 1977, *19*, 241–244.

Davenport-Slack, B., & Boylan, C. H. Psychological correlates of childbirth pain. *Psychosomatic Medicine*, 1974, *36*, 215–223.

Davidson, P. O. Therapeutic compliance. *Canadian Psychological Review*, 1976, *17*, 247–259.

Davidson, P. O. Evaluating life style change programs. In P. O. Davidson & S. M. Davidson (Eds.), *Behavioral medicine: Changing health life styles*. New York: Brunner/Mazel, 1980.

Davidson, P. O., & McDougall, C.E.A. The generality of pain tolerance. *Journal of Psychosomatic Research*, 1969, *13*, 83–89.

Davis, C. D., & Merrone, F. A. An objective evaluation of a prepared childbirth program. *American Journal of Obstetrics and Gynecology*, 1962, *84*, 1196.

Davis, M. S. Predicting non-compliant behavior. *Journal of Health and Social Behavior*, 1967, *8*, 265–271.

Davis, M. S. Variation in patients' compliance with doctors' advice: An empirical analysis of patterns of communication. *American Journal of Public Health*, 1968, *58*, 274–288.

Davison, G. C., & Wilson, G. T. Critique of "Desensitization: Social and cognitive factors underlying the effectiveness of Wolpe's procedure." *Psychological Bulletin*, 1972, *78*, 28–31.

Day, G. The psychosomatic approach to pulmonary tuberculosis. *Lancet*, 1951, *1*, 1025–1028.

Deffenbacher, J. L., Mathis, H., & Michaels, A. C. Two self-control procedures in the reduction of targeted and non-targeted anxieties. *Journal of Counseling Psychology*, 1979, *26*, 120–127.

DeGood, D., Tung, A., & Tenicola, R. *Autogenic training and biofeedback for pain control*. Paper presented at the Second World Congress on Pain, Montreal, Canada, August 1978.

Dekker, E. Youth culture and influences on the smoking behavior of young people. In *Proceedings of the 3rd World Conference on Smoking and Health* (DHEW Publication No. (NIH) 77-1413). Washington, D.C.: U.S. Government Printing Office, 1975.

Dembroski, T. (Ed.). *Proceedings of the forum on coronary-prone behavior* (Publication No. (NIH) 78-1451). Washington, D.C.: U.S. Department of Health, Education & Welfare, 1977.

Dembroski, T. M., Caffrey, B., Jenkins, C. D., Rosenman, R. H., Spielberger, C. D., & Tasto, D. L. Summary statement: Assessment of coronary-prone behavior. In T. Dembroski (Ed.), *Proceedings of the forum on coronary-prone behavior* (Publication No. (NIH) 78-1451). Washington, D.C.: U.S. Department of Health, Education & Welfare, 1977.

Dembroski, T. M., McDougall, J. M., & Shields, J. L. Physiologic reactions to social challenge in persons evidencing the Type A coronary-prone behavior pattern. *Journal of Human Stress*, 1977, *3*, 2–9.

Demjen, S., & Bakal, D. A. A cognitive–behavioral treatment program for chronic pain. *Headache*, 1979, *19*, 249.

Denney, D. R. Self-control approaches to the treatment of test anxiety. In I. G. Sarason (Ed.), *Test anxiety: Theory, research and applications*. Hillsdale, N.J.: Erlbaum, 1980.

Dewe, P., Guest, D., & Williams, R. Methods of coping with work-related stress. In C. Mackay & T. Cox (Eds.), *Response to stress: Occupational aspects.* Guilford, England: IPC Science & Technology Press, 1979.

Dick-Read, G. *Natural childbirth.* London: W. Heinemann, 1933.

Dietrich, S. L. Musculoskeletal problems. In M. W. Hilgartner (Ed.), *Hemophilia in children.* Littleton, Mass.: Publishing Sciences Group, 1976.

Dimsdale, J. E., Hackett, T. P., Catanzano, D. M., & White, P. The relationship between diverse measures for Type A personalities and coronary angiographic findings. *Journal of Psychosomatic Research,* 1979, *23,* 289-293.

Dimsdale, J. E., Hackett, T. P., Hutter, A. M., & Block, P. C. The risk of Type A mediated coronary artery disease in different populations. *Psychosomatic Medicine,* 1980, *42,* 55-62.

Dimsdale, J. E., Hackett, T. P., Hutter, A. M., Block, P. C., Catanzano, D. M., & White, P. J. Type A behavior and angiographic findings. *Journal of Psychosomatic Research,* 1979, *23,* 273-276.

Dodge, D., & Martin, W. *Social stress and chronic illness: Mortality patterns in industrial society.* Notre Dame, Ind.: University of Notre Dame Press, 1970.

Doering, S. G., & Entwisle, D. R. Preparation during pregnancy and ability to cope with labor and delivery. *American Journal of Orthopsychiatry,* 1975, *45,* 825-837.

Doering, S. G., Entwisle, D. R., & Quinlan, D. Modeling the quality of women's birth experience. *Journal of Health and Social Behavior,* 1980, *21,* 12-21.

Doleys, D. M., Meredith, R. L., & Ciminero, A. R. (Eds.). *Behavioral medicine: Assessment and treatment strategies.* New York: Plenum, 1982.

Draspa, L. J. Psychological factors in muscular pain. *British Journal of Medical Psychology,* 1959, *32,* 106-116.

Dubuisson, D., & Melzack, R. Classification of clinical pain descriptions by multiple group discriminant analysis. *Experimental Neurology,* 1976, *51,* 480-487.

Dulaney, D. E. The place of hypotheses and intentions: An analysis of verbal control in verbal conditioning. In C. W. Eriksen (Ed.), *Behavior and awareness.* Durham, N.C.: Duke University Press, 1962.

Dunbar, J. Adhering to medical advice: A review. *International Journal of Mental Health,* 1980, *9,* 70-87.

Dunbar, J., & Stunkard, A. Adherence to diet and drug regimen. In R. Levy, B. Rifkind, & N. Ernst (Eds.), *Nutrition, lipids, and coronary heart disease.* New York: Raven, 1979.

Ebersold, M. J., Laws, E. R., Jr., Stonnington, H. H., & Stillwell, G. K. Transcutaneous electrical stimulation for treatment of chronic pain: Preliminary report. *Surgical Neurology,* 1975, *4,* 96-99.

Egbert, L., Batit, G., Welch, C., & Bartlett, M. Reduction of postoperative pain by encouragement and instruction. *New England Journal of Medicine,* 1964, *270,* 825-827.

Ellis, A. *Reason and emotion in psychotherapy.* New York: Lyle Stuart, 1962.

Elms, R., & Leonard, R. L. Effects of nursing approaches during admission. *Nursing Research,* 1966, *15,* 39-48.

Engel, G. L. Studies of ulcerative colitis: III. The nature of the psychologic processes. *American Journal of Medicine,* 1955, *19,* 231-256.

Engels, W. D., & Wittkower, E. D. Psychophysiological allergic and skin disorders. In A. M. Freedman, H. J. Kaplan, & B. J. Sadock (Eds.), *Comprehensive textbook of psychiatry, II.* Baltimore: Williams & Wilkins, 1975.

Engle, K. B., & Williams, T. K. Effect of an ounce of vodka on alcoholics' desire for alcohol. *Quarterly Journal of Studies on Alcohol,* 1972, *33,* 1099-1105.

Enkin, M. W., Smith, S. L., Dermer, S. W., & Emmet, J. O. An adequately controlled study of the effectiveness of P.P.M. training. In N. Morris (Ed.), *Psychosomatic medicine in obstetrics*. New York: Karger, 1972.

Epstein, L., & Wing, R. Behavioral contracting: Health behaviors. *Clinical Behavior Therapy Review*, 1979, *1*, 1–15.

Erickson, M. H., Hershman, S., & Secter, I. I. *Application of medical and dental hypnosis*. New York: Julian, 1961.

Ericsson, K. A., & Simon, H. A. Verbal reports as data. *Psychological Review*, 1980, *87*, 215–251.

Erickson, D. L., Acharya, A., & Michaelson, M. *Use of problem solving approach in the treatment of chronic pain*. Paper presented at the Second World Congress on Pain, Montreal, Canada, August 1978.

Etzwiler, D. D., & Robb, J. R. Evaluation of programmed education among juvenile diabetics and their families. *Diabetes*, 1972, *21*, 967–971.

Euster, S. Rehabilitation after mastectomy: The group process. *Social Work in Health Care*, 1979, *4*, 251–263.

Evans, M., & Paul, G. L. Effects of hypnotically suggested analgesia on physiological and subjective responses to cold stress. *Journal of Consulting and Clinical Psychology*, 1970, *35*, 362–371.

Evans, R. I., Rozelle, M. B., Mittelmark, M. B., Hansen, W. B., Bane, A. L., & Havis, J. Deterring the onset of smoking in children: Knowledge of immediate physiological effects and coping with peer pressure, media pressure, and parent modeling. *Journal of Applied Social Psychology*, 1978, *8*, 126–135.

Evaskus, D. S., & Laskin, D. M. A biochemical measure of stress in patients with myofascial dysfunction syndrome. *Journal of Dental Research*, 1972, *51*, 1464–1466.

Fagerhaugh, S. Pain expression and control on a burn care unit. *Nursing Outlook*, 1974, *22*, 645–650.

Family doctor vs. chronic pain. *Patient Care*, 1978, *12*, whole issue.

Farquhar, J. W., Maccoby, N., Wood, P. D., Alexander, J. K., Breitrose, H., Brown, B. W., Jr., Haskell, W. L., McAlister, A. L., Meyer, A. J., Nash, J. D., & Stern, M. P. Community education for cardiovascular health. *Lancet*, 1977, *4*, 1192–1196.

Ferguson, J., & Taylor, C. B. (Eds.). *A comprehensive handbook of behavioral medicine*. New York: Spectrum, 1980.

Feuerstein, M., & Skjei, E. *Mastering pain*. New York: Bantam Books, 1979.

Fielding, W., & Benjamin, L. *The case against "natural childbirth."* New York: Viking, 1962.

Finer, B. Clinical use of hypnosis in pain management. In J. J. Bonica (Ed.), *Advances in neurology* (Vol. 4). New York: Raven, 1974.

Finesilver, C. Preparation of adult patients for cardiac catheterization and coronary cineangiography. *International Journal of Nursing Studies*, 1978, *15*, 211–221.

Flowers, C. E. Patient participation in labor and delivery. *Texas Journal of Medicine*, 1962, *58*, 988–993.

Follick, M. J., & Turk, D. C. *Problem specification by ostomy patients*. Paper presented at the 12th annual convention of the Association for Advancement of Behavior Therapy, Chicago, November 1978.

Follick, M. J., Zitter, R. E., & Kulich, R. J. Outpatient management of chronic pain. In T. J. Coates (Ed.), *Behavioral medicine: A practical handbook*. Champaign, Ill.: Research Press, 1981.

Fordyce, W. E. Pain viewed as learned behavior. In J. J. Bonica (Ed.), *Advances in neurology* (Vol. 4). New York: Raven, 1974. (a)

Fordyce, W. E. Treating chronic pain by contingency management. In J. J. Bonica (Ed.), *Advances in neurology* (Vol. 4). New York: Raven, 1974. (b)

Fordyce, W. E. *Behavioral methods for chronic pain and illness.* St. Louis: C. V. Mosby, 1976.

Fordyce, W. E., Fowler, R. S., & DeLateur, B. An application of behavior modification technique to a problem of chronic pain. *Behaviour Research and Therapy,* 1968, *6,* 105-107.

Fordyce, W. B., Fowler, R. S., Jr., Lehmann, J. F., DeLateur, B. J., Sand, P. L., & Trieschmann, R. B. Operant conditioning in the treatment of chronic pain. *Archives of Physical Medicine and Rehabilitation,* 1973, *54,* 399-408.

Fordyce, W., McMahon, R., Rainwater, G., Jackins, S., Questad, K., Murphy, T., & DeLateur, B. Pain complaint-exercise performance relationship in chronic pain. *Pain,* 1981, *10,* 311-322.

Fordyce, W. E., & Steger, J. C. Chronic pain. In O. F. Pomerleau & J. P. Brady (Eds.). *Behavioral medicine: Theory and practice.* Baltimore: Williams & Wilkins, 1979.

Foreyt, J. P., & Rathjen, D. P. (Eds.). *Cognitive-behavior therapy: Research and application.* New York: Plenum, 1978.

Forgione, A. G., & Barber, T. X. A strain gauge pain stimulator. *Psychophysiology,* 1971, *8,* 102-106.

Fortin, F., & Kirouac, S. A randomized controlled trial of preoperative patient education. *International Journal of Nursing Studies,* 1976, *13,* 11-24.

Fotopoulos, S., Graham, C., & Cook, M. Psychophysiologic control of cancer pain. In J. J. Bonica & V. Ventafridda (Eds.), *Advances in pain research and therapy* (Vol. 2). New York: Raven, 1979.

Fowler, R. S., Jr., & Kraft, G. H. Tension perception in patients having pain associated with chronic muscle tension. *Archives of Physical Medicine and Rehabilitation,* 1974, *55,* 28-30.

Fox, C. D., Steger, H. G., & Jennison, J. H. Ratio scaling of pain perception with the submaximum effort tourniquet technique. *Pain,* 1979, *7,* 21-29.

Frank, J. D. *Persuasion and healing: A comparative study of psychotherapy.* New York: Schocken Books, 1961.

Frank, J. D. Psychotherapy: The restoration of morale. *American Journal of Psychiatry,* 1974, *131,* 271-274.

Frank, J. D. Psychotherapy of bodily disease: An overview. *Psychotherapy and Psychosomatics,* 1975, *26,* 192-202.

Frankel, B. L., Patel, C. H., Horowitz, D., Friedwald, W. T., & Gaardner, K. R. Treatment of hypertension with biofeedback and relaxation techniques. *Psychosomatic Medicine,* 1978, *40,* 276-293.

Frankenhaeuser, M. Psychobiological aspects of life stress. In S. Levine & H. Ursin (Eds.), *Coping and health.* New York: Plenum, 1980.

Franks, C. M., Fried, R., & Ashem, B. An improved apparatus for the aversive conditioning of cigarette smokers. *Behaviour Research and Therapy,* 1966, *4,* 301-308.

French, J. R., & Raven, B. The bases of social power. In D. Cartwright (Ed.), *Studies in social power.* Ann Arbor: University of Michigan Press, 1959.

Friedman, E. A., & Sachtleben, M. B. Dysfunctional labor: I. Prolonged latent phase in the nullipara. *Obstetrics and Gynecology,* 1961, *17,* 135-138.

Friedman, M., & Rosenman, R. H. Association of specific overt behavior patterns with blood and cardiovascular findings: Blood cholesterol level, blood clotting time, incidence of arcus senilis, and clinical coronary artery disease. *Journal of the American Medical Association,* 1959, *169,* 1286-1296.

Friedman, S. B., & Glasgow, L. A. Psychological factors and resistance to infectious disease. In P. M. Insel & R. H. Moos (Eds.), *Health and the social environment.* Toronto: D. C. Heath, 1974.

Fromm, E., Brown, D. P., Hurt, S. W., Oberlander, J. Z., Boxer, A. M., & Pfeifer, G. The phenomena and characteristics of self-hypnosis. *International Journal of Clinical and Experimental Hypnosis,* 1981, *21,* 189–246.

Fuller, S. S., Endress, M. P., & Johnson, J. E. The effects of cognitive and behavioral control on coping with an aversive health examination. *Journal of Human Stress,* 1978, *4,* 18–25.

Fulop-Miller, R. *Triumph over pain.* New York: The Literary Guild of America, 1938.

Galeazzi, L., & Minella, E. Statistical assessment of 300 cases of childbirth under hypnosis. *Minerva Medicine,* 1972, *63,* 952–954.

Garrity, T. F. Social involvement and activities as predictors of morale six months after myocardial infarction. *Social Science and Medicine,* 1973, *7,* 199–207. (a)

Garrity, T. F. Vocational adjustment after first myocardial infarctions: Comparative assessment of several variables suggested in the literature. *Social Science and Medicine,* 1973, *7,* 705–717. (b)

Garrity, T. F. Morbidity, mortality, and rehabilitation. In W. D. Gentry & R. B. Williams (Eds.), *Psychological aspects of myocardial infarction and coronary care.* St. Louis: C. V. Mosby, 1975.

Garrity, T. F., & Klein, R. F. A behavioral predictor of survival among heart attack patients. In E. Palmore & F. G. Jeffers (Eds.), *Prediction of life span.* Lexington, Mass.: D. C. Heath, 1971.

Genest, M. *A cognitive-behavioral bibliotherapy to ameliorate pain.* Paper presented at the annual meetings of the American Psychological Association, Toronto, Canada, August 1978.

Genest, M. *Controlling pain: A cognitive-behavioral bibliotherapy approach with experimentally produced pain.* Unpublished master's thesis, University of Waterloo, 1979.

Genest, M. Preparation for childbirth: A selected review of evidence for efficacy. *Journal of Obstetric, Gynecologic and Neonatal Nursing,* 1981, *10,* 82–85.

Genest, M. *Coping with severe disability: Rheumatoid arthritis.* Research in progress at University Hospital, Saskatoon, Saskatchewan, Canada, 1982.

Genest, M., Meichenbaum, D. H., & Turk, D. C. *A cognitive-behavioral approach to the management of pain.* Paper presented at the 11th annual convention of the Association for Advancement of Behavior Therapy, Atlanta, December 1977.

Genest, M., & Turk, D. C. A proposed model for behavioral group theapy with pain patients. In D. Upper & S. M. Ross (Eds.), *Behavioral group therapy: An annual review.* Champaign, Ill.: Research Press, 1979.

Genest, M., & Turk, D. C. Think-aloud approaches to cognitive assessment. In T. V. Merluzzi, C. R. Glass, & M. Genest (Eds.), *Cognitive assessment.* New York: Guilford, 1981.

Gentry, W. D. Preadmission behavior. In W. D. Gentry & R. B. Williams, Jr. (Eds.), *Psychological aspects of myocardial infarction and coronary care.* St. Louis: C. V. Mosby, 1975.

Gessel, A. H., & Alderman, M. M. Management of myofascial pain dysfunction syndrome of the temporamandibular joint by tension control training. *Psychosomatics,* 1971, *12,* 302–309.

Getto, C. J., Franks, R. D., & Willett, A. B. Treatment of chronic pain in the general psychiatric hospital. *International Journal of Psychiatry in Medicine,* 1978–1979, *9,* 247–256.

Gillmore, M. R., & Hill, C. T. Reactions to patients who complain of pain: Effects of ambiguous diagnosis. *Journal of Applied Social Psychology*, 1981, *11*, 14–22.

Gillum, R. F., & Barsky, A. J. Diagnosis and management of patient noncompliance. *Journal of the American Medical Association*, 1974, *228*, 1563–1567.

Girodo, M., & Wood, D. Talking yourself out of pain: The importance of believing you can. *Cognitive Therapy and Research*, 1979, *3*, 23–34.

Glass, D. C. *Behavior patterns, stress, and coronary disease*. Hillsdale, N.J.: Erlbaum, 1977.

Goldfried, M. R. The use of relaxation and cognitive relabeling as coping skills. In R. B. Stuart (Ed.), *Behavioral self-management. Strategies, techniques and outcome*. New York: Brunner/Mazel, 1977.

Goldfried, M. R., & Davison, G. *Clinical behavior therapy*. New York: Holt, Rinehart & Winston, 1976.

Goldfried, M. R., & D'Zurilla, T. J. A behavioral–analytic model for assessing competence. In C. D. Spielberger (Ed.), *Current topics in clinical and community psychology* (Vol. 1). New York: Academic Press, 1969.

Goldfried, M. R., & Trier, C. S. Effectiveness of relaxation as an active coping skill. *Journal of Abnormal Psychology*, 1974, *83*, 348–355.

Goleman, D. Meditation without mystery. *Psychology Today*, 1977, *10*, 54–67; 88.

Gordon, W. A., Freidenbergs, I., Diller, L., Hibbard, M., Wolf, C., Levine, L., Lipkins, R., Ezrachi, O., & Lucido, D. Efficacy of psychosocial intervention with cancer patients. *Journal of Consulting and Clinical Psychology*, 1980, *48*, 743–759.

Gottfredson, D. K. *Hypnosis as an anesthetic in dentistry* (Doctoral dissertation, Brigham Young University). *Dissertation Abstracts International*, 1973, *33* (7-B), 3303.

Gottlieb, H., Strite, L. C., Koller, R., Madorsky, A., Hockersmith, V., Kleeman, M., & Wagner, J. Comprehensive rehabilitation of patients having chronic low back pain. *Archives of Physical Medicine and Rehabilitation*, 1977, *58*, 101–108.

Gottman, J., Notarius, C., Gonso, J., & Markman, H. *A couple's guide to communication*. Champaign, Ill.: Research Press, 1976.

Gracely, R. H. *Psychophysical assessment of human pain*. Paper presented at the Second World Congress on Pain, Montreal, Canada, August 1978.

Graham, C., Bond, S. S., Gerkovich, M. M., & Cook, M. R. Use of the McGill Pain Questionnaire in the assessment of cancer pain: Replicability and consistency. *Pain*, 1980, *8*, 377–387.

Graham, G. W. Hypnotic treatment for migraine headaches. *International Journal of Clinical and Experimental Hypnosis*, 1975, *23*, 165–171.

Green, E., Walters, E. D., Green, A., & Murphy, G. Feedback technique for deep relaxation. *Psychophysiology*, 1969, *6*, 371–378.

Greene, C. S., Lerman, M. D., & Sutcher, H. D. The TMJ pain-dysfunction syndrome: Heterogeneity of the patient population. *Journal of the American Dental Association*, 1969, *79*, 1168–1172.

Greene, R. J., & Reyher, J. Pain tolerance in hypnotic analgesia and imagination states. *Journal of Abnormal Psychology*, 1972, *79*, 29–38.

Greene, R. S. Modification of smoking behavior by free operant conditioning methods. *Psychological Record*, 1964, *14*, 171–178.

Greenhoot, J. H., & Sternbach, R. A. Conjoint treatment of chronic pain. In J. J. Bonica (Ed.), *Advances in neurology* (Vol. 4). New York: Raven, 1974.

Grimm, L., & Kanfer, F. H. Tolerance of aversive stimulation. *Behavior Therapy*, 1976, *7*, 593–601.

Gruen, W. Effects of brief psychotherapy during the hospitalization period on the recovery process in heart attacks. *Journal of Consulting and Clinical Psychology*, 1975, *43*, 223–232.

Grzesiak, R. C. Relaxation techniques in treatment of chronic pain. *Archives of Physical Medicine and Rehabilitation*, 1977, *58*, 270–272.

Grzesiak, R. C. Chronic pain: A psychobehavioral perspective. In L. P. Ince (Ed.), *Behavioral psychology in rehabilitation medicine: Clinical applications*. Baltimore: Williams & Wilkins, 1981.

Grzesiak, R. C., & Zaretsky, H. H. Psychology in rehabilitation: Professional and clinical aspects. In R. Murray & J. C. Kijek (Eds.), *Current perspectives in rehabilitation nursing*. St. Louis: C. V. Mosby, 1979.

Guillemin, R., Vargo, T., Rossier, J., Minick, S., Ling, N., Rivier, C., Vale, W., & Bloom, F. B-Endorphin and adrenocorticotropin are secreted concomitantly by the pituitary gland. *Science*, 1977, *147*, 1367–1369.

Gutmann, M., & Benson, H. Interaction of environmental factors and systemic arterial blood pressure: A review. *Medicine*, 1971, *50*, 543–553.

Hackett, G., & Horan, J. J. Stress inoculation for pain: What's really going on? *Journal of Counseling Psychology*, 1980, *27*, 107–116.

Hackett, G., Horan, J. J., Buchanan, J., & Zumoff, P. Improving exposure component and generalization potential of stress inoculation for pain. *Perceptual and Motor Skills*, 1979, *48*, 1132–1134.

Hackett, T. P., & Cassem, N. H. Psychological management of the myocardial infarction patient. *Journal of Human Stress*, 1975, *1*, 25–38.

Haggard, H. *Devils, drugs and doctors*. New York: Harper, 1929.

Haggerty, K. Changing lifestyles to improve health. *Preventive Medicine*, 1977, *6*, 276–289.

Hall, K., & Stride, E. The varying response to pain in psychiatric disorders: A study in abnormal psychology. *British Journal of Medical Psychology*, 1954, *27*, 48–60.

Hall, S. M., & Hall, R. G. Outcome and methodological considerations in behavioral treatment of obesity. *Behavior Therapy*, 1974, *5*, 59–68.

Halpern, L. M. Psychotropic drugs and the management of chronic pain. In J. J. Bonica (Ed.), *Advances in neurology* (Vol. 4). New York: Raven, 1974. (a)

Halpern, L. M. Treating pain with drugs. *Minnesota Medicine*, 1974, *57*, 176–184. (b)

Hamburg, D. A., & Adams, J. E. A perspective on coping behavior: Seeking and utilizing information in major transitions. *Archives of General Psychiatry*, 1967, *17*, 277–284.

Hamburg, D. A., Coelho, G. V., & Adams, J. E. Coping and adaptation: Steps toward a synthesis of biological and social perspectives. In G. V. Coelho, D. A. Hamburg, & J. E. Adams (Eds.), *Coping and adaptation*. New York: Basic Books, 1974.

Hammonds, W., Brena, S. F., & Unikel, I. P. Compensation for work related injuries and rehabilitation of patients with chronic pain. *Southern Medical Journal*, 1978, *71*, 664–666.

Hanson, R., & Franklin, M. Sexual loss in relation to other functional losses for spinal cord injured males. *Archives of Physical Medicine and Rehabilitation*, 1976, *57*, 291–293.

Hanvik, L. J. MMPI profiles in patients with low back pain. *Journal of Consulting Psychology*, 1951, *15*, 350–353.

Harding, H. C. Hypnosis in the treatment of migraine. In J. Lassner (Ed.), *Hypnosis and psychosomatic medicine*. New York: Springer-Verlag, 1967.

Hardy, J. D., Wolff, H. G., & Goodell, H. Studies on pain: An investigation of some quantitative aspects of the dol scale of pain intensity. *Journal of Clinical Investigation*, 1948, *27*, 380–386.

Hardy, J. D., Wolff, H. G., & Goodell, H. *Pain sensations and reactions*. New York: Hafner, 1952.

Harrell, T. H., & Beiman, I. Cognitive-behavioral treatment of irritable colon syndrome. *Cognitive Therapy and Research*, 1978, *2*, 371-375.

Harris, R., & Monaco, G. Psychology of pragmatic implications: Information processing between the lines. *Journal of Experimental Psychology: General*, 1978, *107*, 1-22.

Hartman, L. M., & Ainsworth, K. D. Self-regulation of chronic pain. *Canadian Journal of Psychiatry*, 1980, *25*, 38-43.

Haynes, R. B., Taylor, D. W., & Sackett, D. L. *Compliance in health care.* Baltimore: The Johns Hopkins University Press, 1979.

Hedberg, A. G., & Schlong, A. Eliminating fainting by school children during mass inoculation clinics. *Nursing Research*, 1973, *22*, 352-353.

Heinrich, R., Cohen, M., Naliboff, B., Collins, G., & Bonebakker, A. *Behavioral and physical therapy treatment of chronic low back pain.* Paper presented at the second general meeting of the American Pain Society, New York, September 1980.

Heinrich, R., & Fuller, M. *Control and modulation of pain in selected chronic pain patients by a guided affective imagery technique.* Paper presented at the First World Congress on Pain, Florence, Italy, September 1975.

Heller, K. The effects of social support: Prevention and treatment implications. In A. P. Goldstein & F. H. Kanfer (Eds.), *Maximizing treatment gains: Transfer enhancement in psychotherapy.* New York: Academic Press, 1979.

Hendrie, H. C., Paraskevas, F., Baragar, F. D., & Adamson, J. D. Stress, immunoglobulin levels, and early polyarthritis. *Journal of Psychosomatic Research,* 1971, *15*, 337-342.

Henry, J. P., & Cassel, J. C. Psychosocial factors in essential hypertension. *American Journal of Epidemiology*, 1969, *90*, 171-210.

Henryk-Gutt, R., & Rees, W. L. Psychological aspects of migraine. *Journal of Psychosomatic Research*, 1973, *17*, 141-153.

Heppner, P. P. A review of problem-solving literature and its relationship to the counseling process. *Journal of Counseling Psychology*, 1978, *25*, 366-375.

Herman, E. *Pain control classes for patients with chronic pain.* Paper presented at the Second World Congress on Pain, Montreal, Canada, September 1978.

Herman, E., & Baptiste, S. Pain control: Mastery through group experience. *Pain*, 1981, *10*, 79-86.

Hersen, M., & Bellack, A. S. (Eds.). *Behavioral assessment: A practical handbook.* Elmsford, N.Y.: Pergamon, 1976.

Higgins, R. L., & Marlatt, G. A. Fear of interpersonal evaluation as a determinant of alcohol consumption in male social drinkers. *Journal of Abnormal Psychology*, 1975, *84*, 644-651.

Hilgard, E. R. The alleviation of pain by hypnosis. *Pain*, 1975, *1*, 213-231.

Hilgard, E. R. *Divided consciousness: Multiple control in human thought and action.* New York: Wiley, 1977.

Hilgard, E. R., Cooper, L., Lennox, J. R., Morgan, A., & Voevodsky, J. The use of pain-state report in the study of hypnotic analgesia to the pain of ice water. *Journal of Nervous and Mental Diseases*, 1967, *114*, 501-513.

Hilgard, E. R., & Hilgard, J. R. *Hypnosis in the relief of pain.* Los Altos, Calif.: Kaufmann, 1975.

Hilgard, E. R., & Morgan, A. H. Heart rate and blood pressure in the study of laboratory pain in man under normal conditions and as influenced by hypnosis. *Acta Neurobiologiae Experimentalis*, 1975, *35*, 741-759.

Hilgard, J. R. *Personality and hypnosis: A study of imaginative involvement.* Chicago: University of Chicago Press, 1970.

Hill, H., Kornetsky, C., Flanary, H., & Wilker, A. Effects of anxiety and morphine on discrimination of painful stimuli. *Journal of Clinical Investigation*, 1952, *31*, 473. (a)

Hill, H., Kornetsky, C., Flanary, H., & Wilker, A. Studies on anxiety associated with anticipation of pain. I. Effects of morphine. *Archives of Neurology and Psychiatry*, 1952, *67*, 612–619. (b)

Hockersmith, V. W. *Biofeedback applications in chronic back pain disability.* Paper presented at the annual meeting of the American Psychological Association, Chicago, August 1975.

Holroyd, K. A. Stress, coping and the treatment of stress related illness. In J. R. McNamara (Ed.), *Behavioral approaches in medicine: Application and analysis.* New York: Plenum, 1980.

Holroyd, K. A., & Andrasik, F. Coping and the self-control of chronic tension headache. *Journal of Consulting and Clinical Psychology*, 1978, *46*, 1036–1045.

Holroyd, K. A., & Andrasik, F. *Do the effects of cognitive therapy endure: A two year follow-up of tension headache sufferers treated with cognitive therapy and biofeedback.* Paper presented at the 14th annual convention of the Association for Advancement of Behavior Therapy, New York, November 1980.

Holroyd, K. A., & Andrasik, F. A cognitive–behavioral approach to recurrent tension and migraine headache. In P. C. Kendall (Ed.), *Advances in cognitive-behavioral research and therapy* (Vol. 1). New York: Academic Press, 1981.

Holroyd, K. A., Andrasik, F., & Westbrook, T. Cognitive control of tension headache. *Cognitive Therapy and Research*, 1977, *1*, 121–133.

Holroyd, K. A., Appel, M. A., & Andrasik, F. A cognitive–behavioral approach to psychophysiological disorders. In D. H. Meichenbaum & M. E. Jaremko (Eds.), *Stress prevention and management: A cognitive-behavioral approach.* New York: Plenum, 1982.

Horan, J. J. *In vivo* emotive imagery: A technique for reducing childbirth anxiety and discomfort. *Psychological Reports*, 1973, *32*, 1328.

Horan, J. J., & Dellinger, J. K. *In vivo* emotive imagery: A preliminary test. *Perceptual and Motor Skills*, 1974, *39*, 359–362.

Horan, J. J., Hackett, G., Buchanan, J. D., Stone, C. I., & Demchik-Stone, D. Coping with pain: A component analysis of stress-inoculation. *Cognitive Therapy and Research*, 1977, *1*, 211–221.

Horan, J. J., Layng, F. C., & Pursell, C. H. Preliminary study of effects of *in vivo* emotive imagery on dental discomfort. *Perceptual and Motor Skills*, 1976, *42*, 105–106.

Horowitz, M. J., Hulley, S., Alvarez, W., Reynolds, H. M., Benfari, R., Blair, S., Borhani, N., & Simon, N. Life events, risk factors, and coronary disease. *Psychosomatics*, 1979, *20*, 586–592.

Houde, R. The use and misuse of narcotics in the treatment of chronic pain. In J. J. Bonica (Ed.), *Advances in neurology* (Vol. 4). New York: Raven, 1974.

Howard, J. H., Rechnitzer, P. A., & Cunningham, D. A. Stress inoculation for managers and organizations. *The Business Quarterly*, 1975, *40*, 73–79.

Hudgens, A. J. Family-oriented treatment of chronic pain. *Journal of Marital and Family Therapy*, 1979, *5*, 67–78.

Hughes, J., Smith, T. W., Kosterlitz, H. W., Fothergill, L. A., Morgan, B. A., & Morris, H. R. Identification of two related pentapeptides from the brain with potent opiate agonist activity. *Nature*, 1975, *258*, 577–579.

Hughey, M. J., McElin, T. W., & Young, T. Maternal and fetal outcome of Lamaze-prepared patients. *Obstetrics and Gynecology*, 1978, *51*, 643–647.

Hulka, B., Kupper, L. L., Cassel, J. C., & Mayo, F. Doctor-patient communication and outcomes among diabetic patients. *Journal of Community Health*, 1975, *1*, 15–27.

Hunt, W. A., & Bespalec, D. A. An evaluation of current methods of modifying smoking behavior. *Journal of Clinical Psychology*, 1974, *30*, 431–438.

Hunt, W. A., & Matarazzo, J. D. Habit mechanisms in smoking. In W. A. Hunt (Ed.), *Learning mechanisms in smoking*. Chicago: Aldine, 1970.

Hunt, W. A., & Matarazzo, J. D. Three years later: Recent developments in the experimental modification of smoking behavior. *Journal of Abnormal Psychology*, 1973, *81*, 107–114.

Hurd, P. D., Johnson, C. A., Pechacek, T., Bast, L. P., Jacobs, D. R., & Luepker, R. V. Prevention of cigarette smoking in seventh grade students. *Journal of Behavioral Medicine*, 1980, *3*, 15–28.

Huttel, F., Mitchell, I., Fischer, W. M., & Meyer, A. E. A quantitative evaluation of psychoprophylaxis in childbirth. *Journal of Psychosomatic Research*, 1972, *16*, 81–92.

Ignelzi, R. J., Sternbach, R. A., & Timmermans, G. The pain ward follow-up analysis. *Pain*, 1977, *3*, 277–280.

Imboden, J. B., Canter, A., & Cluff, L. E. Convalescence from influenza: A study of the psychological and clinical determinants. *Archives of Internal Medicine*, 1961, *108*, 393–399.

Ince, L. P. (Ed.). *Behavioral psychology in rehabilitation medicine: Clinical applications*. Baltimore: Williams & Wilkins, 1981.

Intagliata, J. Increasing the interpersonal problem-solving skills of an alcoholic population. *Journal of Consulting and Clinical Psychology*, 1978, *46*, 489–498.

International Association for the Study of Pain, Subcommittee on Taxonomy. Pain terms: A list with definitions and notes on usage. *Pain*, 1979, *6*, 249–252.

Ischlondsky, N. E. *Brain and behavior*. St. Louis: C. V. Mosby, 1949.

Jacobs, M. A., Spilken, A. Z., Norman, M. M., Wohlberg, G. W., & Knapp, P. H. Interactions of personality and treatment conditions associated with success in a smoking control program. *Psychosomatic Medicine*, 1971, *33*, 545–556.

Jacobson, E. *You must relax* (4th ed.). New York: McGraw-Hill, 1962.

Janis, I. L. Emotional inoculation: Theory and research on effects of preparatory communications. *Psychoanalysis and Social Science*, 1958, *5*, 155–163. (a)

Janis, I. L. *Psychological stress*. New York: Wiley, 1958. (b)

Janis, I. L., & King, B. The influence of role-playing on opinion change. *Journal of Abnormal and Social Psychology*, 1954, *49*, 211–218.

Janis, I. L., & Rodin, J. Attribution, control and decision making: Social psychology and health care. In G. Stone, F. Cohen, & N. Adler (Eds.), *Health psychology*. San Francisco: Jossey-Bass, 1979.

Jaremko, M. E. Cognitive strategies in the control of pain tolerance. *Journal of Behaviour Therapy and Experimental Psychiatry*, 1978, *9*, 239–244.

Javert, C. T., & Hardy, J. D. *Measurement of pain intensity in labor and its physiologic, neurologic and pharmacologic implications*. Paper presented before the New York Obstetrical Society, February 1950.

Jeffery, R. W., Wing, R. R., & Stunkard, A. J. Behavioral treatment of obesity: The state of the art. *Behavior Therapy*, 1978, *9*, 189–199.

Jellinek, E. M. *The disease concept of alcoholism*. New Haven, Conn.: College & University Press, 1960.

Jenkins, C. D. Recent evidence supporting psychologic and social risk factors for coronary disease. *New England Journal of Medicine*, 1976, *294*, 987–994; 1033–1038.

Jenkins, C. D., Zyzanski, S. J., & Rosenman, R. H. Risk of new myocardial infarction in middle-aged men with manifest heart disease. *Circulation*, 1976, *53*, 342-347.

Jenni, M. A., & Wollersheim, J. P. Cognitive therapy, stress management training and the Type A behavior pattern. *Cognitive Therapy and Research*, 1979, *3*, 61-75.

Jessup, B. A., Neufeld, R. W. J., & Merskey, H. Biofeedback therapy for headache and other pain: An evaluative review. *Pain*, 1979, *7*, 225-270.

Johansson, F., & von Knorring, L. A double-blind controlled study of a serotonin uptake inhibitor (Zimelidine) versus placebo in chronic pain. *Pain*, 1979, *7*, 69-78.

Johnson, E. M., & Stark, D. E. A group program for cancer patients and their family members in an acute care teaching hospital. *Social Work in Health Care*, 1980, *5*, 335-350.

Johnson, J. E. Effects of accurate expectations about sensation on the sensory and distress components of pain. *Journal of Personality and Social Psychology*, 1973, *27*, 261-275.

Johnson, J. E., Fuller, S. S., Endress, M. P., & Rice, V. H. Altering patients' responses to surgery: An extension and replication. *Research in Nursing and Health*, 1978, *1*, 111-121.

Johnson, J. E., Kirchhoff, K. T., & Endress, M. P. Altering children's distress behavior during orthopedic cast removal. *Nursing Research*, 1975, *75*, 404-410.

Johnson, J. E., & Leventhal, H. Effects of accurate expectations and behavioral instructions on reactions during a noxious medical examination. *Journal of Personality and Social Psychology*, 1974, *24*, 710-718.

Johnson, J. E., Morrissey, J. F., & Leventhal, H. Psychological preparation for an endoscopic examination. *Gastrointestinal Endoscopy*, 1973, *19*, 180-182.

Johnson, R. F. Q. Suggestions for pain reduction and response to cold-induced pain. *Psychological Record*, 1974, *24*, 161-169.

Jonas, S. *Medical mystery: The training of doctors in the United States.* New York: W. W. Norton, 1978.

Jones, R. A., Wiese, H. J., Moore, R. W., & Haley, J. V. On the perceived meaning of symptoms. *Medical Care*, 1981, *19*, 710-717.

Joyce, C. R. B., Caple, E., Mason, M., Reynolds, E., & Matthews, J. A. Quantification study of doctor-patient communication. *Quarterly Journal of Medicine*, 1969, *38*, 183-194.

Kahn, R. L., Wolfe, R. P., Quinn, R. P., Snoek, J. D., & Rosenthal, R. A. *Organizational stress: Studies in role conflict and ambiguity.* New York: Wiley, 1964.

Kahneman, D. *Attention and effort.* Englewood Cliffs, N.J.: Prentice-Hall, 1973.

Kanfer, F. H., & Goldfoot, D. A. Self-control and tolerance of noxious stimulation. *Psychology Reports*, 1966, *18*, 79-85.

Kanfer, F. H., & Saslow, G. Behavioral diagnosis. In C. Franks (Eds.), *Behavior therapy: Appraisal and status.* New York: Appleton-Century-Crofts, 1969.

Kanfer, F. H., & Seidner, M. L. Self control: Factors enhancing tolerance of noxious stimulation. *Journal of Personality and Social Psychology*, 1973, *24*, 381-389.

Kannel, W. B. Some lessons in cardiovascular epidemiology from Framingham. *American Journal of Cardiology*, 1976, *37*, 269-282.

Kannel, W. B., & Dawber, T. R. Hypertensive cardiovascular disease: The Framingham study. In G. Onesti, K. E. Tim, & J. H. Moyer (Eds.), *Hypertension: Mechanism and management.* New York: Grune & Stratton, 1973.

Kaplan, B. H., Cassel, J. C., & Gore, S. Social support and health. *Medical Care*, 1977, *15*, 47-58.

Karmel, M. *Thank you, Dr. Lamaze.* Philadelphia: J. B. Lippincott, 1959.

Karol, R. L., Doerfler, L. A., Parker, J. C., & Armentrout, D. P. A therapist manual for the cognitive–behavioral treatment of chronic pain. *JSAS Catalog of Selected Documents in Psychology*, 1981, *11*, 15–16. (Ms. No. 2205)

Kasl, S. V. Social-psychological characteristics associated with behaviors which reduce cardiovascular risk. In A. J. Enelow & J. B. Henderson (Eds.), *Applying behavioral science to cardiovascular risk*. New York: American Heart Association, 1975. (a)

Kasl, S. V. Issues in patient adherence to health care regimens. *Journal of Human Stress*, 1975, *1*, 5–17. (b)

Kasl, S. V. Cardiovascular risk reduction in a community setting: Some comments. *Journal of Consulting and Clinical Psychology*, 1980, *48*, 143–149.

Kasl, S. V., & Cobb, S. Health behavior, illness behavior and sick-role behavior. I. Health and illness behavior. *Archives of Environmental Health*, 1966, *12*, 246–266. (a)

Kasl, S. V., & Cobb, S. Health behavior, illness behavior, and sick-role behavior. II. Sick-role behavior. *Archives of Environmental Health*, 1966, *12*, 531–541. (b)

Katz, J. L., Weiner, H., Gallagher, T. G., & Hellman, L. Stress, distress and ego defenses. *Archives of General Psychiatry*, 1970, *23*, 131–142.

Katz, J. L., Weiner, H., Gutmann, A., & Yu, T. F. Hyperuricemia, gout and executive suite. *Journal of the American Medical Association*, 1973, *224*, 1251–1257.

Kazdin, A. E. Covert modeling and the reduction of avoidance behavior. *Journal of Abnormal Psychology*, 1973, *81*, 87–95.

Kazdin, A. E., & Wilcoxon, L. A. Systematic desensitization and nonspecific treatment effects: A methodological evaluation. *Psychological Bulletin*, 1976, *83*, 729–758.

Keefe, F. J. Assessment strategies in behavioral medicine. In J. R. McNamara (Ed.), *Behavioral approaches to medicine: Applications and analysis*. New York: Plenum, 1979.

Keefe, F. J., & Rosenstiel, A. K. *Development of a questionnaire to assess cognitive coping strategies in chronic pain patients*. Paper presented at the 14th annual convention of the Association for Advancement of Behavior Therapy, New York, November 1980.

Keller, M. The disease concept of alcoholism revisited. *Journal of Studies on Alcohol*, 1976, *37*, 1694–1717.

Kendall, P. C. Stressful medical procedures: Cognitive behavioral strategies for stress management and prevention. In D. H. Meichenbaum & M. E. Jaremko (Eds.), *Stress prevention and management: A cognitive–behavioral approach*. New York: Plenum, 1982.

Kendall, P. C., & Hollon, S. D. Cognitive–behavioral interventions: Overview and current status. In P. C. Kendall & S. D. Hollon (Eds.), *Cognitive–behavioral interventions: Theory, research, and procedures*. New York: Academic Press, 1979.

Kendall, P. C., & Hollon, S. D. Assessing self-referent speech: Methods in the measurement of self-statements. In P. C. Kendall & S. D. Hollon (Eds.), *Cognitive–behavioral interventions: Assessment methods*. New York: Academic Press, 1980. (a)

Kendall, P. C., & Hollon, S. D. (Eds.). *Assessment strategies for cognitive–behavioral interventions*. New York: Academic Press, 1980. (b)

Kendall, P. C., Williams, L., Pechacek, T. F., Graham, L. E., Shisslak, C., & Herzoff, N. Cognitive–behavioral and patient education interventions in cardiac catheterization procedures: The Palo Alto medical psychology project. *Journal of Consulting and Clinical Psychology*, 1979, *47*, 49–58.

Kerr, F. W. L. Pain: A central inhibitory balance theory. *Mayo Clinic Proceedings*, 1975, *50*, 685–690.

Khatami, M., & Rush, A. J. A pilot study of the treatment of outpatients with chronic pain. Symptom control, stimulus control and social system intervention. *Pain*, 1978, *5*, 163–172.

Kiesler, D. Some myths of psychotherapy research and the search for a paradigm. *Psychological Bulletin*, 1966, *65*, 110–136.

Kimble, G., & Perlmutter, L. The problem of volition. *Psychological Review*, 1970, *77*, 361–384.

Klein, G. S. *Perception, motives and personality*. New York: Alfred Knopf, 1970.

Klein, R. F. Relationship between psychological and physiological stress in the coronary care unit. In W. D. Gentry & R. B. Williams, Jr. (Eds.), *Psychological aspects of myocardial infarction and coronary care*. St. Louis: C. V. Mosby, 1975.

Klein, R. F., Dean, A., & Willson, M. L. The physician and post-myocardial infarction invalidism. *Journal of the American Medical Association*, 1965, *194*, 123–128.

Klepac, R. K., Dowling, J., Hauge, G., & McDonald, M. *Cognitive strategies for reducing dental avoidance: Preliminary data*. Paper presented at the second annual convention of the Society for Behavioral Medicine, New York, November 1980.

Klepac, R. K., Hauge, G., Dowling, J., & McDonald, M. Direct and generalized effects of three components of stress inoculation for increased pain tolerance. *Behavior Therapy*, 1981, *12*, 417–424.

Klusman, L. E. Reduction of pain in childbirth by the alleviation of anxiety during pregnancy. *Journal of Consulting and Clinical Psychology*, 1975, *43*, 162–165.

Knapp, T. W., & Florin, I. The treatment of migraine headache by training in vasoconstriction of the temporal artery and a cognitive stress-coping training. *Behavioral Analysis and Modification*, 1981, *4*, 267–274.

Knox, V. J. Cognitive strategies for coping with pain: Ignoring vs. acknowledging. *Dissertation Abstracts International*, 1973, *34* (5-B), 2308.

Koenig, P. The placebo effect in patent medicine. *Psychology Today*, April 1973, *7*, 60.

Koestler, A. *Darkness at noon*. London: Jonathan Cape, 1940.

Kotarba, J. A. Chronic pain center. A study of voluntary client compliance and entrepreneurship. *American Behavior Scientist*, 1981, *24*, 786–800.

Krantz, D. S. Cognitive processes and recovery from heart attack: A review and theoretical analysis. *Journal of Stress*, 1980, *6*, 27–38.

Kremer, E., Block, A., Morgan, C., & Gaylor, M. Behavioral approaches to pain management: Social communication skills and pain relief. In D. Osborne & D. Eiser (Eds.), *Psychology and medicine*. New York: Academic Press, 1980.

Kremsdorf, R. B., Kochanowicz, N. A., & Costell, S. Cognitive skills training versus EMG biofeedback in the treatment of tension headaches. *Biofeedback and Self-Regulation*, 1981, *6*, 93–102.

Kristein, M. M. Economic issues in prevention. *Preventive Medicine*, 1977, *6*, 252–264.

Kroger, W. S., & Fezler, W. D. *Hypnosis and behavior modification: Imagery conditioning*. Philadelphia: J. B. Lippincott, 1976.

Kubler-Ross, E. *On death and dying*. New York: Macmillan, 1969.

Kunckle, C. Phasic pains induced by cold. *Journal of Abnormal Physiology*, 1949, *1*, 811–824.

Lack, D. Z., & Bloom, D. M. *Results of treatment of a heterogeneous group of patients with chronic benign pain in a community hospital*. Paper presented at the Second World Congress on Pain, Montreal, Canada, August 1978.

Lader, M. H., & Mathews, A. M. A physiological model of phobic anxiety and desensitization. *Behaviour Research and Therapy*, 1968, *6*, 411–421.

Ladouceur, R., & Carrier, C. *Awareness and pain control*. Paper presented at the annual convention of the Association for Advancement of Behavior Therapy, San Francisco, December 1979.

REFERENCES

401

Lalonde, M. *A new perspective on the health of Canadians.* Ottawa, Ontario: Ministry of National Health & Welfare, 1974.

Lamaze, F. [*Painless childbirth*] (L. R. Celestin, trans.). London: Burke, 1958.

Lambert, W., Libman, E., & Poser, E. The effect of increased salience of a membership group on pain tolerance. *Journal of Personality,* 1960, *28,* 350.

Lando, H. A. *Stimulus control, rapid smoking, and contractual management in the maintenance of nonsmoking.* Unpublished manuscript, Iowa State University, Ames, 1977.

Lange, A., & Jakubowski, P. *Responsible assertive behavior.* Champaign, Ill.: Research Press, 1976.

Langer, E. J., Janis, I. L., & Wolfer, J. A. Reduction of psychological stress in surgical patients. *Journal of Experimental Social Psychology,* 1975, *1,* 155–165.

Laskin, D. M., & Greene, C. S. Influence of the doctor–patient relationship on placebo therapy for patients with myofascial pain-dysfunction (MPD) syndrome. *Journal of the American Dental Association,* 1972, *85,* 892–894.

Lassner, J. (Ed.). *Hypnosis in anesthesiology.* Berlin: Springer-Verlag, 1964.

Lazarus, A. A. *Behavior therapy and beyond.* New York: McGraw-Hill, 1972.

Lazarus, A. A., & Fay, A. Resistance or rationalization? A cognitive–behavioral perspective. In P. L. Wachtel (Ed.), *Resistance: Psychodynamic and behavioral approaches.* New York: Plenum, 1982.

Lazarus, R. S. *Psychological stress and the coping process.* New York: McGraw-Hill, 1966.

Lazarus, R. S. A cognitively oriented psychologist looks at biofeedback. *American Psychologist,* 1975, *30,* 553–560. (a)

Lazarus, R. S. The self-regulation of emotion. In L. Levi (Ed.), *Emotions—Their parameters and measurement.* New York: Raven, 1975. (b)

Lazarus, R. S. A strategy for research on psychological and social factors in hypertension. *Journal of Human Stress,* 1978, *4,* 35–40.

Lazarus, R. S., & Cohen, J. B. Environmental stress. In I. Altman & J. F. Wohlwill (Eds.), *Human behavior and the environment: Current theory and research.* New York: Plenum, 1977.

Lazarus, R. S., & Launier, R. Stress-related transactions between person and environment. In L. A. Pervin & M. Lewis (Eds.), *Perspectives in interactional psychology.* New York: Plenum, 1978.

Lea, P., Ware, P., & Monroe, R. The hypnotic control of intractable pain. *American Journal of Clinical Hypnosis,* 1960, *3,* 3–8.

Ledwidge, B. Cognitive behavior modification: A step in the wrong direction? *Psychological Bulletin,* 1978, *85,* 353–375.

Ledwidge, B. Cognitive behavior modification or new ways to change minds: Reply to Mahoney and Kazdin. *Psychological Bulletin,* 1979, *86,* 1050–1053.

Lefebvre, M. F. Cognitive distortion and cognitive errors in depressed psychiatric and low back pain patients. *Journal of Consulting and Clinical Psychology,* 1981, *49,* 517–525.

Lefer, L. A psychoanalytic view of a dental phenomenon. *Contemporary Psychoanalysis,* 1966, *2,* 135–150.

Leon, G. R. Current directions in the treatment of obesity. *Psychological Bulletin,* 1976, *83,* 557–578.

Leon, G. R., Roth, L., & Hewitt, M. I. Eating patterns, satiety, and self-control behavior of obese persons during weight reduction. *Obesity and Bariatric Medicine,* 1977, *6,* 172–181.

LeShan, L. The world of the patient in severe pain of long duration. *Journal of Chronic Diseases*, 1964, *17*, 119–126.

Levendusky, P., & Pankratz, L. Self-control techniques as an alternative to pain medication. *Journal of Abnormal Psychology*, 1975, *84*, 165–168.

Leventhal, H., Ahles, T., & Butler, L. *Cognitive control of pain: Attention to the sensory aspects of the cold pressor stimulus.* Unpublished manuscript, University of Wisconsin, Madison, 1977.

Leventhal, H., Meyer, D., & Nerenz, D. The common sense representation of illness danger. In S. Rachman (Ed.), *Medical psychology* (Vol. 2). London: Pergamon, 1980.

Leventhal, H., Safer, M. A., Cleary, P. D., & Gutmann, M. Cardiovascular risk modification by community-based programs for life-style change: Comments on the Stanford study. *Journal of Consulting and Clinical Psychology*, 1980, *48*, 150–158.

Levi, L. *Occupational stress: Sources, management, and prevention.* Reading, Mass.: Addison-Wesley, 1979.

Levine, S. B. Sexual dysfunction and diabetes. In B. A. Hambug, L. F. Lipsett, C. E. Inoff, & A. L. Drash (Eds.), *Behavioral and psychosocial aspects of diabetes: Proceedings of a national conference* (NIH Publication No. 80-1993). Washington, D.C.: U.S. Government Printing Office, 1981.

Levy, R., & Carter, R. Compliance with practitioner instructions. *Social Work*, 1976, *21*, 188–193.

Lewin, K. *A dynamic theory of personality: Selected papers.* New York: McGraw-Hill, 1935.

Lichtenstein, E., & Danaher, B. G. Modification of smoking behavior: A critical analysis of theory, research and practice. In M. Hersen, R. M. Eisler, & P. M. Miller (Eds.), *Progress in behavior modification* (Vol. 3). New York: Academic Press, 1976.

Liebeskind, J. C., & Paul, L. A. Psychological and physiological mechanisms of pain. *Annual Review of Psychology*, 1977, *28*, 41–60.

Linehan, M. M. Issues in behavioral interviewing. In J. D. Cone & R. P. Hawkins (Eds.), *Behavioral assessment: New directions in clinical psychology.* New York: Brunner/ Mazel, 1977.

Lloyd, M. A., & Appel, J. B. Signal detection theory and the psychophysics of pain: An introduction and overview. *Psychosomatic Medicine*, 1976, *38*, 79–94.

Locke, E. A. Behavior modification is not cognitive and other myths: A reply to Ledwidge. *Cognitive Therapy and Research*, 1979, *3*, 119–126.

Loftus, E. Leading questions and eyewitness report. *Cognitive Psychology*, 1975, *7*, 560–572.

LoGerfo, J. P. Hypertension: Management in a prepaid health care project. *Journal of the American Medical Association*, 1975, *223*, 245–248.

Loro, A. D., Jr., Levenkron, J. C., & Fisher, E. B., Jr. Critical clinical issues in the behavioral treatment of obesity. *Addictive Behaviors*, 1979, *4*, 383–391.

Louks, J. L., Freeman, C. W., & Calsyn, D. A. Personality organization as an aspect of back pain in a medical setting. *Journal of Personality Assessment*, 1978, *42*, 152–158.

Lovallo, W. The cold pressor test and autonomic function: A review and integration. *Psychophysiology*, 1975, *12*, 268–283.

Ludwig, A. M. On and off the wagon: Reasons for drinking and abstaining by alcoholics. *Quarterly Journal of Studies on Alcohol*, 1972, *33*, 91–96.

Maccoby, N., Farquhar, J. W., Wood, P. D., & Alexander, J. Reducing the risk of cardiovascular disease: Effects of a community-based campaign on knowledge and behavior. *Journal of Community Health*, 1977, *3*, 100–114.

MacKay, C. *Extraordinary popular delusions and the madness of crowds.* New York: The Noonday Press, 1956. (Originally published, 1841.)

Mahoney, M. J. *Cognition and behavior modification.* Cambridge, Mass.: Ballinger, 1974. (a)

Mahoney, M. J. Self-reward and self-monitoring techniques for weight control. *Behavior Therapy*, 1974, *5*, 48–57. (b)

Mahoney, M. J. The obese eating style: Bites, beliefs, and behavior modification. *Addictive Behaviors*, 1975, *1*, 47–53.

Mahoney, M. J. Cognitive therapy and research: A question of questions. *Cognitive Therapy and Research*, 1977, *1*, 5–16. (a)

Mahoney, M. J. On the continuing resistance to thoughtful therapy. *Behavior Therapy*, 1977, *8*, 673–677. (b)

Mahoney, M. J. Reflections on the cognitive-learning trend in psychotherapy. *American Psychologist*, 1977, *37*, 6–13. (c)

Mahoney, M. J. Some applied issues in self-monitoring. In J. D. Cone & R. P. Hawkins (Eds.), *Behavioral assessment: New directions in clinical psychology*. New York: Brunner/Mazel, 1977. (d)

Mahoney, M. J. Cognitive and noncognitive views in behavior modification. In P. O. Sjoden, S. Bates, & W. S. Dockens (Eds.), *Trends in behavior therapy*. New York: Academic Press, 1979.

Mahoney, M. J., & Arnkoff, D. Cognitive and self-control therapies. In S. L. Garfield & A. E. Bergin (Eds.), *Handbook of psychotherapy and behavior change: An empirical analysis*. New York: Wiley, 1978.

Mahoney, M. J., & Kazdin, A. E. Cognitive behavior modification: Misconceptions and premature evaluation. *Psychological Bulletin*, 1979, *86*, 1044–1049.

Mahoney, M. J., & Mahoney, K. *Permanent weight control*. New York: W. W. Norton, 1976.

Mahoney, M. J., Moura, H., & Wade, T. The relative efficacy of self-reward, self-punishment and self-monitoring techniques. *Journal of Consulting and Clinical Psychology*, 1973, *40*, 404–407.

Maiman, L. A., Becker, M. H., Kirscht, J. P., Haefner, D. P., & Drachman, R. H. Scales for measuring health belief model dimensions: A test of predictive value, internal consistency, and relationship among beliefs. *Health Education Monographs*, 1977, *5*, 215–230.

Maisto, S. A., Lauerman, R., & Adesso, V. J. A comparison of two experimental studies of the role of cognitive factors in alcoholics' drinking. *Journal of Studies of Alcohol*, 1977, *38*, 145–149.

Malec, J., Glasgow, R. E., Ely, R., & Kling, J. Coping with pain: A self-management approach. JSAS *Catalog of Selected Documents in Psychology*, 1977, *7*, 113. (Ms. No. 1601)

Malow, R. M., & Dougher, M. J. A signal detection analysis of the effects of transcutaneous stimulation on pain. *Psychosomatic Medicine*, 1979, *41*, 101–108.

Maltzman, I. Orienting in classical conditioning and generalization of the galvanic skin response to words: An overview. *Journal of Experimental Psychology: General*, 1977, *106*, 111–119.

Marbach, J. J., & Dworkin, S. F. Chronic MPD, group therapy and psychodynamics. *Journal of the American Dental Association*, 1975, *90*, 827–833.

Marlatt, G. A. Alcohol, stress, and cognitive control. In I. G. Sarason & C. D. Spielberger (Eds.), *Stress and anxiety* (Vol. 3). Washington, D.C.: Hemisphere, 1976.

Marlatt, G. A. Craving for alcohol, loss of control, and relapse: A cognitive–behavioral analysis. In P. E. Nathan, G. A. Marlatt, & T. Loberg (Eds.), *Alcoholism: New directions in behavioral research and treatment*. New York: Plenum, 1978.

Marlatt, G. A. Alcohol use and problem drinking: A cognitive–behavioral analysis. In P. C. Kendall & S. D. Hollon (Eds.), *Cognitive–behavioral interventions: Theory, research and procedures*. New York: Academic Press, 1979.

Marlatt, G. A., Demming, B., & Reid, J. B. Loss of control drinking in alcoholics: An experimental analogue. *Journal of Abnormal Psychology*, 1973, *81*, 233–241.

Marlatt, G. A., & Gordon, J. R. Determinants of relapse: Implications for the maintenance of behavior change. In P. O. Davidson & S. M. Davidson (Eds.), *Behavioral medicine: Changing health life styles*. New York: Brunner/Mazel, 1980.

Marlatt, G. A., & Rohsenow, D. J. Cognitive processes in alcohol use: Expectancy and the balanced placebo design. In N. K. Mello (Ed.), *Advances in substance abuse: Behavioral and biological research*. Greenwich, Conn.: JAI Press, 1980.

Marmer, M. J. *Hypnosis and anesthesia*. Springfield, Ill.: Charles C Thomas, 1969.

Marmor, J. The psychodynamics of realistic worry. *Psychoanalysis and Social Science*, 1958, *5*, 155–163.

Marston, M. V. Compliance with medical regimens. A review of the literature. *Nursing Research*, 1970, *19*, 312–323.

Martin, M. J. Tension headache, a psychiatric study. *Headache*, 1966, *6*, 47–54.

Martin, P. R. Behavioral management of headaches: A review of the evidence. *International Journal of Mental Health*, 1980, *9*, 88–110.

Martin, P. R., & Mathews, A. M. Tension headaches: Psychophysiological investigation and treatment. *Journal of Psychosomatic Research*, 1978, *22*, 389–399.

Martin, R. W., & Chapman, C. R. Dental dolorimetry for human pain research: Methods and apparatus. *Pain*, 1979, *6*, 349–364.

Maruta, T., Swanson, D. W., & Swenson, W. M. Chronic pain: Which patients may a pain-management program help? *Pain*, 1979, *7*, 321–329.

Mason, J. W. A re-evaluation of the concept of "non-specificity" in stress theory. *Journal of Psychiatric Research*, 1971, *8*, 323–333.

Mason, J. W. Clinical psychophysiology. In M. F. Reiser (Ed.), *American handbook of psychiatry* (Vol. 4). New York: Basic Books, 1975. (a)

Mason, J. W. A historical view of the stress field, part I. *Journal of Human Stress*, 1975, *1*, 6–12. (b)

Mason, J. W. A historical view of the stress field, part II. *Journal of Human Stress*, 1975, *1*, 22–36. (c)

Mason, J. W., Buescher, E. L., Belfer, M. L., Artenstein, M. S., & Mougey, E. H. A prospective study of corticosteroid and catecholamine levels in relation to viral respiratory illness. *Journal of Human Stress*, 1979, *5*, 18–27.

Mattson, A., & Gross, S. Social and behavioral studies on hemophilic children and their families. *Journal of Pediatrics*, 1966, *68*, 952.

McAlister, A., Perry, C., & Maccoby, N. Adolescent smoking: Onset and prevention. *Pediatrics*, 1979, *63*, 650–658.

McBurney, D. H. Acupuncture, pain and signal detection theory. *Science*, 1975, *189*, 66.

McBurney, D. H. Correspondence: Signal detection theory and pain. *Anesthesiology*, 1976, *44*, 355–358.

McCaffery, M. *Nursing management of the patient with pain* (2nd ed.). Philadelphia: J. B. Lippincott, 1979.

McCaffery, M., Morra, M. E., Gross, J., & Moritz, D. A. *Dealing with pain: A handbook for persons with cancer and their families*. New Haven, Conn.: Yale Comprehensive Cancer Center, 1980.

McCreary, C., Turner, J., & Dawson, E. Differences between functional versus organic low back pain patient. *Pain*, 1977, *4*, 73–78.

McCreery, D. B., & Bloedel, J. R. A critical examination of the use of signal detection theory in evaluating a putative analgesic–transcutaneous electrical nerve stimulation. *Sensory Processes*, 1978, *2*, 38–57.

McDaniel, J. V. *Physical disability and human behavior.* Elmsford, N.Y.: Pergamon, 1969.

McDonald, G. W. The diabetes supplement of the national health survey. *Journal of the American Diabetes Association,* 1968, *52,* 118–120.

McGlashan, T. H., Evans, F. J., & Orne, M. T. The nature of hypnotic analgesia and placebo response to experimental pain. *Psychosomatic Medicine,* 1969, *31,* 227–246.

McGuire, W. Inducing resistance to persuasion: Some controversial approaches. In L. Berkowitz (Ed.), *Advances in social psychology* (Vol. 1). New York: Academic Press, 1964.

McKay, C. J., & Cox, T. (Eds.). *Response to stress: Occupational aspects.* London: International Publishing Corporation, 1979.

McLean, A. (Ed.). *Occupational stress.* Springfield, Ill.: Charles C Thomas, 1974.

McLean, A. *Work stress.* Reading, Mass.: Addison-Wesley, 1979.

McLean, A., Black, G., & Colligan, M. (Eds.). *Reducing occupational stress* (DHEW (NIOSH) Publication No. 78-140). Cincinnati: National Institute of Occupational Safety and Health, 1978.

McNamara, J. R. (Ed.). *Behavioral approaches in medicine: Application and analysis.* New York: Plenum, 1979.

Mechanic, D. *Medical sociology.* New York: The Free Press, 1976.

Mechanic, D. Effects of psychological distress on perceptions of physical health and use of medical and psychiatric facilities. *Journal of Human Stress,* 1978, *4,* 26–32.

Meichenbaum, D. H. Examination of model characteristics in reducing avoidance behavior. *Journal of Personality and Social Psychology,* 1971, *17,* 298–307.

Meichenbaum, D. H. A cognitive-behavior modification approach to assessment. In M. Hersen & A. S. Bellack (Eds.), *Behavioral assessment: A practical handbook.* Elmsford, N.Y.: Pergamon, 1976. (a)

Meichenbaum, D. H. Cognitive factors in biofeedback therapy. *Biofeedback and Self-Regulation,* 1976, *1,* 201–216. (b)

Meichenbaum, D. H. Toward a cognitive theory of self control. In G. E. Schwartz & D. Shapiro (Eds.), *Consciousness and self-regulation* (Vol. 1). New York: Plenum, 1976. (c)

Meichenbaum, D. H. *Cognitive-behavior modification: An integrative approach.* New York: Plenum, 1977.

Meichenbaum, D. H. Why does using imagery in psychotherapy lead to change? In J. Singer & K. Pope (Eds.), *The power of human imagination.* New York: Plenum, 1978.

Meichenbaum, D. H. Cognitive behavior modification: The need for a fairer assessment. *Cognitive Therapy and Research,* 1979, *3,* 127–132.

Meichenbaum, D. H. *Coping with stress.* London: Multimedia Publications, in press.

Meichenbaum, D. H., Burland, S., Gruson, L., & Cameron, R. Metacognitive assessment. In S. Yussen (Ed.), *The development of reflection.* New York: Academic Press, 1980.

Meichenbaum, D. H., & Butler, L. Cognitive ethology: Addressing the streams of cognition and emotion. In K. Blankstein, P. Pliner, & J. Polivy (Eds.), *Advances in the study of communication and affect* (Vol. 6: *Assessment and modification of emotional behavior*). New York: Plenum, 1979.

Meichenbaum, D. H., & Cameron, R. *An examination of cognitive and contingency variables in anxiety relief procedures.* Unpublished manuscript, University of Waterloo, 1972. (a)

Meichenbaum, D. H., & Cameron, R. *Stress inoculation: A skills-training approach to anxiety management.* Unpublished manuscript, University of Waterloo, 1972. (b)

Meichenbaum, D. H., & Cameron, R. Cognitive-behavior therapy. In G. T. Wilson & C. M. Franks (Eds.), *Contemporary behavior therapy.* New York: Guilford, 1982.

Meichenbaum, D. H., & Genest, M. A cognitive–behavioral approach: An illustration in the group treatment of anxiety. In G. Harris (Ed.), *The group treatment of human problems: A social learning approach.* New York: Grune & Stratton, 1977.

Meichenbaum, D. H., & Gilmore, J. B. Resistance: From a cognitive–behavioral perspective. In P. L. Wachtel (Ed.), *Resistance in psychodynamic and behavioral therapies.* New York: Plenum, 1982.

Meichenbaum, D. H., & Jaremko, M. E. (Eds.). *Stress prevention and management: A cognitive–behavioral approach.* New York: Plenum, 1982.

Meichenbaum, D. H., & Turk, D. C. The cognitive–behavioral management of anxiety, anger, and pain. In P. O. Davidson (Ed.), *The behavioral management of anxiety, depression and pain.* New York: Brunner/Mazel, 1976.

Meichenbaum, D. H., & Turk, D. C. Stress, coping, and disease: A cognitive behavioral perspective. In R. W. J. Neufeld (Ed.), *Psychological stress and psychopathology.* New York: McGraw-Hill, 1982.

Melamed, B. G., & Siegel, L. J. Reduction of anxiety in children facing hospitalization and surgery by use of filmed modeling. *Journal of Consulting and Clinical Psychology,* 1975, *43,* 511–521.

Melamed, B. G., & Siegel, L. J. *Behavioral medicine: Practical applications in health care.* New York: Springer, 1980.

Melzack, R. *The puzzle of pain.* Harmondsworth, England: Penguin, 1973.

Melzack, R. The McGill Pain Questionnaire: Major properties and scoring methods. *Pain,* 1975, *1,* 277–299. (a)

Melzack, R. Prolonged relief of pain by brief, intense, transcutaneous somatic stimulation. *Pain,* 1975, *1,* 357–373. (b)

Melzack, R. Pain mechanisms and stress. *Stress,* 1980, *1,* 18–23. (a)

Melzack, R. Psychologic aspects of pain. *Pain,* 1980, *9,* 143–154. (b)

Melzack, R., & Casey, K. L. Sensory, motivational and central control determinants of pain: A new conceptual model. In D. Kenshalo (Ed.), *The skin senses.* Springfield, Ill.: Charles C Thomas, 1968.

Melzack, R., & Dennis, S. G. Neurophysiological foundations of pain. In R. A. Sternbach (Ed.), *The psychology of pain.* New York: Raven, 1978.

Melzack, R., Ofiesch, J., & Mount, B. The Brompton mixture: Effects on pain in cancer patients. *Canadian Medical Association Journal,* 1976, *115,* 125–129.

Melzack, R., & Perry, C. Self-regulation of pain: The use of alpha-feedback and hypnotic training for the control of chronic pain. *Experimental Neurology,* 1975, *46,* 452–469.

Melzack, R., & Scott, T. H. The effects of early experience on the response to pain. *Journal of Comparative and Physiological Psychology,* 1957, *50,* 155–161.

Melzack, R., & Torgerson, W. S. On the language of pain. *Anesthesiology,* 1971, *34,* 50–59.

Melzack, R., & Wall, P. Pain mechanisms: A new theory. *Science,* 1965, *50,* 971–979.

Melzack, R., & Wall, P. Psychophysiology of pain. *International Anesthesiology Clinic,* 1970, *8,* 3–34.

Melzack, R., Weisz, A. Z., & Sprague, L. T. Strategems for controlling pain: Contributions of auditory stimulation and suggestion. *Experimental Neurology,* 1963, *8,* 239–247.

Merluzzi, T. V., Glass, C. R., & Genest, M. (Eds.). *Cognitive assessment.* New York: Guilford, 1981.

Merskey, H., & Spear, F. G. The reliability of the pressure algometer. *British Journal of Social and Clinical Psychology,* 1964, *3,* 130–136.

Meyer, A. J., Nash, J. D., McAlister, A. L., Maccoby, N., & Farquhar, J. W. Skills training in a cardiovascular health education campaign. *Journal of Consulting and Clinical Psychology,* 1980, *48,* 129–142.

Meyer, E., & Mendelson, M. Psychiatric consultation with patients in medical and surgical wards: Patterns and processes. *Psychiatry*, 1961, *24*, 197-220.

Meyerowitz, B. E. Psychosocial correlates of breast cancer and its treatments. *Psychological Bulletin*, 1980, *57*, 108-131.

Miller, N. E. Introduction: Current issues and key problems. In D. Shapiro (Ed.), *Biofeedback and self-control, 1973*. Chicago: Aldine, 1974.

Miller, N. E. Application of learning and biofeedback to psychiatry and medicine. In A. M. Freedman, H. I. Kaplan, & B. J. Sadock (Eds.), *Comprehensive textbook of psychiatry*. Baltimore: Williams & Wilkins, 1975.

Miller, N. E. The role of learning in physiological response to stress. In G. Serban (Ed.), *Psychopathology of human adaptation*. New York: Plenum, 1976.

Miller, N. E. Behavioral medicine: New opportunities but serious dangers. *Behavioral Medicine Update*, 1979, *1*, 5-7.

Miller, P. M., Hersen, M., Eisler, R. M., & Hilsman, G. Effects of social stress on operant drinking of alcoholics and social drinkers. *Behaviour Research and Therapy*, 1974, *12*, 67-72.

Mills, R. T., & Krantz, D. S. Information, choice, and reactions to stress-experiment in a blood-bank with laboratory analog. *Journal of Personality and Social Psychology*, 1979, *37*, 608-620.

Mitchell, K. R., & Mitchell, D. M. Migraine: An exploratory treatment application of programmed behavior therapy techniques. *Journal of Psychosomatic Research*, 1971, *15*, 137-157.

Mitchell, K. R., & White, R. G. The control of migraine headache by behavioural self-management: A controlled case study. *Headache*, 1976, *16*, 178-184. (a)

Mitchell, K. R., & White, R. G. Self-management of tension headaches: A case study. *Journal of Behavior Therapy and Experimental Psychiatry*, 1976, *7*, 387-389. (b)

Mitchell, K. R., & White, R. G. Behavioral self-management: An application to the problem of migraine headaches. *Behavior Therapy*, 1977, *8*, 213-222.

Moore, P. A., Duncan, G. H., Scott, D. S., Gregg, J. M., & Ghia, J. N. The submaximal effort tourniquet test: Its use in evaluating experimental and chronic pain. *Pain*, 1979, *6*, 375-382.

Moos, R. H., & Tsu, V. The crisis of physical illness: An overview. In R. M. Moos (Ed.), *Coping with physical illness*. New York: Plenum, 1977.

Morgan, D. C., Kremer, E., & Gaylor, M. The behavioral medicine unit: A new facility. *Comprehensive Psychiatry*, 1979, *20*, 79-89.

Morganstern, K. P. Behavioral interviewing: The initial stages of assessment. In M. Hersen & A. S. Bellack (Eds.), *Behavioral assessment: A practical guide*. Elmsford, N.Y.: Pergamon, 1976.

Mount, B. The problem of caring for the dying in a general hospital: The palliative care unit as a possible solution. *Canadian Medical Association Journal*, 1976, *115*, 122-124.

Murphy, T. Cancer pain. *Postgraduate Medicine*, 1973, *53*, 187-194.

Murphy, T. Evaluating the individual patient with chronic pain: Roundtable discussion. *Patient Care*, 1978, *12*, 28-30; 35; 37; 39-41; 44; 46; 50-51; 55-60.

Murray, H. A. *Explorations in personality*. New York: Oxford University Press, 1938.

Murray, R., & Kijek, J. C. (Eds.). *Current perspective in rehabilitation nursing*. St. Louis: C. V. Mosby, 1979.

Nathan, P. W. The gate-control theory of pain: A critical review. *Brain*, 1976, *99*, 123-158.

Neal, H. *The politics of pain*. New York: McGraw-Hill, 1978.

Neisser, U. *Cognitive psychology*. New York: Appleton-Century-Crofts, 1967.

Nelson, R. O. Methodological issues in assessment via self-monitoring. In J. D. Cone & R. P. Hawkins (Eds.), *Behavioral assessment: New directions in clinical psychology.* New York: Brunner/Mazel, 1977.

Neufeld, R. W. J. The effect of experimentally altered cognitive appraisal on pain tolerance. *Psychonomic Science,* 1970, *20,* 106–107.

Neufeld, R. W. J., & Davidson, P. O. The effects of vicarious and cognitive rehearsal on pain tolerance. *Journal of Psychosomatic Research,* 1971, *15,* 319–325.

Newman, J. E., & Beehr, T. A. Personal and organizational strategies for handling job stress: A review of research and opinion. *Personnel Psychology,* 1979, *32,* 1–43.

Newman, R. I., Seres, J. L., Yospe, L. P., & Garlington, B. Multidisciplinary treatment of chronic pain: Long-term follow-up of low-back pain patients. *Pain,* 1978, *4,* 283–292.

Nisbett, R., & Ross, L. *Human inference: Strategies and shortcomings of social judgment.* Englewood Cliffs, N.J.: Prentice-Hal, 1980.

Nisbett, R., & Wilson, T. D. Telling more than we know: Verbal reports on mental processes. *Psychological Review,* 1977, *84,* 231–259.

Noordenbos, W. *Pain.* Amsterdam: Elsevier, 1959.

Norr, K. L., Block, C. R., Charles, A., Meyering, S., & Meyers, E. Explaining pain and enjoyment in childbirth. *Journal of Health and Social Behavior,* 1977, *18,* 260–275.

Notermans, S. L. H. Measurement of the pain threshold determined electrical stimulation and its clinical application. *Neurology,* 1966, *16,* 1071–1087.

Nouwen, A., & Solinger, J. W. The effectiveness of the EMG biofeedback training in low back pain. *Biofeedback and Self-Regulation,* 1979, *4,* 103–111.

Novaco, R. W. Functions and regulation of the arousal of anger. *American Journal of Psychiatry,* 1976, *133,* 1124–1128. (a)

Novaco, R. W. Treatment of chronic anger through cognitive and relaxation controls. *Journal of Consulting and Clinical Psychology,* 1976, *44,* 681. (b)

Novaco, R. W. A stress inoculation approach to anger management in the training of law enforcement officers. *American Journal of Community Psychology,* 1977, *5,* 327–346.

Novaco, R. W. Anger and coping with stress: Cognitive behavioral interventions. In. J. P. Foreyt & D. P. Rathjen (Eds.), *Cognitive behavior therapy: Research and application.* New York: Plenum, 1978.

Novaco, R. W., Cook, T., & Sarason, I. G. Military recruit training: An area for stress coping skills. In D. H. Meichenbaum & M. E. Jaremko (Eds.), *Stress prevention and management: A cognitive-behavioral approach.* New York: Plenum, 1982.

Noyes, R., Jr. Treatment of cancer pain. *Psychosomatic Medicine,* 1981, *43,* 57–70.

Nuechterlein, K. H., & Holroyd, J. C. Biofeedback in the treatment of tension headache: Current status. *Archives of General Psychiatry,* 1980, *37,* 866–873.

Obrist, P. The cardiovascular-behavioral interaction—As it appears today. *Psychophysiology,* 1976, *13,* 95–107.

Ost, L.-G., & Gotestam, K. G. Behavioral and pharmacological treatments for obesity: An experimental comparison. *Addictive Behaviors,* 1976, *1,* 331–338.

The pain clinic: Boon or boondoggle? *Patient Care,* 1978, *12,* 188–189.

Palmblad, J., Cantell, K., Strander, H., Froberg, J., Karlsson, C., Levi, L., Granstrom, M., & Unger, P. Stressor exposure and immunological response in man: Interferon-producing capacity and phagocytosis. *Journal of Psychosomatic Research,* 1976, *20,* 193–199.

Parsons, T. Illness and the role of the physician: A sociological perspective. *American Journal of Orthopsychiatry,* 1951, *21,* 452–460.

Parsons, T. Definitions of health and illness in the light of American values and social structure. In E. G. Jaco (Ed.), *Patients, physicians, and illness*. New York: The Free Press, 1958.

Patel, C. H., & North, W. R. S. Randomized control trial of yoga and biofeedback in management of hypertension. *Lancet*, 1975, *2*, 93–99.

Pattie, F. A. Methods of induction, susceptibility of subjects, and criteria in hypnosis. In R. M. Dorcus (Ed.), *Hypnosis and its therapeutic applications*. New York: McGraw-Hill, 1956.

Paul, G. L. *Insight vs. desensitization in psychotherapy: An experiment in anxiety reduction.* Stanford, Calif.: Stanford University Press, 1966.

Paulley, J. W., & Haskell, D. J. Treatment of migraine without drugs. *Journal of Psychosomatic Research*, 1975, *19*, 367–374.

Pavlov, I. P. *Conditioned reflexes*. London: Milford, 1927.

Pavlov, I. P. *Lectures on conditioned reflexes*. London: International Publishers, 1928.

Pechacek, T. F., & Danaher, B. G. How and why people quit smoking: A cognitive–behavioral analysis. In P. C. Kendall & S. D. Hollon (Eds.), *Cognitive-behavioral interventions: Theory, research, and procedures.* New York: Academic Press, 1979.

Pechacek, T. F., & McAlister, A. Strategies for the modification of smoking behavior: Treatment and prevention. In J. Ferguson & C. B. Taylor (Eds.), *A comprehensive handbook of behavioral medicine.* New York: Spectrum, 1979.

Pederson, L. L., & Lefcoe, N. M. A psychological and behavioral comparison of ex-smokers and smokers. *Journal of Chronic Disease*, 1976, *29*, 431–434.

Perri, M. G., Richards, C. S., & Schultheis, K. R. Behavioral self-control and smoking reductions. A study of self-initiated attempts to reduce smoking. *Behavior Therapy*, 1977, *8*, 360–365.

Perry, C., Gelfand, R., & Markovitch, P. The relevance of hypnotic susceptibility in clinical context. *Journal of Abnormal Psychology*, 1979, *88*, 592–603.

Peterson, D. *The clinical study of social behavior.* Englewood Cliffs, N.J.: Prentice-Hall, 1968.

Peterson, L., & Shigetomi, C. The use of coping techniques to minimize anxiety in hospitalized children. *Behavior Therapy*, 1981, *12*, 1–14.

Petrie, A. *Individuality in pain and suffering.* Chicago: University of Chicago Press, 1967.

Petrovich, D. V. The Pain Apperception Test: Psychological correlates of pain perception. *Journal of Clinical Psychology*, 1958, *14*, 367–374.

Petrov-Maskakov, M. A. Physiopsychoprophylactic preparation for labor in pathology of pregnancy. In N. Morris (Ed.), *Psychsomatic medicine in obstetrics and gynecology.* New York: Karger, 1972.

Pettingale, K. W., Greer, S., & Tee, D. E. Serum IgA and emotional expression in breast cancer patients. *Psychosomatic Research*, 1977, *21*, 395–399.

Philips, C. A psychological analysis of tension headache. In S. Rachman (Ed.), *Contributions to medical psychology* (Vol. 1). Oxford, England: Pergamon, 1977.

Philips, C. Tension headache: Theoretical problems. *Behaviour Research and Therapy*, 1978, *16*, 249–261.

Phillips, L. W. Training in sensory and imaginal responses in behavior therapy. In R. D. Rubin, H. Fensterheim, A. A. Lazarus, & C. M. Franks (Eds.), *Advances in behavior therapy.* New York: Academic Press, 1971.

Pilowsky, I., Chapman, C. R., & Bonica, J. J. Pain, depression, and illness behavior in a pain clinic population. *Pain*, 1977, *4*, 183–192.

Pilowsky, I., & Spence, N. D. Patterns of illness behaviour in patients with intractable pain. *Journal of Psychosomatic Research*, 1975, *19*, 279–288.

Pilowsky, I., & Spence, N. D. Illness behavior syndromes associated with intractable pain. *Pain*, 1976, *2*, 61–71. (a)

Pilowsky, I., & Spence, N. D. Is illness behavior related to chronicity in patients with intractable pain? *Pain*, 1976, *2*, 167–173. (b)

Pilowsky, I., & Spence, N. D. Pain and illness behaviour: A comparative study. *Journal of Psychosomatic Research*, 1976, *20*, 131–134. (c)

Pinsky, J. J. The behavioral consequences of chronic intractable benign pain. *Behavioral Medicine*, 1980, *7*, 12–20.

Pirat, J. Diabetes mellitus and its degenerative complications: A prospective study of 4,400 patients observed between 1947–1973 (Part 1). *Diabetes Care*, 1978, *3*, 168–188.

Plato. [*Charmides in the dialogues of Plato*] (B. Jowett, trans.). Chicago: Encyclopedia Britannica, 1952.

Pollin, W. Foreword. In M. E. Jarvik (Ed.), *Research on smoking behavior* (DHEW Publication No. (ADM) 78–581). Washington, D.C.: U.S. Department of Health, Education & Welfare, 1977.

Pomerleau, O. F., Adkins, D. M., Pertschuk, M. Predictors of outcome and recidivism in smoking cessation treatment. *Addictive Behaviors*, 1978, *3*, 65–70.

Pomerleau, O. F., & Brady, J. P. (Eds.). *Behavioral medicine: Theory and practice*. Baltimore: Williams & Wilkins, 1979.

Poser, E. G. A simple and reliable apparatus for the measurement of pain. *American Journal of Psychology*, 1962, *75*, 304–305.

Power, L. Placebos and medical research. *San Francisco Chronicle*, March 15, 1978, p. 24.

Pranulis, M. Coping with acute myocardial infarction. In W. D. Gentry & R. B. Williams (Eds.), *Psychological analysis of myocardial infarction and coronary care*. St. Louis: C. V. Mosby, 1975.

Price, K. P., & Tursky, B. The effect of varying stimulus parameters on judgments of nociceptive electrical stimulation. *Psychophysiology*, 1975, *12*, 663–666.

Prieto, E. J., Hopson, L., Bradley, L. A., Byrne, M., Geisinger, K. F., Midax, D., & Marchisello, P. J. The language of low back pain: Factor structure of the McGill Pain Questionnaire. *Pain*, 1980, *8*, 11–19.

Prokop, C. K., & Bradley, L. A. (Eds.). *Medical psychology: Contributions to behavioral medicine*. New York: Academic Press, 1981.

Qualls, P. J., & Sheehan, P. W. Electromyograph biofeedback as a relaxation technique: A critical appraisal and reassessment. *Psychological Bulletin*, 1981, *90*, 21–42.

Rabkin, J. G., & Struening, E. L. Life events, stress and illness. *Science*, 1976, *194*, 1013–1020.

Rachman, S. Systematic desensitization. *Psychological Bulletin*, 1967, *67*, 93–103.

Raft, D., Toomey, T., & Gregg, J. M. Behavior modification and haloperidol in chronic facial pain. *Southern Medical Journal*, 1979, *72*, 155–159.

Raimy, V. *Misunderstanding of the self: Cognitive psychotherapy and the misconception hypothesis*. San Francisco: Jossey-Bass, 1975.

Rapaport, D. On the psychoanalytic theory of motivation. In M. M. Gill (Ed.), *The collected papers of David Rapaport*. New York: Basic Books, 1970. (Originally published, 1960.)

Reading, A. E. The internal structure of the McGill Pain Questionnaire in dysmenorrhea patients. *Pain*, 1979, *7*, 353–358. (a)

Reading, A. E. Short-term effects of psychological preparation for surgery. *Social Science & Medicine—Medical Psychology & Sociology*, 1979, *13A*, 641–654. (b)

Reading, A. E., & Martin, R. The treatment of mandibular dysfunction pain. *British Dental Journal*, 1976, *140*, 201–205.

Reeves, J. EMG-biofeedback reduction of tension headache. *Biofeedback and Self-Regulation*, 1976, *1*, 217–225.

Reid, D. E., & Cohen, M. E. Evaluation of present day trends in obstetrics. *Journal of the American Medical Association*, 1950, *142*, 615–623.

Rimon, R. A psychosomatic approach to rheumatoid arthritis: A clinical study of 100 female patients. *Acta Rheumatologica Scandinavica*, 1969, *13* (Supplement).

Roberts, A. H., & Reinhardt, L. The behavioral management of chronic pain: Long term follow-up with comparison groups. *Pain*, 1980, *8*, 151–162.

Rodin, J. Somatophysics and attribution. *Personality and Social Psychology Bulletin*, 1978, *4*, 531–540.

Rodin, J. *Cognitive behavior therapy for obesity*. New York: BMA Audio Cassettes, 1979.

Rogers, M. P., Dubey, D., & Reich, P. The influence of the psyche and the brain on immunity and disease susceptibility: A critical review. *Psychosomatic Medicine*, 1979, *41*, 147–164.

Rollman, G. B. Signal detection theory measurement of pain: A review and critique. *Pain*, 1977, *3*, 187–211.

Rollman, G. B. Signal detection theory pain measures: Empirical validation studies and adaptation level effects. *Pain*, 1979, *6*, 9–21.

Rook, K. S., & Hammen, C. L. A cognitive perspective on the experience of sexual arousal. *Journal of Social Issues*, 1977, *33*, 7–29.

Rose, R. M. Endocrine responses to stressful psychological events. *Psychiatric Clinics of North America*, 1980, *3*, 251–276.

Rosenbaum, M. Individual differences in self-control behaviors and tolerance of painful stimulation. *Journal of Abnormal Psychology*, 1980, *89*, 581–590. (a)

Rosenbaum, M. A schedule for assessing self-control behaviors: Preliminary findings. *Behavior Therapy*, 1980, *11*, 74–86. (b)

Rosenman, R. H., Brand, R. J., Jenkins, C. D., Friedman, M., Straus, R., & Wurm, M. Coronary heart disease in the Western Collaborative Group Study: Final follow-up experience of 8.5 years. *Journal of the American Medical Association*, 1975, *233*, 872–877.

Rosenman, R. H., Brand, R. J., Sholtz, R. I., & Friedman, M. Multivariate prediction of coronary heart disease during 8.5 year follow-up in the Western Collaborative Group Study. *American Journal of Cardiology*, 1976, *37*, 903–910.

Rosenman, R. H., & Friedman, M. Modifying Type A behaviour pattern. *Journal of Psychosomatic Research*, 1977, *21*, 323–331.

Rosenman, R. H., Friedman, M., Straus, R., Wurm, M., Kositchek, R., Hahn, W., & Werthessen, N. T. A predictive study of coronary heart disease: The Western Collaborative Group Study. *Journal of the American Medical Association*, 1964, *189*, 15–22.

Rosenman, R. H., Rahe, R. H., Borhani, N. O., & Feinlieb, M. Heritability of personality and behavior pattern. *Proceedings of the First International Congress on Twins*, University of Rome, 1975.

Roskies, E. Considerations in developing a treatment program for the coronary-prone (Type A) behavior pattern. In P. O. Davidson & S. M. Davidson (Eds.), *Behavioral medicine: Changing health life styles*. New York: Brunner/Mazel, 1980.

Roskies, E. Stress management for Type A individuals. In D. H. Meichenbaum & M. Jaremko (Eds.), *Stress prevention and management: A cognitive-behavioral approach*. New York: Plenum, 1982.

Roskies, E., Kearney, H., Spevack, M., Surkis, A., Cohen, C., & Gilman, S. Generalizability and durability of treatment effects in an intervention program for coronary-prone (Type A) managers. *Journal of Behavioral Medicine*, 1979, *2*, 195–207.

Roskies, E., & Lazarus, R. S. Coping theory and the teaching of coping skills. In P. O. Davidson & S. M. Davidson (Eds.), *Behavioral medicine: Changing health life styles*. New York: Brunner/Mazel, 1980.

Roskies, E., Spevack, M., Surkis, A., Cohen, C., & Gilman, S. Changing the coronary-prone (Type A) behavior pattern in a nonclinical population. *Journal of Behavioral Medicine*, 1978, *2*, 201–216.

Russell, M. A. H. Cigarette smoking: Natural history of a dependence disorder. *British Journal of Medical Psychology*, 1971, *44*, 1–16.

Russell, R., & Sipich, J. Cue-controlled relaxation in the treatment of test anxiety. *Journal of Behavior Therapy and Experimental Psychiatry*, 1973, *4*, 47–49.

Russo, D. C., Bird, P. O., & Masek, B. J. Assessment issues in behavioral medicine. *Behavioral Assessment*, 1980, *2*, 1–18.

Rybstein-Blinchik, E. Effects of different cognitive strategies on chronic pain experience. *Journal of Behavioral Medicine*, 1979, *2*, 93–101.

Rybstein-Blinchik, E., & Grzesiak, R. C. Reinterpretative cognitive strategies in chronic pain management. *Archives of Physical Medicine and Rehabilitation*, 1979, *60*, 609–612.

Rychtarik, R., & Wollersheim, J. The role of cognitive mediators in alcohol with some implications for treatment. JSAS *Catalog of Selected Documents in Psychology*, 1978, *11*, 203. (Ms. No. 1763)

Sacerdote, P. The use of hypnosis in cancer patients. *Annals of the New York Academy of Sciences*, 1966, *126*, 1011–1019.

Sacerdote, P. Theory and practice of pain control in malignancy and other protracted or recurring painful illness. *International Journal of Clinical and Experimental Hypnosis*, 1970, *18*, 160–180.

Sacerdote, P. Hypnosis and terminal illness. In G. D. Burrows & L. Dennerstein (Eds.), *Handbook of hypnosis and psychosomatic medicine*. New York: Elsevier North-Holland, 1980.

Sachs, L. B., Feuerstein, M., & Vitale, J. H. Hypnotic self-regulation of chronic pain. *American Journal of Clinical Hypnosis*, 1977, *20*, 106–113.

Sackett, D. L., & Haynes, R. B. *Compliance with therapeutic regimens*. Baltimore: The Johns Hopkins University Press, 1976.

Samuels, M., & Samuels, N. *Seeing with the mind's eye: History, techniques, and uses of visualization*. New York: Random House, 1975.

Sarason, I. G. Anxiety and self-preoccupation. In I. G. Sarason & C. D. Spielberger (Eds.), *Stress and anxiety* (Vol. 2). Washington, D.C.: Hemisphere, 1975.

Sarason, I. G., Johnson, J. H., Berberich, J. P., & Siegel, J. M. Helping police officers to cope with stress: A cognitive–behavioral approach. *American Journal of Community Psychology*, 1979, *7*, 593–603.

Sarbin, T. R., & Coe, W. C. *Hypnosis: A social psychological analysis of influence communication*. New York: Holt, Rinehart & Winston, 1972.

Sargent, J., Green, E., & Walters, E. Preliminary report on the use of autogenic feedback training in the treatment of migraine and tension headaches. *Psychosomatic Medicine*, 1973, *35*, 129–135.

Saunders, C. Control of pain in terminal cancer. *Nursing Times*, 1976, *72*, 1133–1135.

Saunders, C. The nature of terminal pain and the hospice concept. In J. Bonica & V. Ventafridda (Eds.), *Advances in pain research and therapy* (Vol. 2). New York: Raven, 1979.

Scherwitz, L. K., Berton, K., & Leventhal, H. Type A assessment and interaction in the Behavior Pattern Interview. *Psychosomatic Medicine*, 1977, *39*, 229–240.

Schofield, A. T. *The force of mind*. London: J. & A. Churchill, 1902.

Schwartz, G. E. Biofeedback as therapy: Some theoretical and practical issues. *American Psychologist*, 1973, *28*, 666–673.

Schwartz, L., & Choyes, L. M. *Facial pain and mandibular dysfunction*. Philadelphia: W. B. Saunders, 1968.

Schwartz, R. M., & Gottman, J. M. Toward a task analysis of assertive behavior. *Journal of Consulting and Clinical Psychology*, 1976, *44*, 910–920.

Scott, D. S. Experimenter-suggested cognitions and pain control: The problem of spontaneous strategies. *Psychological Reports*, 1978, *37*, 122–129.

Scott, D. S., & Barber, T. X. Cognitive control of pain: Effects of multiple cognitive strategies. *Psychological Record*, 1977, *27*, 373–383. (a)

Scott, D. S., & Barber, T. X. Cognitive control of pain: Four serendipitous results. *Perceptual and Motor Skills*, 1977, *44*, 569–570. (b)

Scott, D. S., & Leonard, D. S. Modification of pain threshold by the covert reinforcement procedure and a cognitive strategy. *Psychological Record*, 1978, *28*, 49–57.

Scott, J. R., & Rose, N. B. Effect of psychoprophylaxis (Lamaze preparation) on labor and delivery in primiparas. *New England Journal of Medicine*, 1976, *294*, 1205–1207.

Seeburg, K. N., & DeBoer, K. F. Effects of EMG biofeedback on diabetes. *Biofeedback and Self-Regulation*, 1980, *5*, 289–293.

Seer, P. Psychological control of essential hypertension: Review of the literature and methodological critique. *Psychological Bulletin*, 1979, *86*, 1015–1043.

Seligman, M. E. P. *Helplessness: On depression, development, and death*. San Francisco: W. H. Freeman, 1975.

Selye, H. *The stress of life*. New York: McGraw-Hill, 1956.

Seres, J. L., & Newman, R. I. Results of treatment of chronic low back pain at the Portland Pain Center. *Journal of Neurosurgery*, 1976, *45*, 32–36.

Shacham, S. *Imagery and suggestion in pain reduction*. Unpublished manuscript, University of Wisconsin, Madison, 1977. (Cited in H. Leventhal & D. Everhart. Emotion, pain, and physical illness. In C. E. Izard (Ed.), *Emotion and psychopathology*. New York: Plenum, 1979.)

Shacham, S., & Leventhal, H. *Attention and the control of distress during cold pressor impact*. Unpublished manuscript, University of Wisconsin, Madison, 1978. (Cited in H. Leventhal & D. Everhart. Emotion, pain, and physical illness. In C. E. Izard (Ed.), *Emotion and psychopathology*. New York: Plenum, 1979.)

Shapiro, A. K. Psychological aspects of medication. In H. I. Lief, V. F. Lief, & N. R. Lief (Eds.), *The psychological bases of medical practice*. New York: Hoeber, 1963.

Shapiro, D., Tursky, B., Schwartz, G., & Shnidman, S. Smoking on cue: A behavioral approach to smoking reduction. *Journal of Health and Social Behavior*, 1971, *12*, 108–113.

Shapiro, H. I., & Schmitt, L. G. Evaluation of the psychoprophylactic method of childbirth in primigravida. *Connecticut Medicine*, 1973, *37*, 341–343.

Shawver, M. Pain associated with cancer. In A. Jacox (Ed.), *Pain: A source book for nurses and other health professionals*. Boston: Little, Brown, 1977.

Shealy, C. N. *The pain game*. Millbrae, Calif.: Celestial Arts, 1976.

Shealy, C. N., & Shealy, M. C. Behavioral techniques in the control of pain: A case for health maintenance vs. disease treatment. In M. Weisenberg & B. Tursky (Eds.), *Pain: New perspectives in theory and research*. New York: Plenum, 1975.

Shelton, J. L., & Ackerman, J. M. *Homework in counseling and psychotherapy.* Springfield, Ill.: Charles C Thomas, 1974.

Sherrington, C. S. *The integration action of the nervous system.* London: Constable, 1906.

Shipley, R. H., Butt, J. H., & Horowitz, E. A. Preparation to reexperience a stressful medical examination: Effect of repetitious videotape exposure and coping style. *Journal of Consulting and Clinical Psychology,* 1979, *47,* 485–492.

Shipley, R. H., Butt, J. H., Horowitz, B., & Fabry, J. E. Preparation for a stressful medical procedure: Effect of amount of stimulus preexposure and coping style. *Journal of Consulting and Clinical Psychology,* 1978, *46,* 499–507.

Shontz, F. *The psychological aspects of physical illness and disability.* New York: Macmillan, 1975.

Siegel, S. Morphine tolerance acquisition as an associative process. *Journal of Experimental Psychology: Animal Behavior Processes,* 1977, *3,* 1–13.

Silver, R. L., & Wortman, C. B. Coping with undesirable life events. J. Garber & M. E. P. Seligman (Eds.), *Human helplessness: Theory and applications.* New York: Academic Press, 1980.

Simon, E. J., Hiller, J. M., & Edelman, I. Solubility of a stereospecific opiate–macromolecular complex from rat brain. *Science,* 1975, *190,* 389–390.

Simonton, O., Matthews-Simonton, S., & Sparks, T. Psychological intervention in the treatment of cancer. *Psychosomatics,* 1980, *21,* 226–233.

Singer, J., & Pope, K. (Eds.). *The power of human imagination.* New York: Plenum, 1978.

Sjoberg, L., & Johnson, T. Trying to give up smoking: A study of volitional breakdowns. *Addictive Behaviors,* 1978, *3,* 139–164.

Sjoberg, L., & Persson, L.-O. A study of attempts by obese patients to regulate eating. *Addictive Behaviors,* 1979, *4,* 349–359.

Sjolund, B., Terenius, L., & Eriksson, M. Increased cerebrospinal fluid levels of endorphins after electroacupuncture. *Acta Physiologica Scandinavica,* 1977, *100,* 382–384.

Skyler, J. S. Living with the complications of diabetes. In B. A. Hamburg, L. F. Lipsett, G. E. Inoff, & A. L. Drash (Eds.), *Behavioral and psychosocial issues in diabetes: Proceedings of a national conference* (NIH Publication No. 80-1993). Washington, D.C.: U.S. Government Printing Office, 1981.

Smith, G. M., & Beecher, H. K. Experimental production of pain in man: Sensitivity of a new method to 600 mg of aspirin. *Clinical Pharmacology and Therapeutics,* 1969, *10,* 213–216.

Smith, G. M., Egbert, L., Markowitz, R., Mosteller, F., & Beecher, H. K. An experimental pain method sensitive to morphine in man: The submaximum effort tourniquet technique. *Journal of Pharmacology and Experimental Therapeutics,* 1966, *145,* 324–332.

Snyder, S. H. Opiate receptors and internal opiates. *Scientific American,* 1977, *236,* 44–56.

Sobel, H. J. Projective methods of cognitive analysis. In T. V. Merluzzi, C. R. Glass, & M. Genest (Eds.), *Cognitive assessment.* New York: Guilford, 1981.

Sobel, H. J., & Worden, J. W. *Helping cancer patients cope.* New York: BMA Audio Cassettes, 1981.

Solomon, G. F., Amkraut, A. D., & Kasper, P. Immunity, emotions, and disease. *Annals of Clinical Research,* 1974, *6,* 313–322.

Soule, A. B., Copans, S. A., Standley, K., & Duchowny, M. S. Local regional anesthesia during childbirth: Effect on newborn behaviors. *Science,* 1974, *186,* 634–635.

South India agog at painless birth. *Kitchener-Waterloo Record,* March 15, 1974, p. 12.

Spanos, N. P., Barber, T. X., & Lang, G. Effects of hypnotic induction, suggestions of analgesia, and demands for honesty on subjective reports of pain. *Journal of Abnormal Psychology,* 1974, *83,* 356–363.

Spanos, N. P., & Bodorik, H. L. Suggested amnesia and disorganized recall in hypnotic and task-motivated subjects. *Journal of Abnormal Psychology*, 1977, *56*, 295–305.

Spanos, N. P., & Chaves, J. F. Hypnosis research: A methodological critique of two alternative paradigms. *American Journal of Clinical Hypnosis*, 1970, *13*, 108–127.

Spanos, N. P., & Hewitt, E. C. The hidden observer in hypnotic analgesia: Discovery or experimental creation? *Journal of Personality and Social Psychology*, 1980, *39*, 1201–1214.

Spanos, N. P., Horton, C., & Chaves, J. F. The effect of two cognitive strategies in pain threshold. *Journal of Abnormal Psychology*, 1974, *84*, 677–681.

Spanos, N. P., Radtke-Bodorik, H. L., Ferguson, J. D., & Jones, B. The effects of hypnotic susceptibility, suggestions for analgesia, and the utilization of cognitive strategies on the reduction of pain. *Journal of Abnormal Psychology*, 1979, *88*, 282–292.

Spanos, N. P., Stam, H. J., & Brazil, K. The effects of suggestion and distraction on coping ideation and reported pain. *Journal of Mental Imagery*, in press.

Spanos, N. P., Stam, H. J., D'Eon, J. L., Pawlak, A. E., & Radtke-Bodorik, H. L. Effects of social psychological variables on hypnotic amnesia. *Journal of Personality and Social Psychology*, 1980, *39*, 737–750.

Speers, M. A., & Turk, D. C. Diabetes self-care: Knowledge, beliefs, motivation and action. *Patient Counselling and Health Education*, 1982, *4*, 144–149.

Spielberger, C. D., & De Nike, L. D. Descriptive behaviorism versus cognitive theory in verbal operant conditioning. *Psychological Review*, 1966, *73*, 306–326.

Staats, A. W. (with contributions by C. K. Staats). *Complex human behavior*. New York: Holt, Rinehart & Winston, 1963.

Stahler, F., Stahler, E., & Gutanian, R. Perinatal mortality of the child lowered by psychoprophylaxis. In N. Morris (Ed.), *Psychosomatic medicine in obstetrics and gynecology*. New York: Karger, 1972.

Stam, H. J., & Spanos, N. P. Experimental designs, expectancy effects, and hypnotic analgesia. *Journal of Abnormal Psychology*, 1980, *89*, 751–762.

Stambaugh, E. E., II, & House, A. E. Multimodality treatment of migraine headache: A case study utilizing biofeedback, relaxation, autogenic and hypnotic treatments. *American Journal of Clinical Hypnosis*, 1977, *19*, 235–240.

Staub, E., Tursky, B., & Schwartz, G. E. Self-control and predictability: Their effects on reactions to aversive stimulation. *Journal of Personality and Social Psychology*, 1971, *18*, 157–162.

Steffy, R., Meichenbaum, D. H., & Best, J. A. Aversive and cognitive factors in the modification of smoking behavior. *Behaviour Research and Therapy*, 1970, *8*, 115–125.

Stenn, P. G., Mothersill, K. J., & Brooke, R. I. Biofeedback and a cognitive behavioral approach to treatment of myofascial pain dysfunction syndrome. *Behavior Therapy*, 1979, *10*, 29–36.

Stern, J. A., Brown, M., Ulett, G. A., & Sletten, J. A comparison of hypnosis, acupuncture, morphine, Valium, aspirin, and placebo in the management of experimentally induced pain. *Annals of the New York Academy of Sciences*, 1977, *296*, 175–193.

Sternbach, R. A. *Pain: A psychophysiological analysis*. New York: Academic Press, 1968.

Sternbach, R. A. *Pain patients: Traits and treatment*. New York: Academic Press, 1974. (a)

Sternbach, R. A. Varieties of pain games. In J. J. Bonica (Ed.), *Advances in neurology* (Vol. 4). New York: Raven, 1974. (b)

Sternbach, R. A. Treatment of the chronic pain patient. *Journal of Human Stress*, 1978, *4*, 11–15. (a)

Sternbach, R. A. Clinical aspects of pain. In R. A. Sternbach (Ed.), *The psychology of pain*. New York: Raven, 1978. (b)

Sternbach, R. A., Deems, L. M., Timmermans, G., & Huey, L. I. On the sensitivity of the tourniquet pain test. *Pain*, 1977, *3*, 105–110.

Sternbach, R. A., Murphy, R. W., Akeson, W. H., & Wolf, S. R. Chronic low-back pain: The "low-back loser." *Postgraduate Medicine*, 1973, *53*, 135–138.

Sternbach, R. A., & Rusk, T. N. Alternatives to the pain career. *Psychotherapy: Theory, Research and Practice*, 1973, *10*, 321–324.

Stevens, J. O. *Awareness: Exploring, experimenting, experiencing*. Moab, Utah: Real People Press, 1971.

Stevens, R. J. Psychological strategies for management of pain in prepared childbirth. II: A study of the psychoanalgesia in prepared childbirth. *Birth and the Family Journal*, 1977, *4*, 4–9.

Stevens, R. J., & Heide, F. Analgesic characteristics of prepared childbirth techniques: Attention focusing and systematic relaxation. *Journal of Psychosomatic Research*, 1977, *21*, 429–438.

Stone, C. I., Demchik-Stone, D. A., & Horan, J. J. Coping with pain: A component analysis of Lamaze and cognitive–behavioral procedures. *Journal of Psychosomatic Research*, 1977, *21*, 451–456.

Stone, D. B. A study of the incidence and causes of poor control in patients with diabetes mellitus. *American Journal of the Medical Sciences*, 1964, *241*, 64/436–69/441.

Stone, G. C. Patient compliance and the role of the expert. *Journal of Social Issues*, 1979, *35*, 34–59.

Stone, G. C., Cohen, F., & Adler, N. E. (Eds.). *Health psychology—A handbook*. San Francisco: Jossey-Bass, 1979.

Stoyva, J. Self-regulation and the stress-related disorders: A perspective on biofeedback. In D. I. Mostofsky (Ed.), *Behavior control and modification of physiological activity*. Englewood Cliffs, N.J.: Prentice-Hall, 1976.

Strassberg, D. S., & Klinger, B. I. The effect on pain tolerance of social pressure within the laboratory setting. *Journal of Social Psychology*, 1972, *88*, 123–130.

Stravino, V. D. Nature of pain. *Archives of Physical Medicine and Rehabilitation*, 1970, *51*, 37–44.

Strupp, H. Specific vs. nonspecific factors in psychotherapy and the problem of control. *Archives of General Psychiatry*, 1970, *23*, 393–401.

Stunkard, A. J. The management of obesity. *New York Journal of Medicine*, 1958, *58*, 79–87.

Stunkard, A. J. New therapies for the eating disorders: Behavior modification of obesity and anorexia nervosa. *Archives of General Psychiatry*, 1972, *26*, 391–398. (a)

Stunkard, A. J. The success of TOPS, a self-help group. *Postgraduate Medicine*, 1972, *51*, 143–147. (b)

Stunkard, A. J. Behavioral treatment of obesity: Failure to maintain weight loss. In R. B. Stuart (Ed.), *Behavioral self-management: Strategies, techniques, and outcomes*. New York: Brunner/Mazel, 1977. (a)

Stunkard, A. J. Testimony before select committee on nutrition and human needs: Part II. Obesity. Washington, D.C.: U.S. Government Printing Office, 1977. (b)

Stunkard, A. J., & Mahoney, M. J. Behavioral treatment of eating disorders. In H. Leitenberg (Ed.), *Handbook of behavior modification and behavior therapy*. Englewood Cliffs, N.J.: Prentice-Hall, 1976.

St. Van Eps, L. Psychoprophylaxis in labour. *Lancet*, 1955, *2*, 112–115.

Suinn, R. M., & Bloom, L. J. Anxiety management training for pattern A behavior. *Journal of Behavioral Medicine*, 1978, *1*, 25–37.

Swanson, D. W., Floreen, A. C., & Swenson, W. M. Program for managing chronic pain:

II. Short-term results. *Mayo Clinic Proceedings*, 1976, *51*, 409–411.

Swanson, D. W., Maruta, T., & Swenson, W. M. Results of behavior modification in the treatment of chronic pain. *Psychosomatic Medicine*, 1979, *41*, 55–61.

Swanson, D. W., Swenson, W. M., Maruta, T., & McPhee, M. C. Program for managing chronic pain. I. Program description and characteristics of patients. *Mayo Clinic Proceedings*, 1976, *51*, 401–408.

Swerdlow, M. The value of clinics for the relief of chronic pain. *Journal of Medical Ethics*, 1978, *4*, 117–118.

Syme, S. L. Implications and future prospects. In S. L. Syme & L. G. Reeder (Eds.), Social stress and cardiovascular disease. *Milbank Memorial Fund Quarterly*, 1967, *45*, 175–180.

Syme, S. L. Social and psychological risk factors in coronary heart disease. *Modern Concepts of Cardiovascular Diseases*, 1975, *14*, 17–21.

Szasz, T. S. The psychology of persistent pain. In A. Soulairac (Ed.), *Pain*. London: Academic Press, 1968.

Tamerin, J. S. The psychodynamics of quitting smoking in a group. *American Journal of Psychiatry*, 1972, *128*, 589–595.

Tan, S.-Y., Melzack, R., & Poser, E. G. Arthrogram pain: Cognitive–behavioral skills training and assessment measures. Paper presented at the annual convention of the American Psychological Association, Montreal, September 1980.

Tanzer, D. *The psychology of pregnancy and childbirth: An investigation of natural childbirth*. Unpublished doctoral dissertation, Brandeis University, 1967.

Tavormina, J. B., Kastner, L. S., Slater, P. M., & Watt, S. L. Chronically ill children: A psychologically and emotionally deviant population? *Journal of Child Psychology*, 1976, *4*, 99–110.

Taylor, C. B., Farquhar, J. W., Nelson, E., & Agras, S. Relaxation therapy and high blood pressure. *Archives of General Psychiatry*, 1977, *34*, 339–345.

Taylor, C. B., Zlutnick, S. I., Corley, M. J., & Flora, J. The effects of detoxification, relaxation, and brief supportive therapy on chronic pain. *Pain*, 1980, *8*, 303–318.

Thibaut, J. W., & Kelley, H. H. *The social psychology of groups*. New York: Wiley, 1959.

Thomas, A. N. *Doctor courageous*. New York: Harper & Row, 1957.

Thomas, L. The nature of disease. *The New Yorker*, January 22, 1978, *87*, 125–127; 129–135.

Thorpe, G. L. Desensitization, behavior rehearsal, self-instructional training and placebo effects on assertive-refusal behavior. *European Journal of Behavioral Analysis and Modification*, 1975, *1*, 30–44.

Toomey, T. C., Ghia, J. N., Mao, W., & Gregg, J. M. Acupuncture and chronic pain mechanisms: The moderating effects of affect, personality, and stress on response to treatment. *Pain*, 1977, *3*, 137–145.

Triesman, M. Mind, body and behavior: Control systems and their disturbances. In P. London & D. Rosenhan (Eds.), *Foundations of abnormal psychology*. New York: Holt, Rinehart & Winston, 1968.

Tupper, C. Conditioning for childbirth. *American Journal of Obstetrics and Gynecology*, 1956, *71*, 733–740.

Turk, D. C. *Cognitive control of pain: A skills-training approach*. Unpublished master's thesis, University of Waterloo, 1975.

Turk, D. C. *A coping skills-training approach for the control of experimentally produced pain*. Unpublished doctoral dissertation, University of Waterloo, 1977.

Turk, D. C. Cognitive-behavioral techniques in the management of pain. In J. P. Foreyt & D. P. Rathjen (Eds.), *Cognitive behavior therapy: Research and application*. New York: Plenum, 1978. (a)

Turk, D. C. *The application of cognitive and behavioral skills for pain regulation.* Paper presented at the annual meeting of the American Psychological Association, Toronto, August 1978. (b)

Turk, D. C. Coping with pain: A review of cognitive control techniques. Unpublished manuscript, Yale University, 1978. (c)

Turk, D. C. Unpublished treatment credibility data, Yale University, 1978. (d)

Turk, D. C. Factors influencing the adaptive process with chronic illness. In I. G. Sarason & C. D. Spielberger (Eds.), *Stress and anxiety* (Vol. 6). Washington, D.C.: Hemisphere, 1979.

Turk, D. C. Cognitive learning approaches in health care. In D. M. Doleys, R. L. Meredith, & A. R. Ciminero (Eds.), *Behavioral medicine: Assessment and treatment strategies.* New York: Plenum, 1982.

Turk, D. C., & Genest, M. Regulation of pain: The application of cognitive and behavioral techniques for prevention and remediation. In P. C. Kendall & S. D. Hollon (Eds.), *Cognitive–behavioral intervention: Theory, research, and procedures.* New York: Academic Press, 1979.

Turk, D. C., & Kerns, R. D. *Conceptual issues in the assessment of laboratory and clinical pain.* Paper presented at the annual meeting of the American Psychological Association, Toronto, August 1980.

Turk, D. C., & Kerns, R. D. *A comparison of three nonmedical treatments of chronic pain,* in progress.

Turk, D. C., Kerns, R. D., Bowen, W., & Rennert, K. *An outpatient cognitive–behavioral group approach for the management of chronic pain.* Paper presented at the Second Annual Meeting of the American Pain Society, New York, September 1980.

Turk, D. C., Meeks, S., & Turk, L. M. Factors contributing to teacher stress: Implications for research, prevention, and remediation. *Behavioral Counseling Quarterly,* 1982, *3,* 3–26.

Turk, D. C., Meichenbaum, D. H., & Berman, W. H. Application of biofeedback for the regulation of pain: A critical review. *Psychological Bulletin,* 1979, *86,* 1322–1338.

Turk, D. C., & Rennert, K. S. Pain and the terminally-ill cancer patient: A cognitive–social learning perspective. In H. J. Sobel (Ed.), *Behavior therapy in terminal care: A humanistic approach.* Cambridge, Mass.: Ballinger, 1981.

Turk, D. C., Sobel, H. J., Follick, M. J., Youkilis, H. D. A sequential criterion analysis for assessing coping with chronic illness. *Journal of Human Stress,* 1980, *6,* 35–40.

Turk, D. C., & Speers, M. A. Diabetes mellitus: A cognitive–functional analysis of stress and adherence. In T. Burish & L. Bradley (Eds.), *Coping with chronic disease: Research and applications.* New York: Academic Press, 1982.

Turk, D. C., & Speers, M. A. *Improving diabetic self-care: A problem-solving approach,* in progress.

Turk, D. C., & Wack, J. T. *Development of a classificatory system of strategies for coping with pain.* Invited address presented at the 59th general session of the International Association for Dental Research, Chicago, March 1981.

Turk, D. C., & Waldo, M. *Review and analysis of clinics designed to treat chronic pain.* Paper presented at the annual convention of the Association for Advancement of Behavior Therapy, San Francisco, December 1979.

Turnbull, F. Pain and suffering in cancer. *The Canadian Nurse,* 1971, *67,* 28–30.

Turner, J. A. *Evaluation of two behavioral interventions for chronic low back pain.* Unpublished doctoral dissertation, University of California at Los Angeles, Los Angeles, 1979.

Turner, J. A., & Chapman, C. R. Psychological interventions for chronic pain: A critical review. I. Relaxation training and biofeedback. *Pain*, 1982, *12*, 1–22.

Tursky, B. Physical, physiological, and psychological factors that affect pain reaction to electric shock. *Psychophysiology*, 1974, *11*, 95–112.

Tursky, B. Laboratory approaches to the study of pain. In D. I. Mostofsky (Ed.), *Behavioral control and modification of physiological activity*. Englewood Cliffs, N.J.: Prentice-Hall, 1976.

Twycross, R. Disease of the central nervous system: Relief of pain. *British Medical Journal*, 1975, *4*, 212–214.

Twycross, R. G. The assessment of pain in advanced cancer. *Journal of Medical Ethics*, 1978, *4*, 112–116.

Twycross, R. The Brompton cocktail. In J. J. Bonica & V. Ventafridda (Eds.), *Advances in pain research and therapy* (Vol. 2). New York: Raven, 1979.

United States Department of Health, Education & Welfare. *Recent trends in survival of cancer patients* (U.S. Public Health Service Publication No. 75-767). Washington, D.C.: U.S. Government Printing Office, 1975. (a)

United States Department of Health, Education & Welfare. *Third national cancer survey: Incidence data* (National Cancer Institute Monograph No. 41, U.S. Public Health Service Publication No. 75-787). Washington, D.C.: U.S. Government Printing Office, 1975. (b)

United States Department of Health, Education & Welfare. *Diabetes data compiled 1977.* (NIH Publication No. 79-1468). Washington, D.C.: U.S. Government Printing Office, 1979.

United States Public Health Service. *Adult use of tobacco: 1975*. Washington, D.C.: U.S. Department of Health, Education & Welfare, 1976.

United States Surgeon General. *Healthy people: The Surgeon General's report on health promotion and disease prevention* (U.S. Department of Health, Education & Welfare (PHS) Publication No. 79-55071). Washington, D.C.: U.S. Government Printing Office, 1979.

Van Auken, W. B. D., & Tomlinson, D. R. An appraisal of patient training for childbirth. *American Journal of Obstetrics and Gynecology*, 1953, *63*, 100–105.

Van Egeren, L. F. Psychophysiological aspects of systematic desensitization: Some outstanding issues. *Behaviour Research and Therapy*, 1971, *9*, 65–77.

Varni, J. W. Behavioral medicine in hemophilia arthritic pain management: Two case studies. *Archives of Physical Medicine and Rehabilitation*, 1981, *62*, 183–187. (a)

Varni, J. W. Self-regulation techniques in the management of chronic arthritic pain in hemophilia. *Behavior Therapy*, 1981, *12*, 185–194. (b)

Varni, J. W., Gilbert, A., & Dietrich, S. L. Behavioral medicine in pain and analgesia management for the hemophiliac child with Factor VIII inhibitor. *Pain*, 1981, *11*, 121–126.

Velvovsky, I., Platonov, K., Ploticher, V., & Shugom, E. (Eds.). [*Painless childbirth through prophylaxis*] (D. A. Myshne, trans.). Moscow: Foreign Languages Publishing House, 1960.

Vernon, D. T. A., & Bailey, W. C. The use of motion pictures in the psychological preparation of children for induction of anesthesia. *Anesthesiology*, 1974, *40*, 68–72.

Vincent, P. Factors influencing patient noncompliance: A theoretical approach. *Nursing Research*, 1971, *20*, 509–516.

Visotsky, H. M., Hamburg, D. A., Goss, M. E., & Lebovits, B. A. Coping under extreme stress: Observations of patients with severe poliomyelitis. *Archives of General Psychiatry*, 1961, *5*, 423–448.

Wachtel, P. L. *Psychoanalysis and behavior therapy.* New York: Basic Books, 1977.

Wack, J. T., & Turk, D. C. *Latent structure in strategies for coping with pain.* Paper presented at the second general meeting of the American Pain Society, New York, September 1980.

Wain, H. J. Hypnosis in the treatment of chronic pain. *American Journal of Clinical Hypnosis*, 1980, *23*, 41–46.

Wall, P. D. The gate control theory of pain mechanism: A reexamination and re-statement. *Brain*, 1978, *101*, 1–18.

Wall, P. D. On the relation of injury to pain. *Pain*, 1979, *6*, 253–264.

Walls, R. T., Werner, T. J., Bacon, A., & Zane, T. Behavior check lists. In J. D. Cone & R. P. Hawkins (Eds.), *Behavioral assessment: New directions in clinical psychology.* New York: Brunner/Mazel, 1977.

Watkins, J. D., Roberts, D. E., Williams, T. F., Martin, D. A., & Coyle, I. V. Observations of medication errors made by diabetic patients in the home. *Diabetes*, 1967, *16*, 832–835.

Watkins, J. D., Williams, T. F., Martin, D. A., Hogan, M. D., & Anderson, E. A study of diabetic patients at home. *American Journal of Public Health*, 1967, *57*, 452–459.

Watts, F. N. Behavioral aspects of the management of diabetes mellitus: Education, self-care, and metabolic control. *Behaviour Research and Therapy*, 1980, *18*, 171–180.

Wax, R. H., & Wax, M. L. How people stop smoking: An exploratory study. *Mid-American Review of Sociology*, 1978, *3*, 1–15.

Weiner, H. *Psychobiology and human disease.* New York: American Elsevier, 1977.

Weisenberg, M. Pain and pain control. *Psychological Bulletin*, 1977, *84*, 1008–1044.

Weisenberg, M. Understanding pain phenomena. In S. Rachman (Ed.), *Contributions to medical psychology* (Vol. 2). Oxford, England: Pergamon, 1980.

Weisman, A. D. Misgivings and misconceptions in the psychiatric care of terminal patients. *Psychiatry*, 1970, *33*, 67–81.

Weisman, A. D. *On dying and denying: A psychiatric study of terminality.* New York: Behavioral Publications, 1972.

Weisman, A. D. Early diagnosis of vulnerability in cancer patients. *American Journal of the Medical Sciences*, 1976, *27*, 187–196.

Weisman, A. D. *Coping with cancer.* New York: McGraw-Hill, 1979.

Weisman, A. D., & Sobel, H. J. Coping with cancer through self-instruction: A hypothesis. *Journal of Human Stress*, 1979, *5*, 3–8.

Weisman, A. D., & Worden, J. W. *Coping and vulnerability in cancer patients.* Unpublished research report, Project Omega, Department of Psychiatry, Harvard Medical School, Massachusetts General Hospital, 1977.

Weisman, A. D., Worden, J. W., & Sobel, H. J. *Psychosocial screening and intervention with cancer patients: Research report.* Cambridge, Mass.: Shea Bros., 1980.

Weitzenhoffer, A. M. *General techniques of hypnotism.* New York: Grune & Stratton, 1957.

Wepman, B. J. Biofeedback in the treatment of chronic myofascial pain dysfunction. *Psychosomatics*, 1980, *21*, 157–162.

Wernick, R. L. Stress inoculation in the management of clinical pain: Applications to burn patients. In D. H. Meichenbaum & M. E. Jaremko (Eds.), *Stress prevention and management: A cognitive–behavioral approach.* New York: Plenum, 1982.

Wernick, R. L., Jaremko, M. E., & Taylor, P. W. Pain management in severely burned adults: A test of stress inoculation. *Journal of Behavioral Medicine*, 1981, *4*, 103–109.

Wernick, R. L., Taylor, P. W., & Jaremko, M. E. *Assessment procedures and treatment manual for the use of stress inoculation with burn patients.* Unpublished manuscript, Medical University of South Carolina, Charleston, S.C., December 1978.

Westcott, T. B., & Horan, J. J. The effects of anger and relaxation forms of *in vivo* emotive imagery on pain tolerance. *Canadian Journal of Behavioural Science*, 1977, *9*, 216–223.

White, J. C., & Sweet, W. H. *Pain and the neurosurgeon: A forty-year experience.* Springfield, Ill.: Charles C Thomas, 1969.

White, R. W. Strategies of adaptation: An attempt at systematic description. In G. V. Coelho, D. A. Hamburg, & J. E. Adams (Eds.), *Coping and adaptation.* New York: Basic Books, 1974.

Willard, R. D. Perpetual trance as a means of controlling pain in the treatment of terminal cancer with hypnosis. *Journal of the American Institute of Hypnosis*, 1974, *15*, 111–131.

Williams, T. F., Martin, D. A., Hogan, M. D., Watkins, J. F., & Ellis, E. V. The clinical picture of diabetic control, studied in four settings. American Journal of Public Health, 1967, *57*, 441–451.

Wilson, G. T. *Cognitive factors in life-style changes: A social learning perspective.* Paper presented at the 10th Banff International Conference on Behavior Modification, Banff, Alberta, Canada, March 1978. (a)

Wilson, G. T. Methodological considerations in treatment outcome research on obesity. *Journal of Consulting and Clinical Psychology*, 1978, *46*, 687–702. (b)

Wilson, G. T. Booze, beliefs, and behavior: Cognitive processes in alcohol use and abuse. In P. E. Nathan, G. A. Marlatt, & T. Loberg (Eds.), *Alcoholism: New directions in behavioral research and treatment.* New York: Plenum, 1978. (c)

Wilson, G. T., & Abrams, D. Effects of alcohol on social anxiety and physiological arousal: Cognitive versus pharmacological processes. *Cognitive Therapy and Research*, 1977, *1*, 195–210.

Wilson, G. T., & Lawson, D. M. Expectancies, alcohol, and sexual arousal in male social drinkers. *Journal of Abnormal Psychology*, 1976, *85*, 587–594.

Wilson, J. F. Determinants of recovery from surgery: Preoperative instruction, relaxation training and defensive structure (Doctoral dissertation, University of Michigan, 1977). *Dissertation Abstracts International*, 1977, *38*, 1476–1477B.

Wine, J. Cognitive–attentional theory of text anxiety. In I. G. Sarason (Ed.), *Test anxiety: Theory, research and application.* Hillsdale, N.J.: Erlbaum, 1981.

Winett, R. A. Parameters of deposit contracts in the modification of smoking. *Psychological Record*, 1973, *23*, 49–60.

Wolfer, J. A., & Visintainer, M. A. Pediatric surgical patients' and parents' stress responses and adjustment as a function of psychologic preparation and stress-point nursing care. *Nursing Research*, 1975, *24*, 244–255.

Wolff, B. B. Behavioral measurement of human pain. In R. A. Sternbach (Ed.), *The psychology of pain.* New York: Raven, 1978.

Wolff, B. B., & Jarvik, M. E. Variations in cutaneous and deep somatic pain sensitivity. *Canadian Journal of Psychology*, 1963, *17*, 37–44.

Wolff, B. B., Krasnegor, N. A., & Farr, R. S. Effect of suggestion upon experimental pain response parameters. *Perceptual and Motor Skills*, 1965, *21*, 675–683.

Wolff, B. B., & Langley, S. Cultural factors and the response to pain: A review. *American Anthropologist*, 1968, *70*, 494–501.

Wolff, G. T., Friedman, S. B., Hofer, M. A., & Mason, J. W. Relationship between psychological defenses and mean urinary 17-hydroxycorticosteroid excretion rates: I. A predictive study of parents of fatally ill children. *Psychosomatic Medicine*, 1964, *26*, 576–591.

Wolpe, J. *Psychotherapy by reciprocal inhibition.* Stanford, Calif.: Stanford University Press, 1959.

Wolpe, J. Behavior therapy and its malcontents. I. Denial of its bases and psychodynamic fusionism. *Journal of Behavior Therapy and Experimental Psychiatry*, 1976, *7*, 1–5.

Wolpe, J., & Lazarus, A. *Behavior therapy techniques*. New York: Pergamon, 1966.

Woodforde, J. M., & Fielding, J. R. Pain and cancer. *Journal of Psychosomatic Research*, 1970, *14*, 365–370.

Woodforde, J. M., & Merskey, H. Personality traits of patients with chronic pain. *Journal of Psychosomatic Research*, 1972, *16*, 167–172. (a)

Woodforde, J. M., & Merskey, H. Some relationships between subjective measures of pain. *Journal of Psychosomatic Research*, 1972, *16*, 173–178. (b)

Wooley, S. C., Wooley, O. W., & Dyrenforth, S. R. Theoretical, practical, and social issues in behavioral treatments of obesity. *Journal of Applied Behavior Analysis*, 1979, *19*, 3–25.

Worthington, E. L., Jr. Labor room and laboratory: Clinical validation of the cold pressor as a means of testing preparation for childbirth strategies. *Journal of Psychosomatic Research*, 1982, *26*, 223–231.

Worthington, E. L., Jr., & Shumate, M. Imagery and verbal counseling methods in stress inoculation training for pain control. *Journal of Counseling Psychology*, 1981, *28*, 1–6.

Wortman, C. B., & Dunkel-Schetter, C. Interpersonal relationships and cancer: A theoretical analysis. *Journal of Social Issues*, 1979, *35*, 120–155.

Wright, E. *The new childbirth*. London: Tandem, 1964.

Yahia, C., & Ulin, P. R. Preliminary experience with a psychophysical program of preparation for childbirth. *American Journal of Obstetrics and Gynecology*, 1965, *93*, 942–945.

Yalom, I. D. *Group therapy with the terminally ill.*. Paper presented at the annual meeting of the American Psychiatric Association, Miami, May 1976.

Yates, A. J. *Theory and practice in behavior therapy*. New York: Wiley, 1975.

Youell, K. J., & McCullough, J. P. Behavioral treatment of mucous colitis. *Journal of Consulting and Clinical Psychology*, 1975, *43*, 740–745.

Young, L. D., & Blanchard, E. B. Medical applications of biofeedback training: A selective review. In S. Rachman (Ed.), *Contributions to medical psychology* (Vol. 2). Oxford, England: Pergamon, 1980.

Zax, M., Sameroff, A. J., & Farnum, J. E. Childbirth education, maternal attitudes and delivery. *American Journal of Obstetrics and Gynecology*, 1975, *123*, 185–190.

Zeigler, D. K., Hassarein, R., & Hassarein, K. Headache syndromes suggested by factor analysis of symptom variables in a headache prone population. *Journal of Chronic Disease*, 1972, *25*, 253–263.

Ziesat, H. A., Jr., & Gentry, W. D. The pain apperception test: An investigation of concurrent validity. *Journal of Clinical Psychology*, 1978, *34*, 786–789.

Zimbardo, P. *The cognitive control of motivation: The consequences of choice and dissonance*. Glenview, Ill.: Scott, Foresman, 1969.

AUTHOR INDEX

SUBJECT INDEX